DM Entrance Examination
CARDIOLOGY-2

Dr Apoorv Jain
DM Cardiology (Std.)

PEEPEE
PUBLISHERS AND DISTRIBUTORS (P) LTD.

DM Entrance Examination Cardiology-2

Published by
Pawaninder P. Vij & Anupam Vij

Peepee Publishers and Distributors (P) Ltd.
Head Office: 160, Shakti Vihar, Pitam Pura, Delhi-110 034 (India)

Correspondence Address:
7/31, First Floor, Ansari Road, Daryaganj
New Delhi-110 002 (India)
Ph: 65195868, 9811156083, 23246245
e-mail: peepee160@yahoo.co.in
e-mail: peepee160@rediffmail.com
e-mail: peepee160@gmail.com
www.peepeepub.com

First Edition **2013**

Reprint **2013**

ISBN: 978-81-8445-123-8

PREFACE

The idea of this book came because of lack of a comprehensive question bank on cardiology questions for DM entrance. This book is based on memory recall so there may be some missing options or phrases. The purpose of this book is to help DM Cardiology aspirants, in understanding the nature and variety of questions asked in various entrance examinations. As a beginner it is very hard to get a set of question papers which may help in orientation of mind for different entrance examinations .This book may just help you to find right direction.

All the best!

Apoorv Jain

"Books are infinite in number and timc is short. The secret of knowledge is to take what is essential. Take that and try to live up to it."

–Swami Vivekananda

CONTENTS

1

AIIMS MAY 2011

1. **Interheart study diet:**
   A. Risk factors
   B. Mortality
2. **Accord trial for intensive ↓... 3P control showed reduction in:**
   A. ↓ed mortality
   B. ↓ed MI
   C. ↓ed stoke
   D. ↓ed drug related side effect
3. **Simplicity-2 trial used following intervention for resistant HTN:**
   A. Renal sympathetic denervation
   B. Lumbar sympathectomy
   C. Thoracoscopic thoracic sympathectomy
   D. Moxonidine
4. **......... of Kussmaul sign.**
   A. RVMI
   B. RV failure
   C. Constrictive pericarditis
   D. Tamponade
5. **Tamponade type in which pulsus paradoxus is absent:**
   A. Low pressure tamponade
   B. SLE induced tamponade
   C. Tubercular massive pericardial effusion
   D. Large iatrogenic pericardial effusion
6. **Brugada syndrome all *except*:**
   A. All have at least one episode of cardiac event before reach adulthood
   B. Can be provoked by flecainide
   C. ICD is true only prophylaxis
   D. Rest ECG as MS suggestive of risk than β voked
7. **CPVT typical finding:**
   A. Bidirectional VT
8. **WPW all *except*:**
   A. Can conduct both anterior and retrograde
   B. Typically has decremental conduction
   C. If asterio grade conduction is slower than ECG signs are subtle
   D. Prolonged ERP is high
9. **ST ↑ by all *except*:**
   A. Digoxin
   B. IC
   C. Hyperthermia
   D. Hypercalcemia
10. **Digoxin toxicity shown by all *except*:**
    A. AF regularized
    B. PAT with variable ↓l....
    C. Bidirectional VT
    D. Pregnancy
11. **Patient of ER 30% developed AF new meet pharmacological drug of choice for cardio-vascular:**
    A. Ibutilide **B.** Cotacol
    C. Propafenone **D.** Amiodarone
12. **Digoxin had elevated by all *except*:**
    A. Atrovastation
    B. Bisoprolol
    C. Tetracyclic
    D. Amlodipine
13. **Warfarin levels affected by all *except*:**
    A. Renal failure
    B. Myxoedema
    C. CHF
    D. Alcohol
14. **ACE–I of choice in ......**
    A. Ramipril
    B. Lisinopril
    C. Dolapril
    D. Enalapril

15. **Dabigatran all *except*:**
A. It is a prodrug
B. In RELY trial it was shown to be non–interior to warfarin in presently AF related stroke
C. Amiodarone ↓es its level
D. Quinidine is contraindicated with it

16. **Ivabradin can be used in all *except*:**
A. Can be used as 2nd agent in angina
B. AF with FVR
C. Inappropriate sinus tachycardia
D. CHF

17. **PG infusion is indicated in all *except*:**
A. Pulmonary atresia with intact septum
B. Aortic atresia
C. Interrupted aortic arch
D. Supracardiac obstructed TAPVC

18. **Air embolism and stroke following right heart catheterization wave in children. All can be present *except*:**
A. Partial anomalous pulmonary venous connection
B. Tetralogy of Fallot
C. Ebstein's anomaly
D. Common atrium

19. **Gene of Marfan syndrome:**
A. FBN–1
B. TGF–β
C. TGF–Bk_2

20. **Marfan syndrome with aortic involvement:**
A. Pregnancy contraindicated even if N size
B. β-blocker reduce risk of dilation
C. If aortic size 5 cm surgery is indicated
D. Every 6–12 months screening should be done

21. **Severity of MR with AR is suggested:**
A. Austin flint murmur
B. Wide split S_2
C. LVS_3
D. Absence of peripheral sign of AR

22. **S_x in asymptomatic severe MR is due in all *except*:**
A. EF 0.50
B. LV end systolic diameter 45 mm
C. Flow onset AF
...ope

...**MS differentiated from austin flint**

...***except*:**

B. Tricuspid regurgitation velocity > 4 m/s
C. Annular thickening
D. Doming

25. **Most unusual presentation of aortic dissection:**
A. Status epilepticus
B. Syncope
C. Paraply
D. ST ↑ in II, III

26. **Incorrect method:**
A. Egg on side : TGA
B. Snowman : Supracardiac TAPVC
C. Hill waterfall sign : CCTGA
D. 3 Sign : Coarctation

27. **Mismatch drug:**
A. Liraglutide : Amylin analogs
B. DPP IV Sitagliptin
C. Repaglinide : Non-sulfonylurea secretagogues
D. Pioz PPAR–γ inhibiter pioglitaone

28. **Type IV respiratory failure is done:**
A. Hypoperfusion of respiratory muscle
B. Atelactasis
C. Dyselectrolytemia

29. **A–α gradient is normal in:**
A. Hypoventilation
B. ↓ed diffusion
C. V–Q mismatch
D. R–SL shunt

30. **PH : 7.32, PaO_2: 82, PCO_2: 32 HCO_5: 18, SDO_2: 95%:**
A. Mixed acid base
B. Partially compensated met–acidosis
C. Fully compensated met–acidosis
D. Partially compensate respiratory acidosis

31. **Ischemic preconditioning attenuated by:**
A. Sildenafil
B. Glyburide
C. Nicorandil

32. **LV remodeling. All are true *except*:**
A. Myocyte elongation
B. Myocyte hypertrophy
C. Capillary proliferation
D. Fibrosis

33. **SERCA all *except*:**
A. Gene therapy is promising
B. Unregulated in HF
C. Attached with endoplasmic reticulum
D. Take back Ca++ from cytosol to endoplasmic reticulum

34. Which cause taking back of calcium from cytosol to sarcoplasmic reticulum?
A. SERCA 2

35. Early repolarization syndrome all *except*:
A. More common in limb lead
B. Exercise has no effect
C. Isoproterenol /↑es ST
D. Is associated with idiopathic VF

36. DSA all *except*:
A. Twice as common in female
B. 5–10 mm rise of BP
C. 40% ↑se of stroke rate
D. ↑insulin resistance even without obesity

37. All are risk factors of hemorrhagic stroke *except*:
A. Obesity
B. Dyslipidemia
C. Alcohol
D. HTN

38. Most common substrate used by heart of normal resting fasting stroke:
A. Glucose
B. Ketones
C. FFA
D. Proteins (Amino acids)

39. Dilated coronary sinus is seen in:
A. Persistent left SVC
B. Kawasaki
C. Obstructed IVC

40. Drug given in vasovagal all *except*:
A. Paroxetine
B. Levodopa
C. Midodrine
D. β-blocker

41. Aortoarteritis all *except*:
A. Thoracic aortic involvement is most common in India
B. Steroid 1st line of R_x in active state
C. ESR/CRP are poor indicator of activity
D. Intervention in quiescent stage only

42. Renal artery stenosis in all *except*:
A. Turner's
B. Williams
C. Retsum
D. NF

43. Post MI septal rupture all *except*:
A. Parasternal thrill is present
B. Most common with IWMZ
C. Best diagnosis with right heart catheter
D. Seen with in 48 hours in thrombolytic CVA

44. Fever not seen in:
A. Aortoarteritis
B. Carcinoid
C. Rhabdomyoma
D. Myxoma

45. Most common auscultatory finding in atrial myxoma:
A. Diastolic rumble
B. P_2 loud
C. Tumor plop
D. MR

46. Best D_x for post cardiac allograft vasculopathy:
A. IVUS
B. MRA
C. CTA
D. Debutants stress echo

47. First retrograde left heart catheterization done by:
A. Sonnet
B. Grossman

48. Mitral annulus calcification all *except*:
A. Common in art. leaflet
B. Common in elderly leaflet
C. Impaired subannular ventricular contraction
D. Progress to CHB

49. St. Jude valve is:
A. Ball and cage
B. Bileaflet
C. Porcine

50. Mesenchymal stem cells ...... from.
A. Bone marrow
B. Blood
C. Spleen
D. Placenta

51. Endothelial progenitor cell markers all *except*:
A. VEGF
B. CD 3
C. CD 34
D. CD 133

52. HIV with cardiac disease all *except*:
A. CABG not done
B. Cardiac tamponade is rare
C. Endocarditis is treated conventionally
D. PAH is seen

53. HF at birth A/F:
A. HLHS
B. Vein of galen malformation
C. VSD

54. **Brain abscess seen in all *except*:**
A. Pulmonary artery fistula
B. Ebstein
C. PAPVC
D. Truncus arteriosus with Eisenmenger

55. **All are seen with massive BT *except*:**
A. Thrombocytosis
B. Hyperkalemia
C. Hypofibrinogenemia

56. **Central aortic pressure all *except*:**
A. Better predictor of outcome than office
B. Applanation tonometry in radial artery is used for measurement
C. β-blocker better than amlodipine
D. Massive ratio of augmentation pressure to systolic person

57. **Pulses alternans all *except*:**
A. Best seen in carotids
B. Best appreciated during transient breath holding
C. Marker of changes in LVEDP
D. Confirmed by sphygmomanometer

58. **Bezold Jarisch reflex mediated by:**
A. Atrial stretch receptors
B. J–receptors with mechanoreceptors
C. Mechano + chemoreceptors
D. Baro + chemoreceptors

59. **Pheochromocytoma all *except*:**
A. Dopamine is marker of malignancy
B. Most common present with constant HTN
C. 24 hours urinary metanephrines is not a good sensitive test for screening
D. In children extradural involvement is common

60. **Rheumatic fever all *except*:**
A. M–protein provides proactive antibody
B. Myosin content is all with more damage
C. MR ↓es on follow-up
D. Valvulopathy is more important than myocardial damage

61. **S. bovis endocarditis is a/w *except*:**
A. GI malignancy
B. Dental extraction
C. Gynae procedure
D. Urinary tract infection

62. **X-ray chest PA view showing dextrocardia with right sided tendus, which is probably seen?**
A. Normal cardiac anatomy
B. CC TGA
C. Left isomerism
D. Right isomerism

63. **JVP tracing:**
A.
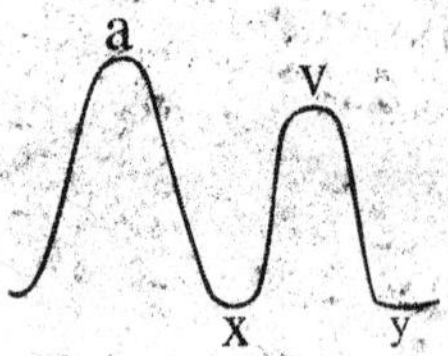

B.
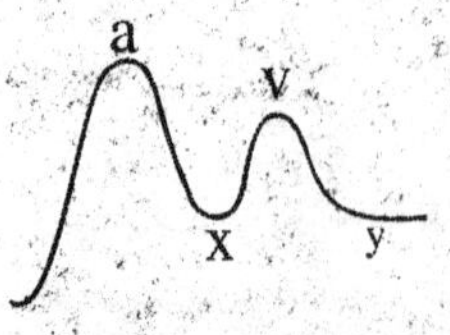

C. Normal (A) with TS in (B)

64. **6 days old infant associated with shock X-Ray Sherry egg on side:**
A.
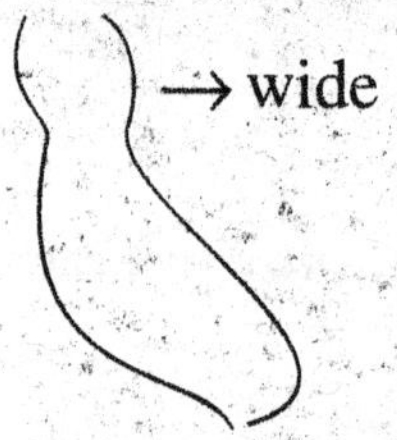

B. Obstructed Q TAPVC
C. TGA
D. TOF

65. **Multiple pneumatoceles in a 60 years male on X-ray:**
A. Biopsy
B. IV antibiotics
C. Pneumonectomy
D. Antifungal

66. **PSAX showing thickened mitral valve. Ruptured mitral valve R_x of choke:**
A. Mitral valvuloplasty
B. CIIP
C. Cast penicillin prophylaxis
D. Cardiac S_x

67. **High pressure TR. Which cannot be a cause?**
A. ASD
B. IE
C. Severe PS
D. PAH

68. **CT chest showing RV, LV and descending aorta with white sodium following post surface of RV, LV presentation will be of:**
A. ↑ed JVP
B. Angina
C. Aortic dissection type A
D. Multiple stab

69. JTF, TWMJ with CHB show on ECA all *except*:
- **A.** Dominant RCA can be involved
- **B.** Patient needs permanent pacemaker on dischy
- **C.** R 10 PCI better than thrombolysis

70. LV pressure tracing:
- **A.**

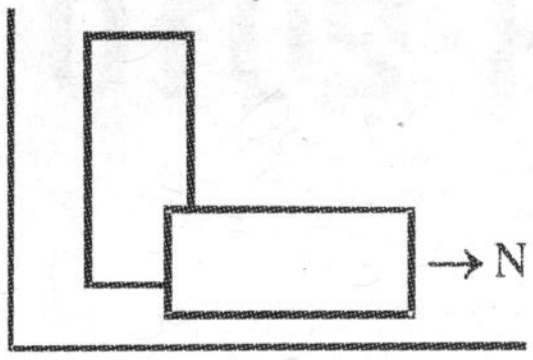

- **B.** Cardiac amyloids
- **C.** HOCM
- **D.** Hypertrophy
- **E.** DCMP

71. J–wave in ECG of a destitute R_x of chest:
- **A.** Re-warming

72. 40 years O→P/W chest pain for 2 days. ECG shows ST ↑ from $V_2 \rightarrow V_6$ and lead II, is intersentia of choice:
- **A.** 10 PCI
- **B.** Echo
- **C.** Stress ECG

73. Holter of a Patient P/W palpitations showing:
- **A.**

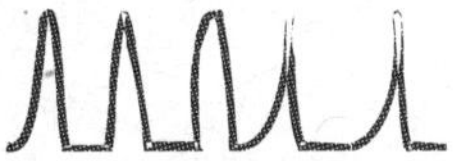

- **B.**

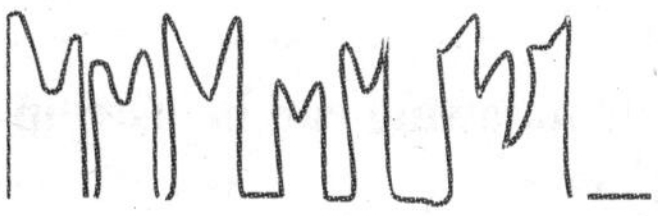

- **C.** RFA
- **D.** β-blocker
- **E.** Amlodipine
- **F.** Nitrate

74. Severe AS patient undergoing right heart catheterization rhythm strip showing ..... .
- **A.**

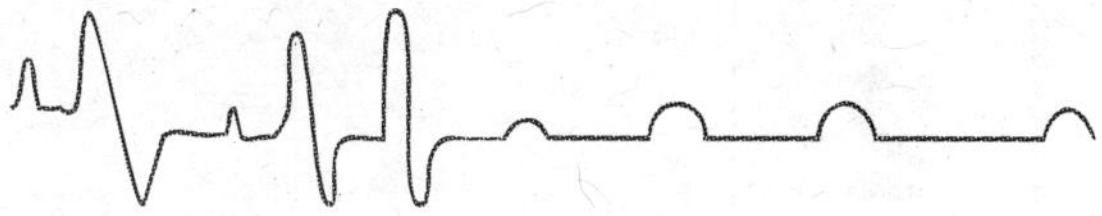

- **B.** Which is ture?
- **C.** Right heart catheterization on should not be due
- **D.** AVR with PPI
- **E.** Patient may not need PPI
- **F.** RB right bundle branch may be diseased

75. LV pressure tracing with catheter pullback showing:
- **A.**

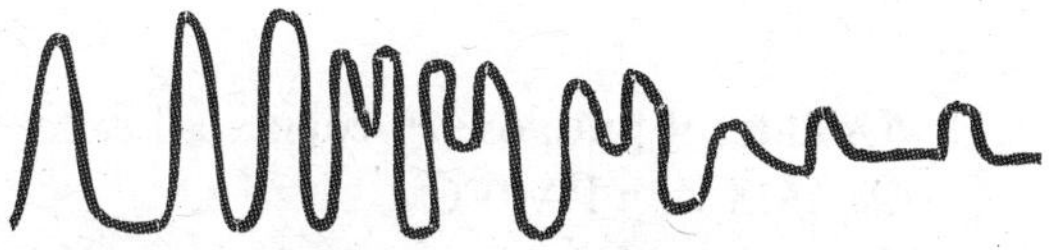

- **B.** Supravalvular AS
- **C.** Coarctation of aorta
- **D.** Subaortic membrane

76. CT head showing SOL in Balal Gaylis with SAH presentation is:
- **A.** Thunder clap headed
- **B.** Cyanosis
- **C.** Aortic vegetation
- **D.** MS

77. A drug given where $t^{1/2}$ B 4 Ins. and given every 4 hours. How many hours needed for steady state?
- **A.** 20 hours
- **B.** 90 hours
- **C.** 48 hours

78. AF and AFL all *except*:
- **A.** Rate control can be tried in AFI
- **B.** RFA is cases in AF then typical AFI
- **C.** Anti-coagulation in both

79. Hardware not used in balloon valvuloplasty:
- **A.** Fogarty catheter
- **B.** Mullin
- **C.** Inoue balloon
- **D.** Brokenbrough needle

2

AIIMS DECEMBER 2010

1. **Unilateral pulmonary edema all *except*:**
   A. MS with PAPVC
   B. MI in Mcleod syndrome
   C. Dilatation with peripheral pul art stenosis
   D. ASD correction in old patient

2. **Fetal hydrops:**
   A. Ebstein's B. TOF
   C. TGA D. PAC

3. **ASD thrill in 2nd ICS all *except*:**
   A. MS B. MR
   C. PS D. TAPVC

4. **All true *except*:**
   A. Ao SpO2 is 90% or less Eisenmenger
   B. Ao SpO2 <90% in TOF
   C. Coronary sinus 88% -TAPVC to coronary sinus
   D. PA 82% in cardiogenic shock

5. **X-Ray →cyanosis ↑PBF and cardiomegaly:**
   A. TGA
   B. TAPVC with IVC obstr.
   C. TOF

6. **Continuous murmur all *except*:**
   A. MS with restrictive ASD
   B. RSOV →LV
   C. Peripheral pulmonary art stenosis
   D. BT shunt

7. **BNP – raised in all *except*:**
   A. RF
   B. CHF
   C. Obesity
   D. Cirrhosis

8. **SCD – feature of all *except*:**
   A. RCM
   B. Non obst HOCM
   C. LCX from RCA
   D. Takotsubo

9. **PPH all are true *except*:**
   A. BMPPR-2 in majority
   B. Pathology like Eisenmenger
   C. ASD may be patient
   D. CCB's may be contraindicated

10. **Ph 7.41, HCO_3 - 25 PO_2 – 90:**
    A. Compensated RTA
    B. CHF with diuretics
    C. Chronic diarrhoea
    D. Ketoacidosis

11. **BNP – raised in all *except*:**
    A. RF
    B. CHF
    C. Obesity
    D. Cirrhosis

12. **Which of the following can be used in CHF?**
    A. Neem Bark
    B. Arjuna terminalis
    C. Strichnine
    D. Gingo biloba

13. **Proven therapy all *except*:**
    A. Ig in myocarditis
    B. Bosentan in Eisenmenger's
    C. Prasugrel in CSA
    D. Low dose dopamine in renal failure

14. **Load independent marker of contractility:**
    A. ESPV - relationship
    B. Corrected EF
    C. O_2 consumption of tissue
    D. Velocity of circumferential fibre

15. **Cardiac tamponade all *except*:**
    A. BP normal or ↑
    B. Diuretics C.I. even if hepatomegaly patient
    C. Pulsus paradoxus always (if carefully looked)
    D. 2D echo finding preceeds clinical findings

16. Inf. endocarditis poor prognosis:
A. Staph aureus in hemodialysis
B. Staph epidermidis
C. Enterococcal in pregnancy
D. Strep viridans in pneumonia

17. Echo velocity 5 cm/sec. BP - 140/80 Cal. RVSP:
A. Cannot be done B. 25
C. 40 D. 10

18. Definition of MI all *except*:
A. SCD may be due to MI
B. Post CABG Trop > 3 times
C. Re-infarction trop T increases 5-7% on serial
D. New RWMA

19. UA/NSTEMI true all *except*:
A. Previous CAD history and risk factors positive
B. Red thrombi common
C. Women NSTEM I > STEM I
D. 10-15% CAG-normal

20. Patient comes within 1 hr of MI; PCI > thrombolysis all *except*:
A. Young smoker
B. Elderly with anterior wall MI
C. Middle age male with inf. wall MI with prev. CABG
D. Women with cardiogenic shock

21. Post thrombolysis all true *except*:
A. High risk patient routinely transformed for PCI
B. Clopidogrel to all patients
C. LMWH better than UFH in case of fibrinolysis with fibrin spec
D. Low dose prehospital fibrinolysis + Gp 2B/3A into in high risk cases

22. Goal of revascularization all *except*:
A. T1 M 1 - 3 not T1 M1 - 2 is goal
B. Infarct related artery - occlusion
C. Spontaneous late patency of IRA
D. OAT trial benefits after 3 days

23. Patient with MI – chest clear, hypoxia increased cause could be:
A. RVMI B. VSD
C. Infarct extension D. MR

24. CCU – in MI all true *except*:
A. LVEDP - 12-18
B. K - 3.8
C. Mg - 2
D. H.R. - 60-80

25. ECG – ST ↑in aVR > V1 ST ↓I, aVL, V4-V6, II, aVF artery involved is:
A. LMCA
B. LCX
C. LAD after SC
D. Post lateral branch of RCA

26. TMT – LBBB at peak exertion is S/o of:
A. TVD with left main
B. TMT should not be done
C. May not indicate ischemia
D. VT

27. Statin therapy reduces mortality by 33% (72% vs 8%) no. of subjects needed to reduce one death:
A. 25 B. 33
C. 100 D. Not possible to cal.

28. HIT – all *except*:
A. Warfarin B. Danaperoid
C. Lepuridin D. Argatoban

29. Ankle brachial index is associated with:
A. <0.5 - critical limb ischemia
B. Smoking more with PVD > CAD
C. ABI doesnot change with exercise
D. Arginine definitely useful

30. AC-MI not suggested:

		RA	RV	PCWP	CI
A.	12	30/6	10	1.8	
B.	10	50/12	20	2.1	
C.	6	30/6	22	2.2	
D.	15	50/15	10	1.8	

31. Asympt AS with – 60 mmHg gradient at rest. TMT at 11 min – stopped due to fatigue. MgX:
A. CAG B. Med follow up
C. AVR D. Ballooning

32. Matching for dose reduction all *except*:
A. Nefidipine - liver failure
B. Lidocaine - CHF
C. Sotalol - RF
D. Metoprotol - RF

33. Matching all *except*:
A. HIT - PO_4
B. Mg Receptors - NMDA
C. Congenital long QT - SCN5A
D. Malignant hyperthermia - heat shock proteins

34. Stem cell marker:
A. CD45 B. CD3
C. CD34 D. CD135

35. SCD – is associated with all *except*:
A. Morning
B. Winter
C. White
D. Monday

36. **Regarding metabolism of drugs all correct *except*:**
A. Digoxin - P - glycoprotein
B. Carvedilol - CY2D6
C. Simvastatin-Glucoronide conjugation
D. CCB-CYP3A4

37. **In elderly true:**
A. Physiological anemia present commonly
B. Law of parisomny may not apply
C. Bacteremia may not indicate UTI
D. Digoxin toxic normal level

38. **False combination:**
A. Moyamoya - Aortic aneurysm
B. Neurofibroma - RAS
C. Marfan's ductal ectasia
D. Mullbery sign - CCP

39. **Eosinophilia with ARF all *except*:**
A. CIN
B. Renal art embolism
C. PAN
D. Drug induced

40. **Hypothermia all *except*:**
A. ASO in TGA
B. CABG - off pump
C. Post operative junct. cardia
D. Prevent neuronal damage

41. **Adenosine all *except*:**
A. Chest pain
B. VT/VF rarely
C. Pulmonary vasoconstriction
D. Take up endothelum

42. **AF-paroxysmal with EF - 30% drug to be used:**
A. Amiodarone B. Sotalol
C. Ibutilide D. Propafenone

43. **ARVD least characteristic:**
A. T ↓V1 – V3 in 14 yrs old
B. Epsilon wave
C. VT = LBBB with sup - axis

44. **All *except*:**
A. Ivabradine ika
B. Ranolazine is Ca++ sensitizer
C. Rotophyline at A1
D. Torcetrapib – CE TP inhibitor

45. **Syncope 20 years with ECG - RBBB - coving with ST elevation:**
A. Beta-blocker
B. ICD
C. Sympathetic ganglionectony
D. Isoprenaline

46. **Pulsus alternans in ECG – intervention done patient improved – diagnosis could be:**
A. Massive P.E. B. LVF
C. Acute AR D. MI with CHF

47. **Correct match are all *except*:**
A. Gall 67 - sarcoidosis
B. Tc99 for osteomyelitis
C. Th-201 - myocarditis

48. **New onset DM treatment given all *except*:**
A. Losartan B. Atorva statin
C. Atenolol D. Enalapril

49. **HIE – earliest effect is seen at:**
A. Hippocampus
B. Mammilary body
C. Cerebellar cortex
D. Pons RAS

50. **In ARDS useful is:**
A. Prone ventilation
B. High frequency ventilation
C. Low tidal volume
D. Inhaled N_2O

51. **Amyloidosis true is:**
A. Macroglossia may be present in familial TTR
B. Low voltage limb lead and precordial leads
C. Angina uncommon in absence of athero-sclerosis
D. Liver transplant in elderly

52. **Suggestive of respiratory pump failure:**
A. Auto PEEP
B. ↓vital capacity
C. High pressure shallow breathing index
D. ↓inspiratory pressure

53. **Hemorrhagic stroke associated with all *except*:**
A. Alcohol
B. Smoking
C. Hyperlipidermia
D. ↑waist-hip ratio

ANSWERS

1	A	2	A	3	A	4	D	5	A	6	B	7	C
8	C	9	A	10	B	11	C	12	B	13	D	14	A
15	A	16	A	17	A	18	B	19	B	20	A	21	D
22	D	23	A	24	B	25	A	26	A	27	A	28	B
29	A	30	D	31	B	32	D	33	D	34	C	35	C
36	C	37	C	38	A	39	C	40	B	41	C	42	C
43	C	44	B	45	B	46	C	47	C	48	B	49	A
50	C	51	A	52	D	53	D						

3

AIIMS DECEMBER 2009

1. **All of the following ↓se in pulmonary embolism *except*:**
   A. A–a gradient (↑sed)
   B. ↓ed MVO_2
   C. ↓ed CO_2 arterial
   D. ↓ed arterial O_2 – hypoxemia (765)

2. **Wrong treatment in pulmonary embolism:**
   A. STK 1.5 million over 2 hours
   B. Tpa 100 mg over 2 hours
   C. Urokinase 4,400/kg bolus + 4,400/kg infusion–F_2
   D. Heparin 5000–10000 bolus + infusion acc. to wt

3. **Air embolism ECG:**
   A. St. ↑ in II, III, AVF
   B. Q in I, a VL, V_1–V_6
   C. ST ↑ in V_1–V_6
   D. ST ↓ in AVR

4. **EST what slow respiratory diseases?**
   A. THR 95%
   B. Desaturation < 90%
   C. ↓ed maximum O_2 consumption
   D. ↓ed anaerobic threshold

5. **THR:**
   A. 220 –age
   B. 180 –age
   C. 100 +age
   D. 85% of 200 –age

6. **Loud ESM at base:**
   A. Eisenmenger
   B. ASD + MR
   C. MVP with RML prolapse
   D. Sub pulmonic VSD supracoastal

7. **High pitched decrescendo EDM in:**
   A. Eisenmenger PDA
   B. MS with PAH
   C. Post op TOF
   D. Paravalvular AR

8. **Wide splint S2 all *except*:**
   A. PPI
   B. PS
   C. Fasting RV
   D. Coronary sinus ASD

9. **Post MI EF < 40 after 1 week. What to do?**
   A. AICD
   B. CAG
   C. MRI for hibernating myocardium

10. **Risk factor for 2° VF all *except*:**
    A. IVCD (intraventricular conduction)
    B. Persistent sinus tachycardia
    C. Treatment requiring pacemaker
    D. AIVR > 6 hours

11. **TPI in MI all *except*:**
    A. LAFB with ↑PR
    B. Alternating BBB
    C. New bifascicular block true
    D. RVMI with CHB

12. **All *except*:**
    A. TIMI 2 flow endpoint in thrombolytic trial
    B. Thrombolysis is reinfarction at 6 weeks → 9-10%
    C. Accelerated tPA causes rapid lysis than infusion
    D. Reteplase better than r–tpa in prehospital thrombolysis (< 4 hours)

13. **Takotsubo all *except*:**
    A. Common in elderly females
    B. Delayed Trop–T elevation
    C. Shock in 15%
    D. Good prognosis

14. **Aurora trial →statin not better in:**
    A. Hemodialysis patients
    B. Elderly
    C. Females
    D. Stoke

15. **Hollenhorst plaque in:**
A. CA myxoma
B. Carotid A stenosis
C. DCMP
D. Crohn's disease

16. **Cotton-wool spots:**
A. Micro hemorrhage
B. Nerve infarct
C. Choroid edema
D. Lipid deposition

17. **All in HDL metabolism disease:**
A. Tangier (↓HDL)
B. CETP def. ↑HDL
C. LCAT def. (Low HDL)
D. Sitosterolemia

18. **Lipid disease in DM:**
A. TG↑, HDL↓
B. LDL↑
C. Hyperchylomicronemia
D. ↓ed Lp a

19. **Which retards diabetic nephropathy (*except*)?**
A. Low protein diet
B. Treatment of mild HTN
C. Smoking cessation
D. Vitamin E supplementation

20. **HTN all *except*:**
A. Blacks have ↓ed PRA and improved response to diuretics
B. Some degree of HTN females ↓ed morbidity than males
C. Both excessive dippers and non dippers have high risk of CAD
D. Exercise induced HTN do not develop HTN in 5 years

21. **SLE all *except*:**
A. CAD is the biggest cause of mortality in females
B. APLA may be protective
C. > 2 years steroid R_x ↑ses CAD risk
D. Associated with coronary A aneurysm

22. **Takayasu arteritis:**
A. Thoracoabdominal involvement common in Indians
B. Pulmonary A involvement may be associated with massive hemoptysis
C. Pregnancy is tolerated well in chronic takayasu
D. Steroids R_x can be given for 8 weeks in active disease

23. **Marfan's major criteria all *except*:**
A. Dural ectasia B. Ectopic lentis
C. MVP D. F/H/O Marfan's

24. **PAN associated with all *except*:**
A. Eosinophilia
B. High ESR
C. CNS vasculitis
D. Mono neuritis multiplex

25. **NF–1 all *except*:**
A. Acoustic neuroma
B. Optic glioma
C. Pheochromocytoma
D. Café au lait spots

26. **Down's syndrome all *except*:**
A. HOCM
B. TOF
C. Congenital hip dislocation
D. Duodenal atresia

27. **eNOS endogenous inhibitors:**
A. Asymmetric Dimethyl Arginine (ADMA)
B. SOD
C. Phosphodiasterase inhibitors
D. Nitroprusside

28. **All have bad prognosis in spinal anesthesia. Which is relatively better?**
A. CAD
B. TOF
C. HOCM
D. Severe valvular disease

29. **ECMO post op in:**
A. ASD with left lung agenesis
B. Late arterial switch
C. MVR for MS
D. Coronary sinus TAPVC

30. **Homograft in all *except*:**
A. Ross (Auto graft)
B. Rastelli
C. Arterial switch
D. VSD with pulmonary atresia

31. **CABG mortality with CPB:**
A. 1% B. 5%
C. 7% D. 10%

32. **Elderly avoided all *except*:**
A. Diazepam
B. Amitriptyline
C. Indomethacin
D. Propoxyphene

33. **Hypoxic pulmonary vasoconstriction by which receptor?**
A. Adenosine
B. Rho
C. Serotonin
D. K^+

34. **β-blocker avoided in CKD–all *except*:**
A. Carvedilol
B. Atenolol
C. Sotalol
D. Nadolol

35. **PT and aPTT ↑ed in def. of factor–all *except*:**
A. 2
B. 5
C. 10
D. 13

36. **Pregnancy class B drug all *except*:**
A. Torseamide
B. Statin
C. Sotalol
D. I.V magnesium sulfate

37. **Regarding anti-coagulation all *except*:**
A. RMP potentiates warfarin
B. Thrombolysis inc. PT
C. Dysfibrinogenemia ↑ses clinical bleeding
D. Lupus anti-coagulant inc. PT without bleed

38. **Amphoterecin B:**
A. Not affected by hepatic and renal failure
B. Liposomal AMB does not cause febrile R_x
C. Effective in histoplasmosis
D. It cause RTA

39. **ASD closure devices used in:**
A. Pregnancy
B. Jehoviah's witness
C. AF
D. Poor patient

40. **Chronic AF treatment:**
A. Pulmonary vein isolation
B. PLATO devices
C. Carotricuspid isthmic ablation

41. **Echo feature of tamponade all *except*:**
A. RV systolic collapse
B. RA diastolic collapse
C. Rocking motion of heart
D. ↑ed tricuspid vel. in inspiration

42. **Young 45 years male inted with STEMI, all true all *except*:**
A. PML rupture more common
B. Basal septal rupture worse prognosis than apical rupture in AWMI
C. Pseudoaneurysm better progress than true aneurysm
D. TR in RVMI is not common

43. **Thrombolysis all *except*:**
A. Gp II6/IIIa started pre pci and given for 12–24 hours post pci

44. **Units all *except*:**
A. BP → Torr
B. MRI → Hounsfield
C. Viscosity → Poise
D. SVR → Wood

45. **Hyperosmolar hyponatremia all *except*:**
A. Hyperlipidemia
B. Cirrhosis
C. Nephrotic syndrome
D. CHF

46. **Post op functional tachycardia treatment:**
A. Adenosine
B. Digoxin
C. Cooling blanket
D. Milrinone

47. **Left foot gangrene with preserved pulses:**
A. Abdominal aortic aneurysm
B. Buerger's
C. Multiple myeloma
D. PVD

48. **Raynaud's in A/O:**
A. Ageing in females
B. Atherosclerosis of upper limb
C. RA
D. PPH

49. **Which oximetry shows PPHN?**

	A	B	C	D
A. Right Leg	90	80	70	80
B. Right Arm	80	90	90	80

50. **IE in old ages >70 years in young/old patients:**
A. Risks associated with ↑sing ages
B. Females higher risk than males
C. Abd source common
D. Mortality ↑ses with age

51. **Methicillin sensitive IE all *except*:**
A. Vancomycin dose 3 gm
B. Pencillin better than vanco if no hypersensitivity
C. It s/s > 3 months give treatment for 6 weeks
D. Genta can be given if initial 3-5 days

52. **E/E' >8 IN:**
A. CCP
B. Cardiac amyloidosis
C. CAD
D. RCMP

53. **V_1 qr with V_2–N R wave:**
A. RAE
B. Double chambered right ventricle
C. RVMI
D. Mahaim fibres

54. **Carcinoid syndrome all *except*:**
A. Wet beriberi
B. Pellagra
C. Hypoproteinemia
D. ↑ed 5–HIAA

55. **Incidence ↑sing in all *except*:**
A. CRF
B. Endo fibro elastosis
C. Dresslers
D. EMF

56. **CXR increased sized heart with pulmonary edema all *except*:**
A. Multivalvular disease
B. Acute MI
C. Acute myocarditis
D. Severe HTN

57. **Same patient in previous ques, pH-6.3, PO_2-60, PCO_2-51, HCO_3-20, treatment:**
A. Ventilation
B. IABP
C. CAG
D. CABG

58. **VT with LBBB morphology:**
A. ARVD
B. RVOT VT
C. LV VT
D. Ischemic VT

59. **Severe As with CHB during right heart catheterization, treatment:**
A. AVR
B. AVR + PPI
C. PPI
D. EPS

60. **Electrical alternans → ECG shown, patient will present as:**
A. Hypotension
B. Seizures
C. Stroke

61. **Best investigation:**
A. 2D Echo
B. CAG
C. Electrolytes
D. ABG

62. **ECG showing AF with fast ventricular rate–WPW Best acute management:**
A. DC shock
B. Diltiazem
C. Lignocaine
D. Magsulf

63. **Best chronic treatment:**
A. Amiodarone
B. RF ablation
C. AICD

64. **Pre procedure ECG →wide QRS, Post procedure ECG-biv. spikes with n. QRS. What procedure?**
A. Pacemaker
B. ICD
C. CRT

65. **CXR→ Egg on side appearance with oligemic lung fields all *except*:**
A. Ebstein
B. Lutembacher
C. PS with TR
D. Pericardial effusion

66. **CXR does not show:**
A. RAE
B. Pulmonary venous HTN
C. Narrow pedicle
D. Pulmonary oligemia

67. **Continuous Doppler along mitral valve treatment:**
A. Balloon dilation
B. Alcohol septal ablation

68. **Echo showing thickened IVS most common:**
A. Syncope

69. **LA–LV diastolic gradient on cath. all *except*:**
A. Pulmonary vein stenosis
B. CA myoma
C. Supramitral ring
D. Acute AR

70. **Thickened radial a. shows all *except*:**
A. Pseudo HTN
B. ↑ed CAD
C. Calcified vessel
D. ISH

71. **CT scan with SDH:**
A. Arnold Chiari
B. Aortic valve endocarditis
C. Amyloidosis
D. NPH

ANSWERS

1	B	2	A	3	A	4	B	5	A	6		7	A
8		9	B	10	D	11	D	12		13	B	14	A
15	B	16	B	17	D	18	A	19	D	20		21	B
22		23	C	24	A	25	A	26	A	27	A	28	
29		30	A	31		32		33	D	34	A	35	D
36	B	37	A	38		39	D	40	A	41	A	42	C
43	A	44	B	45	A	46	C	47	A	48	A	49	A
50	A	51	A	52	A	53	A	54	A	55	C	56	A
57	B	58	A	59		60	A	61	A	62	A	63	B
64	C	65		66		67		68	A	69		70	
71													

4

AIIMS MAY 2009

1. **Pulsus paradoxus all *except*:**
   A. Pulmonary embolism
   B. Effusive constrictive pericarditis
   C. Nonobst HCM
   D. Marked obesity

2. **30-day mortality in USA:**
   A. 2% B. 10%
   C. >NSTEMI D. >STEMI

3. **Least likely to develop IHD:**
   A. Eruptive
   B. Tuberoeruptive
   C. Tendon xanthoma
   D. Palmar xanthoma

4. **65-year-old, male executive, non DM, non IHD, asymptomatic, no history, TC = 220, HDL = 38, LDL = 128, BP = 130/80, has come for routine health checkup and TMT. Your opinion informed about:**
   A. Do a TMT and repeat every 5 years
   B. Not routinely recommended
   C. EBCT better than TMT
   D. CT angio better because TMT give false result due to HTN

5. **Female patient 65 years with exercise after rest develops perfusion defect in Ant wall in thallium scan most common cause:**
   A. Attenuation artefact
   B. High dose of thallium
   C. Hybernating myocardium + SCD
   D. Absence of collateral

6. **Dobutamine stress echo to right coronary for viable myocardium done in:**
   A. Low dose
   B. With dopamine
   C. With PET
   D. With exercise

7. **Investigation to diagnosis viable myocardium in patient with history of AWMI, 60 years, all *except*:**
   A. Exercise TMT
   B. Dobuta echo
   C. C MRI
   D. PET with FDG

8. **Elderly 60 years with AWMI. Thrombolysis with STK, at 2 hours repeated ECG at 90 minutes with relief of pain 50% and 2-3 mm ST elevation in V_2-V_4 and next step:**
   A. Rescue angioplasty
   B. Repeat STK
   C. Medical Mx
   D. Urokinase

9. **HR = 120/mm, BP = 90/70, ECG Q wave in V_1-V_6 and ST elevation in I, aVL with 8 hours chest pain. Not done all *except*:**
   A. IV metoprolol 5 mg
   B. 1° PCI
   C. Thrombolysis with STK
   D. Atorvas 80 mg

10. **USA early intervention in all *except*:**
    A. Trop T +ve
    B. Prior CABG
    C. HF
    D. Recent onset angina

11. **BMS better than DES true in:**
    A. Diabetic
    B. Tortuous OM
    C. Mid RCA 40 mm lesion
    D. Prox LAD 15 mm leison with 2.5 mm diameter

12. **Ischemic stroke decrease by all *except*:**
    A. Amlodipine
    B. Atenolol
    C. Thiazide
    D. Perindopril

13. **Female with ischemic stroke with BP of 240/145 Treatment preferred is:**
A. Sodium nitroprusside
B. NTG
C. Labetalol
D. Furosemide

14. **40 years female with PPH on Rx with sildenafil, develops chest pain and hospitalised with disprin; nitrite O_2 and β B LMWH found dead 2 days after:**
A. Iatrogenic
B. VT/VF
C. Dyselectrolytemia
D. Pulm embolism

15. **RVMI all *except*:**
A. Prominent Y descent
B. ST elevation disappear within 48 hours in V4R
C. ST elevation in V_1-V_3
D. AV sequential pacing may be hazardous

16. **Prehospital fibrinolytics:**
A. Reteplase B. STK
C. Urokinase D. rtPA

17. **Stable angina with HR 56/min class II anti-arrythmic is:**
A. Ivabradine B. Verapamil
C. Amlodipine D. β blocker

18. **Ranolazine all *except*:**
A. Increase QT
B. (–) delayed Na+ channel
C. Used in UA
D. Does not change HR

19. **Highest cholesterol found in:**
A. Indian with MI
B. Chinese with stroke
C. Japanese asymptomatic
D. Nigerian with asymptomatic HIV

20. **Old man with fatigue from 2:00 pm and presented at 8 pm. Next investigation:**
A. ECG B. RBS
C. Echo D. Electrolyte

21. **Nuns Health Study : Women on Estrogen Rx were found to have RR of CAD 0.56 (P = <0.05) Cf 95% (0.40-0.80) s/o:**
A. The chance of Null hypothesis being wrong 115%
B. RR of CAD decrease is 56%
C. 40-80% will have risk reduction

22. **Brown fat all *except*:**
A. Absent in adult
B. Highly vascular
C. Thermogenesis

23. **BP is 130/80 Echo – EF is 55% ECG, sinus tachycardia with pedal edema Ix for diagnosis:**
A. BNP
B. D-dimer
C. RBC trans ketolase
D. S. sodium

24. **Worse prognosis after MI with HF true:**
A. MI with RBBB
B. RVMI
C. AF
D. Diffuse ST elevation

25. **Abdominal aortic aneurysm all *except*:**
A. May be familial
B. Pulsation below umblicus s/o aneurysm
C. More common in Asian > whites
D. Pain radiating to flank and genitalia s/o rupture

26. **E/E of 15 s/o:**
A. Normal B. Diastolic dysfunction
C. Severe MS D. Ischemia

27. **Venous press in dorsal foot vein in, standing posture is normally:**
A. 5 mm Hg B. 10 mm Hg
C. 15 mm Hg D. 90 mm Hg

28. **ALLAHAT trial all included *except*:**
A. Pravastatin
B. Chlortholidone
C. Hydrochlor thiazides
D. Amlodipine

29. **40 years male with uncomplicated HTN, Rx not given is:**
A. Ramipril + Telmisartan
B. Ramipril + HCZ
C. β B + HCZ
D. β B + Amlodipine

30. **Worse prognosis following exertional syncope:**
A. AS B. PPH
C. Eisenmenger D. HOCM

31. **25 years female with breathlessness with hoarseness of voice least likely:**
A. Severe MS
B. ASD with 4 : 1 shunt
C. PPH
D. Eisenmenger

32. **Post indentation of esophagous an barium seen in all *except*:**
A. Double aortic arch with dextrocardia
B. Pulmomary artery sling
C. Anomalous right subclavian artery
D. Double aortic arch

33. Palpable P2 is seen in all *except*:
A. Ebstein B. Juvenile MS
C. PVOD D. PPH

34. Afterload increase with:
A. Stiff aorta
B. LVH
C. Increase filling pressure
D. Bradycardia

35. Patient of TOF repaired and developed CHB, biventricular pacing done. All seen *except*:
A. TR murmur due to lead
B. Wide split S2
C. PR residual
D. Murmur due to residual VSD

36. William syndrome definitive for Dx:
A. FISH
B. Calcineuron level in serum
C. Arterial biopsy
D. Cardiac catheterization

37. Sodium channelopathy all *except*:
A. Brugada syndrome
B. Long QT interval
C. CPVT
D. Infantile febrile seizure

38. Dopamine causes tachycardia by:
A. Reflex tachycardia
B. Splanchic and renal vasodilation
C. Direct dopaminergic action in heart
D. Increase cardiac NE

39. True all *except*:
A. Lidocaine dose (loading) decrease in CHF
B. Sotalol dose decrease in hepatic dysfunction
C. Amiodarone serum level not helpful in toxicity management
D. Lithium excretion depends on renal blood flow

40. AVNRT @ 200/min cause could be:
A. Mahaim fibre
B. Antegrade slow fibres
C. Fast conduction thru both pathway
D. Slow thru retrograde

41. 70 years male with AF. No risk factor for thromboembolism. Goal for INR is:
A. 1.5 2.0 B. 1.75 2.0
C. 2-3 D. 2.5-3.5

42. Young 20 years male with 2nd degree AV block, reverse with atropine site is:
A. AV node
B. Bundle of HIS
C. Bundle branch
D. Information not enough

43. TCA overdose with wide ops of 0.14 sec and 7 HR > 100 with seizure with vomiting, gastric lavage done. Next step:
A. IV lidocaine B. Amiodarone
C. Phenytoin D. $NaHCO_3$

44. CRT lead placed in:
A. CS B. PL vein
C. Anti-cardiac vein D. LV

45. Brugada patient young child with ICD develops arrythmic storm Rx:
A. I.V. procainamide B. I.V. quinidine
C. I.V. flecainide D. I.V. metoprolol

46. CBF is 100 ml/min/100 gm and aorta and RA PO_2 difference 0.2 ml/min/calculated MVO_2 of myocardium / 100 gm/ min:
A. 2 B. 20
C. 200 D. Cannot be calculated

47. Androgen in athletes causes all *except*:
A. MI
B. Pleosis hepatitis
C. Gyanecomastia
D. Fanconi's anemia

48. All true *except*:
A. Venous hum decrease in supine position
B. Star Edward opening sound louder than St Jude
C. Angina can produce S4
D. Heart sound diminished in MI

49. Contraindicated in pregnancy all *except*::
A. Ramipril
B. Sodium nitroprusside
C. Torsemide
D. Spiromolactone

50. 2 years child with diarrhoea with TG = 25, TC = 12, negligible LDL. Diagnosis is:
A. Tangier
B. Gaucher
C. CETP def
D. A betalipoproteinemia

51. Elderly ladies on warfarin with AF, develops, headache, confusion, CT s/o ICH with INR of 5.4: planned for neuro surgery step to reverse warfarin:
A. FFP
B. Vit. K
C. Clotting factor ppt
D. PRBC

52. Marfan's syndrome surgery may be:
A. Bentel B. DOR procedure
C. Maze procedure D. CoA repair

53. **Chronic anaemia all *except*:**
A. Erythropoietin disease decrease mortality in HF
B. Ferritin level increase in anaemia of chronic disease
C. Increase cyanotic spell in TOF
D. 2.3 DPG level increase in RBC

54. **Most common infection after splenectomy:**
A. Strep. pneumoniae
B. N. meningitides
C. H. influenzae
D. Pseudomonases

55. **Met. syndrome a/w all *except*:**
A. Decrease serum viscosity
B. PCOD
C. OSA
D. Hyperuricemia

56. **Cortical infarct s/o by:**
A. Hemiparesis
B. Homonymous hemianopia
C. Confusion
D. Syncope

57. **1 mmHg increase CO_2 in chromic respiratory acidosis compensated by ____ increase in HCO_3:**
A. 0.1 B. 0.4
C. 0.9 D. 2.5

58. **Lipoprotein associated with Alzheimer's disease:**
A. Apo A B. Apo B
C. Apo C D. Apo E

59. **RTA with sternal fracture and fracture of 1st left rib with mediastinal widening with stable vitals. Next appropriate step:**
A. Repeat X-ray before discharge
B. Aortogram
C. Analgesic and reassurance
D. Manage fracture

60. **CIN prevented by:**
A. IV frusemide
B. Biplane angiography
C. Metformin
D. <200 ml dye

61. **Dopamine receptor implicated in all *except*:**
A. Migraine
B. Preclampsia
C. Neuroleptic malignant syndrome
D. Renal vasodilation

62. **Rx of malignant hyperthermia all *except*:**
A. Amlodipine
B. Dantrolene
C. Cardiac pulmonary bypass
D. Procainamide

63. **Migraine:**
A. 5-HT antagonist safe in post MI
B. Patient with PFO and migraine no benefit of closure of PFO
C. Methysergide used for Rx causes valvular fibrosis
D. Syncope can occur

64. **Palpable purpura seen in:**
A. HSP
B. ITP
C. HIT

65. **Most common cause of sudden cardiac death:**
A. CAD B. HOCM
C. Long QT interval D. ARVD

66. **1st open heart surgery:**
A. Bailey B. Kirkillm
C. Gross D. Lilihee

67. **Hyperkalemia (K^+) all *except*:**
A. NSAID + ACE
B. Hyperthermia
C. Rhabdomyolysis
D. Pernicious anemia Rx with Vit B_{12}

68. **Hypokalemia (K^+) all *except*:**
A. Digoxin toxicity B. β-agonist
C. Amphotericin D. Decrease Mg++

69. **Rx of warfarin induced skin necrosis all *except*:**
A. Heparin B. Vitamin K
C. Protein C D. Bivaluridin

70. **Increase eNOS all *except*:**
A. Increase blood flow
B. Increase cardiac load
C. Acetylcholine
D. Bradycardia

71. **Side effect of clopidogrel:**
A. Post CABG infection
B. Aspirin resistance
C. Nephropathy
D. Coronary artery aneurysm

72. **Malignancy with propensity to metastasise to heart:**
A. Malignant melanoma
B. Ileum carcinoid
C. Adeno Ca lung
D. Stomach Ca

73. **Drug used in TAD (Buerger's disease):**
A. Atorvastatin
B. Prusugrel
C. Nicotine
D. Iloprost

74. Amyloidosis least seen in echo:
- **A.** Diastolic dysfunction
- **B.** Systolic dysfunction
- **C.** Pericardial tamponade
- **D.** IAS hypertrophy

75. Adenosine preferred over verapamil for SVT in all *except*:
- **A.** Patient on theophylline
- **B.** Neonate
- **C.** HF
- **D.** Patient on β blocker

76. IV Phenylephrine decrease all *except*:
- **A.** Murmur of TOF
- **B.** AS
- **C.** Late synoptic murmur of MVP
- **D.** HR

77. Post fontan surgery, patient develops protein loosing enteropathy characterise by all *except*:
- **A.** Lymphocytosis
- **B.** Decrease albumin
- **C.** Decrease gammaglobulin
- **D.** Decrease α-anti trypsin in plasma

78. Only indication for percutaneous pulm valve replacement is:
- **A.** TOF with absent PV
- **B.** Post operative TOF with severe PR
- **C.** Pulmonary artery trifurcation severe stenosis
- **D.** Truncus arteriosus

79. Large ASD with MS all *except*:
- **A.** Loud ejection murmur at 2nd right ICS
- **B.** Diastolic flow murmur of TR
- **C.** Loud diastolic rumble at apex
- **D.** Loud P2

80. Development of heart all true *except*:
- **A.** III arch common carotid A
- **B.** I arch maxillary sinus
- **C.** V left arch of aorta
- **D.** VI left ductus arteriosus

81. Swine flu:
- **A.** Oeltamavir decrease efficiency due to resistance
- **B.** Not have high case fatality rate
- **C.** Mainly human humor transmur
- **D.** HINI

82. Bypass tract seen in all *except*:
- **A.** CC-TGA
- **B.** Ebstein
- **C.** HCM
- **D.** Inlet VSD

83. Least likely to cause early, PVE:
- **A.** Hacek
- **B.** Enterococcus
- **C.** Coagulase negative staph
- **D.** Candida

84. Penicillin for rheumatic fever prophylaxis all *except*:
- **A.** Without carditis - 5 years or 21 years age
- **B.** Before dental extraction
- **C.** Also given after double valve replacement
- **D.** Also given in PRSA

85. Left stellate sympathetic ganglionectomy done in:
- **A.** Brugada
- **B.** Congenital LQT
- **C.** Carotid hypersensitivity
- **D.** Supine hypotension

86. Advance and accord trial true:
- **A.** Decrease stroke
- **B.** Decrease microvascular complication in accord
- **C.** Target HBA1C < 5
- **D.** Decrease cardiovascular mortality

87. Post IWMI at an Rx with statin; Ramipril metoprolol, nitrate, asymptomatic. One month after ECG follow-up s/o occasional VPC. Next step is:
- **A.** Amiodarone
- **B.** Observation
- **C.** Sotatol
- **D.** Procainamide

88. Angiography with 60% LMCA, 80% RCA, diabetic, EF = 35%, chest pain class II, treatment is:
- **A.** CABG
- **B.** Medical
- **C.** PCI of RCA
- **D.** PCI of both

89. Match trials all *except*:
- **A.** COURAGE - CAS
- **B.** OAT - primary PCI
- **C.** ICTUSLTUSA - USA
- **D.** SYNTAX - CABG vs DES

90. 5 kg infant underwent cardiac cath developed absent peripheral pulses and limb ischemia Rx:
- **A.** Fogarty cath. embolectomy
- **B.** Thrombolytic Rx
- **C.** Alpha blocker
- **D.** Surgery embolectomy

91. Linked angina:
- **A.** Post MI
- **B.** Cardioesophageal reflux
- **C.** Post surgery
- **D.** Cluster of PVC

ANSWERS

1	C	2	A	3	A	4	B	5	A	6	A	7	A
8	A	9	A	10	D	11	B	12	B	13	C	14	A
15	D	16	A	17	C	18	C	19	A	20	A	21	
22	A	23	C	24	A	25	B	26	B	27	D	28	C
29	A	30	D	31	B	32	B	33	A	34	A	35	A
36	A	37	C	38	D	39	B	40	B	41	C	42	A
43		44	B	45	B	46	B	47	D	48	A	49	C
50	D	51	A	52	A	53	A	54	A	55	A	56	C
57	B	58	D	59	B	60	B	61	B	62	C	63	C
64	A	65	A	66	D	67	D	68	A	69		70	C
71	A	72	A	73	D	74	C	75	A	76	A	77	C
78	B	79	C	80		81	A	82	D	83	A	84	B
85	B	86	D	87	B	88	A	89	D	90	B	91	B

5

AIIMS DECEMBER 2008

1. **Erythema nodosum seen in all *except*:**
   A. Acute rheumatic fever
   B. Sarcoidosis
   C. GCA
   D. Takayasu
2. **A patient with severe MS, without any history of acute rheumatic fever present is:**
   A. Aschoff nodules
   B. Subcutaneous nodules
   C. Carey Coomb murmur
   D. Erythema marginatum
3. **About MVP true are all *except*:**
   A. PML commoner to prolapse
   B. No click in PML prolapse
   C. PML easier to repair
   D. Eccentric jet in echo
4. **Streptococcus viridans IE not seen is:**
   A. Proliferative GN
   B. Increase ASLO titer
   C. RA factor
   D. Backache
5. **Post PV replacement, early IE seen in all *except*:**
   A. Enterococci
   B. Diphtheroids
   C. Candida
   D. Staph. epidermidis
6. **Hacek endocarditis – Drug of choice:**
   A. Ceftriaxone
   B. Ampicillin sulbactum
   C. Linezolid
   D. Imipenem
7. **Broad spectrum antibiotics associated with all *except*:**
   A. Diarrhea with clostridium difficile
   B. Vancomycin resistant enterococcal IE
   C. Pneumonia due to erythromycin resistant S. pneumoniae
   D. Pharyngitis due to beta-hemolytic streptococci resistant to penicillin
8. **hsCRP : level doesn't signify the ACS (mg/L):**
   A. 1 B. 2
   C. 4 D. 20
9. **HOCM, all are true *except*:**
   A. Screening can be done by fetal edema
   B. Myosin heavy chain mutation
   C. Myocardial disarray
   D. AD with variable penetrance
10. **Best prognosis in infants with LVH:**
    A. Infants of DM mother
    B. PKD disease
    C. Noonan's syndrome
    D. Pompe disease
11. **Least myocardial depression by:**
    A. Ivabridine B. Carvedilol
    C. Dilzem D. Nebibulol
12. **Compensated CHF is decompensated by all *except*:**
    A. Aspirin B. NSAIDs
    C. Trastuzumab D. Pioglitazone
13. **CHF, all used *except*:**
    A. Vasopressin B. Nesiritide
    C. Eplerenone D. Levosimendan
14. **Severe AS + No symptoms surgery not done in all *except*:**
    A. Painless ischemia
    B. AVR 1.0 cm^2
    C. Arrhythmias (persistent)
    D. LV dysfunction in TMT
15. **AR is seen in all *except*:**
    A. HTN
    B. Psoriasis
    C. AS
    D. Twin to twin transfusion

16. **Thoracic aneurysm in a tall, thin female, least likely is:**
A. Takayasu arteritis
B. CMN
C. Marfan's syndrome
D. Familial homocystinuria

17. **RCMP versus CCP, RCMP is favored by:**
A. BNP < 50 pg/ml
B. Septal bounce
C. PASP > 50 mmHg
D. Normal E/A velocity on strike Doppler

18. **Acute rheumatic fever, all true *except*:**
A. IV Ig decreases severe chorea
B. IV methyl prednisolone useful in severe carditis
C. Untreated acute rheumatic fever resolve within 12 weeks
D. Pauciarticular arthritis may be seen in recurrence

19. **Supravalvular AS mutation:**
A. Elastin B. Vimentin
C. Proteoglycan D. MMP-2

20. **Dicrotic pulse all *except*:**
A. HOCM B. Post AVR
C. Cardiac tamponade D. Severe CHF

21. **Chronic MR with RHD IE prophylaxis given in:**
A. Tatoo B. TEE
C. Colonoscopy D. Delivery

22. **Bicuspid AV all *except*:**
A. Commissural fusion
B. Pure AR may be seen
C. Single coronary artery from RCS may be present
D. Aortic dissection increased

23. **Hepatojugular reflux is indicative of all *except*:**
A. TR
B. RHF
C. Decrease afterload
D. Increase PCWP

24. **AV area in cardiac cath. lab by:**
A. Gorlin formula
B. Continuity equation
C. Cournards formula
D. Strass formula

25. **HOCM all *except*:**
A. Post VPC there is decrease PR
B. Phase IV valsalva increases murmur
C. Spike and dome in art. pulse

26. **In STEMI; 30 days mortality is:**
A. 1.5% B. 5%
C. 10% D. 16%

27. **After 5 days of acute MI, HR should not exceed on TMT is:**
A. 70 B. 75
C. 80 D. 85

28. **Mismatch:**
A. Madit II : prior MI with EF < 30%
B. Companion : Severe HF
C. Definite : Non-ischaemic CMP
D. SCD-HeFT : QRS > 130 msec

29. **Statins blocks conversion of HMGCoA to:**
A. Mevalonate
B. Squalene
C. Fernasyl pyrophosphate
D. HMG – Pyrophosphate

30. **Statin induced myopathy is seen in all *except*:**
A. Diabetic renal failure
B. Old age
C. Along with fibrate
D. Obese male

31. **Statins C/I in all *except*:**
A. Pregnancy
B. DM-nephropathy on dialysis
C. CPK > 10 times
D. Severe liver dysfunction

32. **68 years female, asymptomatic DM with LDL = 165, HDL = 45, TG = 185 according to NCEP ATP III guidelines:**
A. Life style mod. only
B. Atorva + Ezetimibe
C. Atorva
D. Atorva + fibrates

33. **Mismatch:**
A. HDL = A2
B. LDL = B100
C. VLDL = B100
D. Chylomicron = ApoE

34. **All increases HDL *except*:**
A. Trans FA
B. Pravastatin
C. Torcetrapib
D. Fibrates

35. **Accord and Advance trial in DM: True are all *except*:**
A. Decrease microvascular complication with tight blood sugar control
B. No decrease macrovascular complication with tight blood sugar control
C. No decrease in total mortality
D. $HbA_1C < 5$

36. 42-year-old male with preoperative evaluation for thyroid mass with HTN. No other heart disease family history of (to brother) similar tumor surgery with no other details, what to do next?

A. Control BP and give fitness
B. ECG, Holter
C. Secondary HTN evaluation
D. No further evaluation

37. 65 years male, planned for inguinal hernia surgery, TMT normal, rest ECG normal, what next to do?

A. Dobutamine stress
B. CT-angiography
C. No further evaluation, proceed to surgery
D. EBCT

38. CAD epidemiology all are true *except*:

A. In Japan there is increase CAD incidence despite fish consumption
B. Decrease mortality in Mediterranean country despite equal cholesterol
C. Southeast Asia: Met. syndrome more than native American
D. China: More stroke than India

39. Post MI, most predictive of SCD:

A. LVEF
B. T wave alternans
C. Signal average ECG
D. Non sust. VT

40. Acute MR on day 4 of MI on NTG, digoxin, diuretics becomes restless and cyanotic PH = 7.2, PaO_2 = 90, PCO_2 = 20, HCO_3^- = 13, treatment is:

A. MVR
B. Captopril for nitrate tolerance
C. IV methylene blue

41. Most common coronary anomaly:

A. ALCAPA
B. LCx from RCA
C. Left main from RCs
D. RCA from LCs

42. Courage trial: (50 years patient with angina class II; on angio TVD normal LAD, distal OM, good LV funct) Mx is:

A. Trial didn't include patient like this
B. Medical Mx
C. PCI with DES
D. CABG

43. DM female presented within 2 hours with chest pain along with ST depression and T inversion in V_1 to V_6, I, aVL and ST elevation in aVR BP 90/60 PR = 120, AVR best Mx:

A. Coronary angiography
B. CT-angio
C. Beta-blocker
D. STK

44. AWMI with LV aneurysm, diagnosis of myocardial viability is with:

A. Rest reinjection of thallium
B. Pyrophosphate scan
C. Metoprolol spect
D. CECT

45. TURP in previous MI, postop 3rd day to confirm ACS ideal investigation is:

A. Cardiac troponin T
B. CPK-MB fraction
C. Echo
D. ECG

46. Troponin T increase in patient not due to myocardial damage:

A. Renal failure **B.** Myocarditis
C. NSTEMI **D.** PTE

47. All *except*:

A. Increase BNP in diastolic dysfunction
B. Normal BNP in acute MI
C. ACE–I decreases BNP
D. Increase BNP in PTE

48. Sequence of events in coronary artery occlusion:

A. Diastolic dysfunction
B. Systolic dysfunction
C. ECG
D. Angina

49. Enoxaparin true is:

A. Partially reversible with protamine
B. NO HIT
C. Monoclonal ab.
D. Acts by vWF

50. All are true *except*:

A. Stable angina class-III angina – Aspirin + clopidogrel
B. Aspirin + Clopidogrel for 1 year after DES
C. Warfarin + Aspirin after PV thrombosis
D. Aspirin for 6 months in ASD – device closure

51. Acute MR after MI all *except*:

A. More with inferior wall MI
B. Indicate TVD
C. Soft and short duration murmur can be seen
D. TR in right sided PMD

52. 2 days post MI all are increased *except*:

A. HDL
B. CPK MB
C. TLC
D. CRP

53. **Pulmonary venous occlusive disease, all *except*:**
A. Normal PCWP
B. Increase PAP
C. LV dysfunction not present
D. Intravascular fibrosis present

54. **Which is not seen in severe ischemia?**
A. Increase lung uptake
B. Decrease LV cavity
C. Increase LV thickness in systole
D. Hypokinesia on stress

55. **Most significant factor for CAD:**
A. Increasing age
B. Homocystinuria
C. Obesity (BMI 25-30)
D. HTN

56. **Most common cyanotic disease in newborn:**
A. TGA
B. Pulmonary AV fistula
C. Pulmonary atresia
D. Ebstein's anomaly

57. **Cleft mitral valve in:**
A. Down's syndrome
B. MVP
C. Repaired MV

58. **PGE_2 infusion not helpful in:**
A. CaO
B. Pulmonary atresia
C. HLHS
D. AV septal defect with MR

59. **In 4 years old child post BT shunt done at 2 years of age has vague history of unconsciousness. All are causes continuous murmur on auscultation:**
A. VT
B. Bradyarrhythmia
C. Seizure
D. Cyanotic spell

60. **8 years old child with history of surgery for CHD in infancy with left upper limb pulses weak diagnosis is:**
A. Double aortic arch
B. TGA
C. CoA
D. Cervical rib

61. **Increase K+ with CRF, ECG finding not present is:**
A. Decrease QT
B. Absent P wave
C. Narrow base T
D. Interventricular conduction delay

62. **Conduction block responding to antibiotic:**
A. Lyme disease
B. Congenital syphilis
C. Diphtheria
D. Acute rheumatic fever

63. **AF in 78 years old male with HR 80/min. Drug to be given is:**
A. Aspirin
B. Warfarin
C. Diltiazem
D. Amiodarone

64. **AF not associated with:**
A. AAI pacing
B. Esophageal surgery
C. Submassive PTE
D. Atrial infarction

65. **True is:**
A. Dronadarone has no iodine
B. Dronadarone decreases HF mortality
C. Amiodarone decreases mortality in SCD-HeFT (V/s placebo)
D. d-sotalol decreases mortality after acute MI

66. **18 years old boy with palpitation with giddiness. Holter at 2:45 AM. SVT for 25 beats. Also dropped 'P' beat. 4 beat prior to dropped beat there was increase in PR of 40 msec with baseline PR of 160 msec. Best Mx:**
A. Atropine with rhythm strip
B. No need of further AVN and Purkinje system
C. Need for pacemaker
D. Infrahisian conduction block should be evaluated

67. **Sympathetic stimulation causes:**
A. Increase ERP in AVN
B. Increase functional Ref. P. in AVN
C. Decrease ERP in atrial in
D. Decrease slope of phase-4 of SAN

68. **Best prognosis VPC:**
A. V_6 VPC with qR morphology
B. Parasystolic VPC
C. Bundle branch rentry VPC
D. VPC in descending limb of T wave

69. **SVT and VT are differentiated by all *except*:**
A. History of previous MI
B. qRS in V_6
C. Fusion beat
D. AV dissociation

70. **All are true *except*:**
A. QT measured in lead II
B. U-wave in V_2-V_4
C. Volt-criteria are less sensitive in adults
D. In V_1 T inversion, after 2 years of age is normal

71. **Not worsened by exercise:**
A. VT from RV in normal adult
B. VT after MI
C. Brugada syndrome
D. HOCM

72. **Accessory pathway can present in infants *except*:**
A. Tachycardia in fetus
B. Delta wave disappearance in TMT SCD increases
C. May present without abnormal wave on ECG

73. **Reperfusion arrhythmia all *except*:**
A. Primary VF
B. NSVT
C. VPC
D. Slow junctional arrhythmia

74. **Pulmonary artery, mixed O_2 saturation is:**
A. 75 B. 85
C. 25 D. 55

75. **Maximum O_2 consumption:**
A. 50 ml/kg/min B. 30 ml/kg/min
C. 14 ml/kg/min D. 10 ml/kg/min

76. **In Kartagener's syndrome which is seen most commonly?**
A. CC-TGA
B. TGA
C. Scimitar syndrome
D. Struc. normal heart

77. **BP measurement 150/94 mmHg should be repeated after (with repeated measurements):**
A. Within 1 week
B. Within 2 months
C. Within 2 weeks
D. Within 6 months

78. **Ambulatory BP monitoring in all *except*:**
A. Masked HTN
B. Pseudo HTN
C. Refractory HTN
D. White coat HTN

79. **All are seen within myocardial wall *except*:**
A. Amyloid
B. Chagas disease
C. Toxoplasma
D. Coxsackie B

80. **All are true *except*:**
A. Increase mortality in male with digoxin (DIG trial)
B. ARB improves mortality equivalent to ACE-I
C. Amiodarone decreases mortality versus placebo in HF

81. **68 years old male with dizziness and fatigue on walking with BP 90/40, HR = 70/min, and on standing HR = 74/min, BP 80/50 all *except*:**
A. Shy-Drager syndrome
B. Parkinsonism
C. Sick sinus syndrome
D. Carotid sinus HS

82. **Difficult to see in perfusion scan investigation:**
A. Inferior B. Anterior
C. Posterior D. Lateral

83. **pH = 7.4, PCO_2 40 mmHg, PaO_2 94, Cl– 80 meq/l, HCO_3 – 25 meq/L. A lady with vague complaint with above parameters diagnosis:**
A. Normal ABG patient malingering
B. Mixed acid base disorder
C. PTE on O_2 therapy
D. Alkali treatment

84. **Renal failure which drug dose modification require?**
A. Atenolol
B. Pravastatin
C. INH
D. Amiodarone

85. **Which acts on DCT?**
A. Torsemide B. Metalozone
C. Bumetinide D. Spirolactone

86. **Increase uric acid all *except*:**
A. Severe hepatocellular failure
B. Pulmonary HT
C. Chronic renal failure
D. Metabolic syndrome

87. **Flash pulmonary edema seen in:**
A. CaO B. RAS
C. PIH D. Conn's syndrome

88. **Increase renin seen in all *except*:**
A. Conn's syndrome
B. Single RAS
C. Accelerated HTN
D. Estrogen

89. **Metabolic syndrome A/W all *except*:**
A. PCOD
B. Hypothyroidism
C. DSA
D. Hypercoagulability

90. **Lacunar infarct all *except*:**
A. Pure motor unilateral - weakness
B. Pure sensory L/L loss
C. Homonymous hemianopia
D. Ataxia with hemiparesis of left unilateral

91. Which decreases recurrence of stroke?
A. β-blocker
B. ACE-I
C. Aldosterone antagonist
D. Central sympathetic inhibitor

92. Interventricular interdependence seen in:
A. CCP
B. PAH (primary)
C. EMF

93. All are matched *except*:
A. Thallium in sarcoplasmic membrane
B. Tecnitiium in mitochondrial integrity
C. TDI in tissue characterization
D. Myocardial contrast for microvascular integrity

94. All are used in PET *except*:
A. Rb_{82}
B. O_{15} water
C. N_{13} Ammonia
D. Tc_{99}

95. Migratory polyarthritis is seen in all *except*:
A. RF
B. Lyme disease
C. SLE
D. Gonococcal arthritis

96. Scleroderma with HTN, DOC to prevent target organ damage:
A. CCB
B. ACE-I
C. β-blocker
D. α blocker

97. 24 years female with glomerulonephritis, fever, hemoptysis. Mediastinal mass compressing right PA with increase ANCA, diagnosis:
A. Wegener's granulomatosis
B. NHL
C. Sarcoidosis
D. Acute inf. endocarditis

98. Limb torniquet on lower limb for 2 hours for orthopaedic surgery. After torniquet release which is seen?
A. Increase venous return
B. Increase CO
C. No significant change in CO
D. Decrease in blood pressure

99. About tension pneumothorax all are true *except*:
A. No needle before X-ray
B. No lung margin may be seen in X-ray
C. Common in ventilation
D. Can cause electromechanical dissociation

100. Chronic respiratory alkalosis all *except*:
A. Permissive hypercapnia
B. G –VE septicemia
C. Pregnancy
D. Cirrhosis

101. Drugs not causing HTN:
A. Levodopa
B. EPO
C. Tacrolimus
D. Indomethacin

102. HES not used in (along with steroids):
A. Anti IL-5
B. Cyclosporine
C. Imatinib
D. Hydroxyurea

103. Sickle cell anaemia treatment:
A. Hydroxyurea
B. Hypotonic saline
C. Vitamin E
D. PPAR-<

104. Cirrhosis patient with no past history of heart disease dev. with cyanosis, diagnosis is done by:
A. TEE
B. Contrast echo
C. Intracardiac echo
D. Hb-electrophoresis

105. N acetyl cyteine I.V. can cause:
A. Anaphylactoid reaction
B. Seizure
C. HTN
D. Renal failure

106. ACE-I with moderate renal failure increase K^+ by:
A. Digoxin
B. NSAIDs
C. Alkali treatment
D. Salbutamol

107. Stress imagining, poor prog, in all *except*:
A. Decrease LV size
B. Decrease systolic thickening
C. Increase lung uptake

108. Absolute indication of surgery in CAD patient is:
A. Asymptomatic pseudoaneurysm associated with IWMI
B. MR with severe LV dysfunction
C. Apical thrombus with AWMI
D. Subacute stent thrombosis

ANSWERS

1	A	2	C	3	B	4	B	5	B	6	A	7	
8	A	9	A	10	A	11	A	12	A	13	A	14	B
15	B	16	D	17	C	18	B	19	A	20	A	21	C
22	C	23	D	24	A	25	B	26	B	27	C	28	D
29	A	30	D	31	B	32	C	33	D	34	A	35	D
36		37	C	38	A	39	A	40	C	41		42	B
43	C	44	A	45	A	46		47	B	48		49	A
50	A	51	B	52	A	53	A	54		55	A	56	A
57	A	58	D	59	D	60	C	61	A	62	A	63	B
64	A	65	A	66		67		68	B	69	B	70	
71	C	72	B	73		74		75		76	D	77	B
78	B	79	A	80	A	81	C	82	A	83		84	A
85	D	86	A	87	B	88	A	89	B	90	C	91	B
92		93	C	94	D	95	A	96	B	97	A	98	
99		100		101	A	102	B	103	A	104	B	105	A
106	A	107	A	108	A								

6

AIIMS JUNE 2008

1. **Statin causes ↑myotoxicity in all *except*:**
   A. Renal failure with DM
   B. Elderly
   C. with fibrate
   D. Obese male
2. **Statin therapy on 2° prevention mortality ↓ per 1000 population:**
   A. 75
   B. 100
   C. 150
3. **NSTEMI, mortality at 30 days:**
   A. 15%
   B. 20%
   C. 5%
4. **No added salt diet:**
   A. 0.5–1gm
   B. 2–3 gm
   C. 6–7 gm
5. **Inter heart study compared:**
   A. Risk
6. **OAT study, PCI not useful time interval included:**
   A. 0–24 hours
   B. 3–28 days
   C. No time criteria
7. **Irrational combination in patient with rec. VT:**
   A. Mexiletine procainamide, amiodarone
   B. Procainamide, sotalol, amiad
   C. Procaine, metoprolol, amiad
8. **Boventan produces:**
   A. Pedal edema
   B. Anemia
   C. Liver toxicity (transaminases inc.)
   D. Headache
9. **Combined in patient with DM and ACS:**
   A. Fondaparinux + bivalirudin
   B. Clopigel + abciximab
   C. Aspirin + fragmn
10. **Study demonstrating that ARI as efficacious as ACE–I in heart failure:**
    A. Valiant
11. **MAC useful in R_x:**
    A. Pulmonary fibrosis
    B. Crohn's disease
    C. M. sclerosis
12. **Brain death:**
    A. Bilateral cortical infarct
    B. Sagittal thrombosis
    C. Basilar thrombosis
    D. No cerebral perfusion
13. **Bosentan S/E all *except*:**
    A. ↑ QT interval
    B. Liver toxicity
    C. Anemia
    D. Pedal edema
14. **PTMC all used *except*:**
    A. Brockenbosyl needle
    B. Fogarty catheter
    C. Inoue balloon
    D. Muller transseptal sheath
15. **PG E2 infusion causes all *except*:**
    A. Hypothermia
    B. Seizure
    C. Apnea
    D. Bradycardia
16. **PICA/ROI equally effective in all the following *except*:**
    A. Door– needle time < 30 mt
    B. Door–balloon < 90 mt
    C. Killing class III
17. **All true in HIV *except*:**
    A. Cardiac tamponade is rare
    B. IE R_x same as gen population
    C. CABG not done

18. **Indication for CAG in U/A all *except*:**
A. Trop T > 0.1
B. GRACE score > 70
C. PCI 6 month sback
D. CABG 2 years back

19. **Rheumatic fever true all *except*:**
A. Myosin in cardiac valves decides degree of damage
B. Antibody to M protein is protective
C. Valvular lack [MR] may disappear with time

20. **All are indication of surgery on IE *except*:**
A. Fever > 15 days
B. CHF
C. Mobile veg > 10 mm
D. ESR > 100

21. **Dose of I/V right PA in ischemic shock:**
A. 0.9 mg/kg, 10% of 10 ml dose as bolus and remainder over 1 hour
B. 5

22. **Endothelial have following markers *except*:**
A. CD_3 B. CD_{34}
C. CD 133 D. VEGF

23. **Mesenchymal stem cells are derived from:**
A. Bone marrow B. Spleen
C. Placenta D. Peripheral blood

24. **Aortic mitral continuity in all *except*:**
A. DORV B. Truncus
C. TOF D. VSD with PS

25. **Conotruncal abnormality in all *except*:**
A. Retinoic acid B. Rubella
C. Alcohol D. 22q deletion

26. **2 days infant with umbilical vein catheter suddenly develop HF with absent femoral pulse. Echo doesn't show coarctation R_x of choice:**
A. Streptokinase
B. Exchange transfusion
C. Ballooning

27. **Massive hemoptysis in VSD with infective endocarditis of 3 mm duration inv. of choice:**
A. CT angio
B. MR angio
C. Echo
D. Hematologic evaluation

28. **Mitral annular calcification in all *except*:**
A. Marfan's
B. Renal failure
C. Dilated CM
D. Hyperparathyroidism

29. **Complete block by all *except*:**
A. Lithium
B. Hypokalemic
C. Hypermagnesemia
D. Yellow oleander poisoning

30. **R_x of vasovagal syncope all *except*:**
A. Midodrine B. β–blocker
C. Paroxetine D. Levodopa

31. **Echo pulmonary valve velocity > 4 seen in:**
A. Hyperthyroidism B. Eisenmenger
C. Muscular VSD D. TOF

32. **Echo continuity equation used to diagnose:**
A. EF
B. Aortic valve area
C. dp/dt

33. **Echo ↑ LVEDP seen in as:**
A. B bump
B. Paradoxical septal motion
C. Normal E/A
D. ↓ EF

34. **A/C MI diagnosed in presence of LBBB all *except*:**
A. ST↑ V_1–V_3 of 1 mm
B. Slurring of S wave in V_1-V_2
C. V_5–V_6 q wave

35. **TMT ST↑ in inf. lead does not suggest:**
A. Coronary artery spasm
B. Transmural ischemia
C. LV aneurysm
D. Right dominance

36. **Stroke–MI:**
A. Finland B. Rural India
C. China D. Japan

37. **Euthanasia was first legal in:**
A. Netherlands B. Finland
C. USA D. Italy

38. **Essential HT in pregnancy all *except*:**
A. Abruptio placentae
B. Syncope
C. Perinatal mortality
D. Inc. incidence of pre-eclampsia

39. **All suggest morphological RV *except*:**
A. Moderator band
B. Apical leaflet attachment
C. Pulmonary artery origin

40. **Pulmonary artery O_2 saturation:**
A. 30 B. 60
C. 80

41. **Max. oxygen saturation in fetus:**
A. Ductus venosus

B. Ductus arteriosus
C. SVC
D. Asc. aorta

42. **Regular cannon wave in all *except*:**
A. CHB B. VT
C. AVRT D. AVNRT

43. **TMT in young asymptomatic persons:**
A. Not indicated
B. Indicated before surgery
C. Indicated for assessment

44. **RBBB with recurrent syncope in old men. indication for PPI:**
A. A-H interval > 150 sec
B. HV interval 100 sec
C. SNRT > 500
D. Carotid sinus massage pause > 2.6 sec

45. **Ryanodine receptor in:**
A. Catecholamine poly VT
B. Brugada syndrome
C. Jarvel Lange Neil syndrome
D. Romano Ward syndrome

46. **Mortality benefit in heart failure demonstrated in all *except*:**
A. Atenolol B. Metoprolol
C. Carvedilol D. Spironolactone

47. **All are normal change in elderly *except*:**
A. RBBB
B. Systolic HT
C. ↓ heart rate variability
D. ↑ maximal heart rate

48. **ICD in all *except*:**
A. CAD with angina with stable VT
B. LT fascicular VT
C. HOCM with MSVT with thickness 30 mm
D. LQT with QT interval 550 ms

49. **Cocaine HTN:**
A. Mitiglinide B. NTG
C. Diltiazem D. Metoprolol

50. **Cardiovascular effect of thyroid hormone all *except*:**
A. LDL↑
B. ↓ vascular resistance
C. ↑ CO
D. ↑ diastolic relaxation

51. **More common in female than male all *except*:**
A. AS B. Alzheimer's
C. PHT D. Biliary cirrhosis

52. **PND not seen in:**
A. AR
B. Constrictive pericarditis
C. LA myxoma

53. **Enoxaparin true is:**
A. Does not cause HIT
B. Partial reversal with protamine

54. **Abciximab all *except*:**
A. Pig-mouse chimeric antibody
B. Given as bolus followed by infusion

55. **BMPR–2 with PPH can coexist with:**
A. SLE
B. Osler Weber-Rendu syndrome/hereditary hemorrhagic telangiectasia
C. Pheochromocytoma

56. **In NHI_N PPH associated with adverse prognosis all *except*:**
A. ↑ right atrial press
B. Inc. pulmonary artery press
C. ↑ Age
D. ↓ Cardiac output

57. **↑HDL is seen in:**
A. Tangier B. Gaucher
C. Hurler D. Pompe

58. **Best outcome in pregnancy:**
A. MVP with mild MR
B. AS with mild LV dysfunction

59. **All following favour c poorer RCD *except*:**
A. PA pressure < 50
B. Pericardial knock
C. BNP level 1000

60. **Cyanosis in premature infants is caused by ingestion by mother of:**
A. Methylene blue
B. Well water
C. Tobacco
D. Alcohol

61. **ABG of hypoxic patient shows $PaCO_2$ 50, (A–a) O_2 gradient 12 diagnosis is:**
A. Pulmonary edema
B. Atelectasis
C. Respiratory MS paralysis

62. **Gondolium enhanced contrast in MR angio causes:**
A. Dec. sperm count
B. Pancreatitis
C. Nephrogenic systemic fibrosis

63. **Aortic dissection least common manifestation:**
A. Paraplegia
B. Status epilepticus
C. ST ↑ II, III, IV

64. **Metabolized by CYP:**
A. Pravastatin B. Erythromycin
C. Digoxin D. Hydralazine

65. **Hypertension with stroke BP–250/120, all can be used *except*:**
A. S/C nifedipine B. I/V MTG
C. I/V labetalol D. Fenoldopam

66. **Atrial flutter true all *except*:**
A. R_x by RF ablation
B. Rate control easier than in AF
C. C/C anti-coagulation needle

67. **Re-entry is a mechanism for which arrhythmic:**
A. Atrial flutter

68. **Pulse difference right arm more than left in all *except*:**
A. Coarctation juxtadural
B. PDA with Eisenmenger
C. Takayasu type I
D. Williams

69. **Inferior wall MI with papillary MS rupture all *except*:**
A. Short systolic murmur
B. Indicates severe TVD
C. More common in inf. MI

70. **Inferior well MI worst prognosis indicated by:**
A. CHB B. ST ↑ CVR
C. Pre depression D. ST ↓ V_1–V_3

71. **Asymptomatic AS with peak instantaneous gradient > 40:**
A. No R_x B. AV repair
C. Ballooning D. Ross procedure

72. **Reverse split seen in all *except*:**
A. PPI B. PDA
C. Angina D. TOF after repair

73. **4 years body who had palliative shunt at 2 years of age has continuous murmur all *except*:**
A. Modified BT B. Central
C. Glenn D. Pott

74. **Diagnosis of angina score:**
A. Framingham B. Rose
C. Minnesota D. Borg

75. **Complement levels normal in all *except*:**
A. Hypertension B. Wegener's
C. IE

76. **Janeway lesions most common in:**
A. Staph. aureus B. Strep epidermidis
C. Hacek

77. **St. Jude's valve is:**
A. Ball and cage B. Bileaflet
C. Bio prosthetic

78. **Persistent prominent U waves in ECG indicator:**
A. Susceptibility to torsades
B. Ischemia
C. Hypocalcemia

79. **Effect of aspirin decreased by:**
A. Ibuprofen B. Cilostazol
C. Warfarin D. Rosiglitazone

80. **Volume control ventilation true all *except*:**
A. Less chance of barotrauma

81. **Constrictive pericarditis not seen:**
A. Hypothyroidism
B. Dressler syndrome
C. TB
D. Pyogenic

82. **Pulsus paradoxus not seen on:**
A. Iatrogenic tamponade
B. Tubercular massive effusion
C. Low pressure tamponade

83. **All are true *except*:**
A. Pulsus alternans better felt in brachial than in carotid
B. Pulsus parvus et tardus better felt in carotid
C. Sphygmomanometer can detect early pulsus paradoxus
D. Dicrotic pulse has prominent pressure wave

84. **BNP level in disease of cardiac origin:**
A. 0.1 B. 1
C. 10 D. 100 pg/ml

85. **Calcium released by SR reabsorbed by:**
A. SERCA

86. **Duration of ventricular APD from origin of QRS complex to:**
A. End of S wave B. End of T wave

87. **Troponin attaches to:**
A. Tropomyosin B. Ca
C. Actin D. Myosin

88. **β-blocker contraindicated due to fear of cardiogenic shock in extensive anterior MI in all *except*:**
A. BP < 100 mm Hg
B. HR basal 80/m
C. Age > 75 years
D. ↑duration from symptoms onset

89. **ACE gene DD polymorphism is associated with all *except*:**
A. ↑ Response to β blocker
B. ↓ Response to ACE (–)
C. Better survival in CHF
D. ↑ Incidence of CAD in the population

90. **Amyloidosis due to multiple myeloma all *except*:**
A. LVH in limb leads
B. Speckled appearance of septum
C. Thickening of vent. wall

91. **Metabolic regulator of coronary blood flow:**
A. Adenosine B. NO

92. **Brain abscess seen in all *except*:**
A. TAPVC
B. Ebstein
C. TGA
D. Pulmonary atresia

93. **Murmur of ASD inc. in all *except*:**
A. MS B. MR
C. HT D. RV MI

94. **In TOF, ESM ↓in:**
A. Amyl nitrite inhalation
B. Valsalva phase IV
C. Large VSD

95. **Warfarin causes all following in fetus *except*:**
A. Macrosomia
B. Mental retardation
C. Optic atrophy
D. Chondrodysplasia punctata

96. **Ischemic preconditioning is attenuated by K^+/ ATP channel inhibited by sulphonylureas:**
A. Glyburide B. Serotonin
C. Sildenafil D. Nicorandil

97. **Acromegaly with LA myxoma:**
A. Men I
B. Carney
C. Men II

98. **Incorrect match:**
A. ENHAME–Ezetimibe
B. OMTARGET–Telmisartan
C. ADVANCE–Atorvastatin
D. HOPE–Ramipril

99. **30 years female with cardiac mass disappears on chemo:**
A. Choriocarcinoma
B. Angiosarcoma
C. Melanoma
D. Rhabdomyoma

100. **30 years female with hypercoagulable state, all possible *except*:**
A. Homocysteinemia
B. Thrombocytosis
C. VWF deficiency
D. PNH

101. **SCD can occur in all *except*:**
A. LCX from RCA
B. Left main from right sinus
C. Coronary disease
D. ALCAPA

102. **Least common Down's:**
A. TOF
B. Cleft mitral valve
C. PDA
D. TGA

103. **Hypocalcemia is caused by all *except*:**
A. Thiazide
B. Hyperphosphatemia
C. Acute respiratory alkalosis

104. **Total electrical alternans in:**
A. Tamponade

ANSWERS

1	D	2		3	C	4	B	5	A	6	B	7	B
8		9	A	10	A	11	C	12		13	A	14	B
15		16	C	17	C	18	B	19	A	20	D	21	
22	A	23	A	24	A	25	B	26	A	27	A	28	C
29	B	30	D	31	D	32	B	33	A	34	B	35	D
36	C	37	A	38	B	39	C	40		41	A	42	A
43	A	44		45	A	46	A	47	A	48	B	49	D
50	A	51	A	52	B	53	B	54	A	55	B	56	C
57	A	58	A	59	C	60	B	61	C	62	A	63	B
64	B	65	A	66	B	67	A	68	B	69	B	70	D
71	A	72	D	73	C	74	B	75	C	76	A	77	B
78	A	79	A	80		81	B	82	C	83	D	84	D
85	A	86		87	A	88	B	89	C	90	A	91	A
92	A	93	D	94	A	95	A	96	A	97	B	98	C
99	A	100	C	101	A	102	D	103		104	A		

7

AIIMS MAY 2008

1. **Which is to be used in aortic dissection?**
   A. Nitroprusside
   B. Nitroglycerine
   C. IV esmolol
   D. Diazoxide

2. **Bidirectional tachycardia is seen in:**
   A. Digoxin toxicity
   B. CPVT
   C. Anderson syndrome
   D. All of the above

3. **Best prognosis is seen in:**
   A. Peripartum cardiomyopathy
   B. Alcoholic cardiomyopathy
   C. Amyloid cardiomyopathy
   D. HIV cardiomyopathy

4. **Regular cannon waves are seen in all *except*:**
   A. CHB
   B. Ventricular tachycardia
   C. AVNRT
   D. AVRT

5. **CHB is not seen in:**
   A. Lithium toxicity
   B. Hypermagnesemia
   C. Yellow oleander poisoning
   D. Hypokalemia

6. **All are reperfusion induced arrhythmia *except*:**
   A. Primary VF
   B. NSVT
   C. Slow junctional rhythm
   D. Multiple VPC

7. **In a diabetic patient having NSTEMI, which of the following is an irrational combination?**
   A. Bivaluridin + Fondaparinux
   B. Prasugrel + Eptifibatide
   C. Enoxaparin + Abciximab
   D. Clopidogrel + Eptifibatide

8. **Which is not used in PTMC?**
   A. Fogarty balloon
   B. Inoue balloon
   C. Mullins sheath
   D. Brokenbrough needle

9. **'No added' salt diet refers to a daily salt in take of:**
   A. 0.5 to 1 gm /day
   B. 3-4 gm/day
   C. 6-8 gm/day
   D. 8-10 gm/day

10. **In a patient who develops ST segment elevation in inferior leads during TMT, all are true *except:***
    A. Ventricular aneurysm
    B. MI
    C. Coronary spasm
    D. RCA dominance

11. **Which shunt is unlikely to be associated with continuous murmur/**
    A. Modified BT
    B. Glenn shunt
    C. Potts shunt
    D. Waterson shunt

12. **Maximum oxygen saturation in a fetus is seen in:**
    A. Ductus venosus
    B. Ductus arteriosus
    C. Ascending aorta
    D. Descending aorta

13. **OASIS 6 trial involved patients with:**
    A. Unstable angina B. STEMI
    C. CHF D. VT

14. **Earliest marker of myocardial ischemia:**
    A. ProBNP
    B. Ischemia modified albumin
    C. Choline
    D. Myoglobin

15. **β blockers have underperformed in recent hypertension trials because of:**
A. ↓ contractility
B. Reflected waves
C. Diabetes
D. Impotency

16. **Which of the following is not useful in ischemic preconditioning?**
A. Nicorandil B. Serotonin
C. Sildenafil D. Glyburide

17. **2-day-old neonate having umbilical artery catheterization develops circulatory collapse; the next intervention would be:**
A. STK
B. CABG
C. Balloon septostomy
D. I.V. fluid

18. **Epidemiologic transition among population founded by:**
A. Braunwald B. Omran
C. Olmansky D. Salim Yusuf

19. **Euthanasia has been legalized in which country?**
A. Holland B. Finland
C. Scotland D. Greenland

20. **Stroke mortality is more than CAD mortality in which country?**
A. China B. Africa
C. India D. Scotland

21. **Mutation in BMPR2 gene is also associated with:**
A. Osler-Rendu disease
B. Goodpasture's syndrome
C. Systemic sclerosis
D. SLE

22. **High HDL level is seen in:**
A. Tangier's disease
B. Gaucher's disease
C. LCAT deficiency
D. Niemann-Pick disease

23. **Which of the following is a side effect of prostaglandin infusion?**
A. Apnea B. Seizure
C. Hypothermia D. Hypotension

24. **All are used in vasovagal syncope *except:***
A. β blockers B. Midodrine
C. Paroetine D. L-Dopa

25. **OAT trial in PCI vs TLT, patient recruitment was done between:**
A. 0-24 hours B. 3-21 days
C. >30 days D. 21-30 days

26. **Interheart study was:**
A. Multiple risk factors
B. Target lipid lowering
C. Mortality
D. Effect of intervention

27. **N-acetyl cysteine used in:**
A. PVD B. IPF
C. Mitral sclerosis D. Crohn's

28. **Aspirin effect on platelets ↓ by:**
A. Brufen B. Cilostazol
C. Rosiglitazone D. Warfarin

29. **Left arm radial pulse weaker than right all *except:***
A. Takayasu arteritis
B. Juxta ductal CoA
C. Supra valvular AS
D. PDA with Eisenmenger

30. **NSTEMI 30-day mortality:**
A. 1.5% B. 5%
C. 10% D. 16%

31. **Statins in secondary prevention trial, mortality ↓ per 1000 patients:**
A. 70 B. 32
C. 150 D. 100

32. **BNP in cardiac dyspnea to differentiate from respiratory dyspnea by:**
A. >0.1 pg/ml B. >10
C. >1 D. >100

33. **CCP vs RCM evidence of CP are all *except*:**
A. Septal bounce
B. PASP<50
C. BNP 1000 pg/ml
D. Pericardial knock

34. **All are bosentan adverse effect *except*:**
A. Anemia
B. Liver dysfunction
C. QT↑
D. Pedal edema

35. **Brain abscess is least likely in:**
A. Pulmonary AV fistula
B. PAPVC NO IE
C. Truncus arteriosis
D. Ebstein's anomaly

36. **Dose of t-PA in stroke:**
A. 0.9 mg/kg B. 10 mg/kg
C. 15 mg/kg D. 5 mg/kg

37. **Pulmonary artery PaO_2:**
A. 20 B. 40
C. 60 D. 80

38. **Not correct:**
A. ENHANCE - Ezetimibe
B. HOPE - Ramipril
C. ON TARGET - Telmesarta
D. ADVANCE - Atorvastation

39. **Post MI patient the same effect of ARB v/z. ACEI was seen in:**
A. Consensus B. Valiant
C. GISSI-3 D. ISIS-4

40. **Cyanotic CHD palliative surgery at 2 years of age. Now at 4 years continuous murmur is positive, least likely is:**
A. Glenn shunt
B. Pott shunt
C. Modified BT shunt
D. Waterson shunt

41. **Central cyanosis in a baby is due to maternal ingestion of:**
A. Methylene blue
B. Tobacco
C. Alcohol
D. Water from well

42. **Cocaine induced unstable angina which one of the following is contraindicated?**
A. β blocker B. NTG
C. Nitroprusside D. Dilzem

43. **ASD shunt increased in all *except*:**
A. MS B. MR
C. RVMI D. HTN

44. **High risk IWMI which is true?**
A. ST↓ V_1-V_3 B. CHB
C. ST↑ in aVR D. PR↑

45. **AICD given in all *except*:**
A. QT >540 msec in LQTS
B. Post MI, hemodynamically stable VT
C. Idiopathic left fascicular VT
D. HCM with septum 30 mm with NSVT

46. **↑ LVEDP is indicated by:**
A. B-bump (M-mode)
B. E-a normal
C. ↓ EF
D. Paradoxical septal movement

47. **Continuity equation used for:**
A. Aortic valve area
B. PA systolic pressure
C. Ejection fraction
D. Trans pulmonary gradient

48. **Re-entry in:**
A. AFL B. CPVT
C. Jewel lange D. TdP

49. **Rayonidine receptor:**
A. CPVT B. Brugada
C. Romanoward D. JLN

50. **Trop T binds with:**
A. Calcium B. Actin
C. Tropomyosin D. Calmodulin

51. **ACE gene polymorphism DD all *except:***
A. ACE inhibitor ↓ed effect
B. β blockers ↑ed effect
C. Good prognosis in HF
D. ↑ risk of CAD

52. **Hypocalcemia in all *except:***
A. DiGeorge syndrome
B. Thiazide
C. Hyperphosphatemia
D. Acute compensated respiratory alkalosis

53. **Cardiovascular effect of thyroid hormone all *except:***
A. ↓ SVR
B. ↑ LDL
C. Improved diastolic function
D. ↓ Cardiac output

54. **In hypoadrenal shock ↓ *except:***
A. AVO_2 diff
B. Cardiac output
C. Central venous press
D. Systemic venous return

55. **Acromegaly with LA myxoma:**
A. Carney syndrome
B. MEN-I
C. MEN-II
D. Noonan

56. **Cardiac mass in 30 years female disappeared on chemotherapy:**
A. Rhabdomyoma
B. Hemangiosarcoma
C. Choriocarcinoma
D. Melanoma

57. **PND seen in all *except:***
A. Chronic constrictive pericarditis
B. LA myxoma
C. AR
D. Hypertensive heart failure

58. **Treatment of ischemic stroke with 210/120 mmHg includes all *except:***
A. Nitroprusside
B. Sublingual nifedipine
C. Fenoldopam
D. Labetalol

59. **30 years female with MI all *except:***
A. Essential thrombocythemia
B. PNH
C. vWF deficiency
D. Hyperhomocysteinemia

60. **ABG PaO_2=40, SpO_2 – 89%, $PaCO_2$-50, Aa-12 mmHg:**
A. Respiratory muscle paralysis
B. Pulmonary edema
C. Atelectasis
D. TOF

61. **Volume controlled ventilation all *except*:**
A. Fixed minute volume ventilation
B. ↓ Risk of barotrauma
C. Benefit in variable pulmonary pathology
D. It delivers fixed volume irrespective of compliance

62. **Metabolic regulation of coronary flow:**
A. Adenosine B. NO
C. Lactic acid D. Fatty acid

63. **Pulmonary valve systolic velocity 4 m/sec:**
A. TOF
B. Hyperthyroidism
C. Eisenmenger
D. Muscular VSD

64. **Gadolinium contrast in MRI causes:**
A. Nephrogenic systemic fibrosis or nephrogenic fibrosing dermatopathy
B. ↓ Sperm count
C. Medullary cancer thyroid
D. Pancreatic cancer

65. **All are endothelial progenitor stem cell *except:***
A. CD3 B. CD133
C. CD34 D. VEGF

66. **Mesenchymal stem cells are produced from:**
A. Bone marrow B. Spleen
C. Peripheral blood D. Placenta

67. **Tamponade with absent paradoxus:**
A. Low-pressure tamponade
B. Iatrogenic tamponade
C. Large tubercular effusion
D. SLE pericardial effusion

68. **In effusion, which does not lead to CCP?**
A. Dressler B. Pyogenic
C. Hypothyroid D. Radiation

69. **HIV patient all *except:***
A. CABG not to be done
B. Tamponade is unusual
C. Causes PAH
D. IE is treated conventionally

70. **Normal serum complement in cardiac disease with renal involvement:**
A. Infective endocarditis
B. Wegener's
C. Atheroembolism
D. Malignant hypertension

71. **Total electrical alternans:**
A. Severe LVD
B. Tamponade
C. 2:1 AV block
D. Constrictive pericarditis

72. **Tall R in VI:**
A. Duchenne
B. Keans Seare syndrome
C. Freidrich ataxia
D. Myotonic dystrophy

73. **Myeloma + cardiac amyloidosis all *except:***
A. Speckled appearance of septum in 2 D echo
B. LVH on limb leads
C. Macroglossia
D. Orthostatic hypotension

74. **Best tolerated in pregnancy:**
A. MVP with mild MR
B. MS with 1.3 cm^2 MVA
C. TOF with SaO_2 82%
D. AS with mild LV dysfunction

75. **More common in female all *except:***
A. Alzheimer's
B. AS
C. Multiple sclerosis
D. Primary biliary cirrhosis

76. **Mitral annual calcification is seen in all *except:***
A. Marfan
B. Hyperparathyroid
C. DCM
D. Renal failure

77. **Very prominent U wave:**
A. Susceptibility to develop torsade de pointes
B. Hypercalcemia
C. Ischemia
D. Artefact

78. **All are physiologic in ageing *except:***
A. RBBB B. Sys HTN
C. ↓ Max HR D. ↓ HR variability

79. **Chronic essential HTN in pregnancy causes all *except:***
A. Pre eclampsia
B. Abruptio placentae
C. ↑ Perinatal mortality
D. Syncope

80. **Warfarin side effects are all *except:***
A. Macrosomia
B. Chondrodysplasia
C. Optic atrophy
D. Mental retardation

81. **MI in LBBB patient is diagnosed by all *except*:**
A. Q in I aVL V_6
B. ST ↑ 1mm in V_5
C. ST ↑ V_1-V_3
D. Slurred S in V_2, V_3

82. **Post MI recurrent HTN irrational combination:**
A. Amiodarone, Sotalol, Procainamide
B. Amiodarone, Metoprolol, Procainamide
C. Amiodarone, Mexiletene, Metoprolol
D. Amiodarone, Procainamide, Mexiletene

83. **Young asymp adult – TMT to screen CAD true is:**
A. Not indicated
B. Can be done after CT angio
C. Prior to hernia repair
D. Female

84. **Reverse split S2 in all *except:***
A. PDA B. Post Op TOF
C. PPI D. Angina pectoris

85. **Rarely seen in Downs:**
A. TGA B. TOF
C. Cleft mitral valve D. PDA

86. **Conotruncal abnormality are due to all *except*:**
A. Retinoic acid
B. Alcohol binges in pregnancy
C. 22q deletion
D. Rubella in 1st trimester

87. **All *except:***
A. Pulsus pavus et tardus best in carotid
B. Pulses alternans in brachial better than carotid
C. Early paradoxus by sphygmomanometer
D. Percussion wave ↑ in dievotic pulse

88. **Janeway lesion seen in:**
A. Staph IE B. Fungal IE
C. Brucellosis D. Late PVE

89. **St Jude valve is:**
A. Caged ball
B. Bileaflet disc
C. Xenograft porcine
D. Pericardial

90. **Strep viridans IE early surgery index in all *except:***
A. CHF
B. ESR > 100
C. Fever > 15 d
D. >10 m vegetations

91. **NSTEMI early intervention are indicated in all *except:***
A. Trop I >1ng ml
B. GRACE score - 70
C. DES last 6 months
D. CABG done 2 years back

92. **Within 3 hours, PCI or TLT can be given in all *except:***
A. Killip III
B. Age 58 years
C. Door needle <30 mm
D. Door balloon <90 min

93. **75-year-old AWMI, all are risk factors for cardiogenic shock, thereby precluding IV β blocker Rx *except*:**
A. Age > 70 years
B. Basal HR – 80 min
C. SBP <120 mmHg
D. Late presentation

94. **In CHF, mortality ↓ by all *except:***
A. Spironolactone
B. Bisoprolol
C. Atenolol
D. Metoprolol

95. **RBBB with recurrent syncope indication for PPI:**
A. AH 180 msec
B. HV 100
C. SNRT 500
D. 2.4 sec pause on carotid sinus massage

96. **Morphological feature RV on echo are all *except*:**
A. Trabeculated apex
B. Origin of pulmonary artery
C. Septal attachment of AV valve
D. Moderator band

97. **Acute rheumatic fever all *except:***
A. Myosin content in valve decides involvement
B. M-protein produces protective antibodies
C. Valve damage is more important than myocardial damage
D. Murmur of MR ↓es in long term

98. **The drug metabolized by CYP is:**
A. Hydralazine B. Pravastatin
C. Erythromycin D. Digoxin

99. **In NIH registry predictors of mortality in PPH were all *except:***
A. RA pressure
B. PA pressure
C. Age
D. Cardiac output

100. Statin myopathy ↑ risk all *except:*
A. DM + Renal failure
B. With fibrates
C. Elderly
D. Obese male

101. Abciximab all are correct *except:*
A. Longer t½
B. Bolus + infusion
C. Pig mouse chimeric ab
D. Cross reacts with other vasc. cells

102. Enoxaparin - true:
A. Effect partially reversed by protamine
B. Does not cause HIT
C. Mech of action by vWF
D. Small mole antibody

103. Action potential duration in ECG from beginning of QRS to:
A. Apex of R B. Nadir of S
C. End of S D. End of T

104. Atrial flutter all *except:*
A. VR in AFL better controlled than in AF
B. Typical AFL treated by RFA
C. Can cause SCD
D. Anti-coagulation required in atrial flutter

105. SCD least likely in:
A. LCx from RCA
B. ALCAPA
C. LMCA from right sinus
D. LMCA dissection

106. Aorto mitral continuity in all *except:*
A. DORV
B. Truncus arteriosus
C. TOF
D. VSD +CoA

107. In MI, all ↑ after 2 days *except:*
A. hs-CRP B. HDL↑
C. Leucocyte D. Ck-MB

108. Papillary muscle rupture all are true *except:*
A. IWMI associated more than AWMI
B. Almost always associated with triple vess disease
C. Right sided rupture - TR
D. Murmur may be silent/short

109. Calcium re-uptake by:
A. SERCA
B. Ca dependent pump
C. Calmodulin
D. Ca/Na pump

110. Asympt 40 years male with AS normal LV function instantaneous gradient 40 mmHg:
A. No intervention
B. AVR
C. ROSS
D. Balloon valvuloplasty

111. Dilated coronary sinus seen in:
A. Persistent left SVC
B. Interrupted IVC
C. Kawasaki disease
D. ASD

112. Aortic dissection most unlikely presentation is:
A. Paraplegia
B. Status epilepticus
C. Syncope
D. ST ↑ in II, III, aVF

113. Brain death:
A. Bilateral cerebral infarction
B. Sagittal sinus thrombosis
C. Basilar artery thrombosis
D. Absent cerebral perfusion

ANSWERS

1	C	2	D	3	A	4	A	5	D	6	A	7	A
8	A	9	B	10	A	11	B	12	A	13	B	14	D
15	B	16	D	17	A	18	C	19	A	20	A	21	A
22	B	23	C	24	D	25	B	26	A	27	B	28	A
29	D	30	B	31	B	32	D	33	C	34	C	35	A
36	A	37	B	38	D	39	B	40	A	41	D	42	A
43	C	44	C	45	C	46	A	47	A	48	A	49	A
50	C	51	C	52	B	53	C	54	A	55	A	56	C
57	A	58	A	59	C	60	A	61	B	62	A	63	A
64	A	65	A	66	A	67	A	68	C	69	A	70	D
71	B	72	A	73	B	74	A	75	B	76	C	77	A
78	A	79	B	80	A	81	C	82	A	83	A	84	B
85	A	86	D	87	A	88	A	89	B	90	B	91	B
92	A	93	B	94	C	95	B	96	B	97	A	98	C
99	C	100	D	101	C	102	A	103	D	104	A	105	
106	A	107	B	108	B	109	A	110	A	111	A	112	B,D
113	D												

8

AIIMS DECEMBER 2007

1. **Reverse pulsus paradoxus is seen in:**
   A. HOCM
   B. Negative pressure ventilation
   C. Pericardial effusion
   D. Absent pericardium

2. **All are seen in neurofibromatosis I *except*:**
   A. Optic glioma
   B. Schwannoma
   C. Lisch nodule
   D. Skeletal dysplasia

3. **ABG pH = 7.55, PCO_2 46, PaO_2 88, HCO_3 = 35 diagnosis is:**
   A. Narcotic overdose
   B. Diuretic therapy
   C. CRF
   D. Pulmonary embolism

4. **ABG pH 7.4, PCO_2 40, PaO_2 88, CL- 80, HCO_3 25 diagnosis is:**
   A. Mixed acid base disorder
   B. Normal
   C. Acute fully compensated respiratory alkalosis
   D. Compensated metabolic acidosis

5. **Cath data RA mean pressure 8 RV 60/7 78% aortic saturation all are possible *except*:**
   A. Pulmonary AV fistula
   B. TAPVC
   C. TOF
   D. Comatrium (common atrium)

6. **Cath data RA=18 a↑v↑RV=90/12 LV=110/8, PCWP – a-24, V – 28, mean 26:**
   A. CP B. MS
   C. Eisenmenger D. RVMI

7. **In patient of MS, LVEDP of 2 mmHg suggest:**
   A. Hypotension
   B. Dehydration
   C. AR
   D. Tight MS

8. **Drug S/E all are correct matches *except*:**
   A. Amiodarone - Lung fibrosis
   B. Abciximab - Bleeding
   C. Statin - Rhabdomyolysis
   D. Torsades - Cisapride

9. **For amyloidosis all are true *except*:**
   A. Tall T wave in lateral lead
   B. Atrial stand still
   C. Atrial fibrillation
   D. Q wave in II, III, aVF

10. **Amyloid treatment include all *except*:**
    A. Senile amyloidosis – NO treatment
    B. SSA chemotherapy
    C. AL – Bone marrow stem cell transplantation
    D. Transthyretin–Liver transplant

11. **Deceleration time 75 msec on mitral valve Doppler suggest:**
    A. CCP B. MR
    C. AF D. CHD

12. **P ½ time is affected by all *except*:**
    A. MR
    B. Poor LV compliance
    C. Low CO
    D. Duration of diastole

13. **RVOT VT at the rate of 160/m clinical finding will be:**
    A. ESM at base
    B. MDM at apex
    C. Reverse S_2 splitting
    D. Wide pulse pressure

14. **True about gene all *except*:**
    A. Apo A1 associated with amyloid cerebral angiopathy
    B. Adducin gene with stroke and diuretic
    C. BMPR2 familial PPH
    D. CYP20 as with warfarin

15. **Rimonabant all are true *except*:**
    - **A.** Cannabinoid 1 stimulant
    - **B.** Can reduce blood pressure
    - **C.** Used to improve insulin sensitivity
    - **D.** Causes weight loss

16. **Drug used in patient going for PCI:**
    - **A.** Bivaluridin **B.** tPA 1/2 dose
    - **C.** Reteplase **D.** Heparin

17. **PCI would be better than thrombolysis in all *except*:**
    - **A.** 1 hour after presentation
    - **B.** 5 days after hip replacement surgery
    - **C.** Kilip class IV
    - **D.** Shock

18. **Eptifibatide induced bleding – complete reversal can be done with:**
    - **A.** Platelet transfusion
    - **B.** Hemodialysis
    - **C.** Antibodies to eptifibatide
    - **D.** Aprotinin

19. **LMWH all are true *except*:**
    - **A.** Molecular weight 4500
    - **B.** Alkaline denaturation of heparin benzyl ester
    - **C.** Protamine completely reverses its effects
    - **D.** Effect is due to anti XA (factor)

20. **Acute anti wall MI is actively least likely with:**
    - **A.** ST ↑aVR **B.** ST ↑aVL
    - **C.** New onset RBBB **D.** ↓QT

21. **Constrictive pericarditis ECG changes include all *except*:**
    - **A.** 50% normal
    - **B.** AF 5-10%
    - **C.** ST-T changes are most common
    - **D.** Low voltage

22. **β blocker all *except* (post MI):**
    - **A.** 13% reduction in mortality
    - **B.** 3% increase in CHF
    - **C.** 2% increase in shock
    - **D.** 1% myocardial rupture

23. **Ryanodine repron are present in:**
    - **A.** Sarcoplasmic reticulum
    - **B.** Sarcolemma
    - **C.** Mitochondria
    - **D.** Nuclear membrane

24. **Action potential duration prolongation in phase 2 is seen with:**
    - **A.** Hypercalcemia
    - **B.** Hyperkalemia
    - **C.** Quinidine
    - **D.** Amiodarone

25. **Diastasis wave:**
    - **A.** H wave **B.** D wave
    - **C.** A wave **D.** C wave

26. **Idiopathic pulmonary fibrosis may be treated by:**
    - **A.** Roxithromycin
    - **B.** Selenium
    - **C.** Vitamin E
    - **D.** Perfinidone

27. **In child most common cause of SVT:**
    - **A.** Ectopic atrial tachycardia
    - **B.** Atrial flutter
    - **C.** AVNRT
    - **D.** AVRT

28. **Arterial switch operation best done in:**
    - **A.** Neonate **B.** Infant
    - **C.** Weight >5 kg **D.** 1-3 months

29. **Left ventricular dysfunction is seen at birth in all *except*:**
    - **A.** ALCAPA **B.** AS
    - **C.** Birth asphyxia **D.** SVT

30. **Cardiac transplant most important matching:**
    - **A.** Age <65
    - **B.** Pulmonary vascular resistance < 7 unit
    - **C.** ABO and body size
    - **D.** ABO and HLA

31. **VT mechanism in post MI setting:**
    - **A.** Reentry
    - **B.** Enhanced automaticity
    - **C.** Triggered activity
    - **D.** Phase 2 reentry

32. **Non-significant murmur may be heard in all of the following *except*:**
    - **A.** Gerbode **B.** Eisenmenger
    - **C.** Ebstein **D.** Ac MR

33. **In adult least common feature of Turner's syndrome is:**
    - **A.** Bicuspid aortic valve
    - **B.** Aortic root dilated
    - **C.** Hepatic cyst
    - **D.** Deafness

34. **In congenital rubella all are seen *except*:**
    - **A.** Macrocephaly
    - **B.** Myocarditis
    - **C.** Peripheral pulmonary stenosis
    - **D.** Deafness

35. **Kartagener's syndrome all are true *except*:**
    - **A.** Splenic hypofunction
    - **B.** Mirror image branching pattern of venous arch
    - **C.** Inverted P in lead
    - **D.** Infertility

36. **Treatment of choice in mild to moderate persistent asthma:**
A. Inhaled steroids
B. Long acting β agonists
C. Theophylline
D. Na cromoglycate

37. **CT can be used in diagnosis of all *except*:**
A. Double aortic arch
B. Pulmonary embolism
C. In stent restenosis
D. Aortic dissection

38. **EBCT in 50 years male, non-diabetic, asymptomatic shows calcification (coronary), first to be done:**
A. EBCT follow up at 2 years if no symptoms
B. Angiography
C. Rest thallium redistribution
D. Risk factor modification

39. **CT true all *except*:**
A. Epicardial fat detected
B. Pericardial thickness 1-2 mm
C. Pericardial effusion is not diagnosed
D. Contrast CT in SVC thrombosis

40. **In MR tissue characterization can be done by all *except*:**
A. Na^{23} B. C^{12}
C. O^{17} D. F^{19}

41. **For ARVD true statement is:**
A. Pathologically LV can be involved
B. RBBB during VT
C. RFA can be successful
D. Common in females

42. **ECG in Brugada syndrome:**
A. ST ↑ V_1V_2
B. LBBB morphology
C. Repolarization is the cause
D. Associated with WPW syndrome - type B

43. **Provocation of Brugada syndrome by all *except*:**
A. Flecainide B. Ajunaline
C. Procainamide D. Amiodarone

44. **In V_1 tall 'R' waner in all *except*:**
A. CTGA B. dTGA
C. Severe PS D. Situs inversus

45. **Follow up medically done in asymptomatic MR in all *except*:**
A. LVEF >65%
B. LVED <55
C. LVES <45
D. Effective regurgitant orifice >40

46. **Aortic dilatation associated with AR procedure of choice is:**
A. Maze
B. Debakey
C. Bental
D. Wringberg

47. **LV mass in (n) adult male in gm/m²:**
A. 25-50 B. 50-86
C. 120-150 D. 150-186

48. **Activated protein C used in:**
A. Sepsis B. Jaundice
C. COPD D. MI

49. **Infective endocarditis false is:**
A. Diphtheroid is commonly contaminants
B. Staph lugdunensis is coagulase positive and causes leyendensis valve destruction
C. Enterococcal resistance is reported with vancomycin
D. Staph aureus resistant to penicillin upto 90%

50. **Infective endocarditis all are true *except*:**
A. ↑ESR in 80-90%
B. ↓C3 – C4 in 5-40%
C. Leukocytosis in 60-80%
D. Rh factor positive in > 50%

51. **True of mitral annular calcification are all *except*:**
A. HOCM
B. Juvenile MS
C. Hyperparathyroidism
D. Marfan's

52. **In pregnancy all are high risk *except*:**
A. TGA repair after atrial switch
B. Marfan
C. Severe AS
D. Eisenmenger

53. **In pregnancy changes seen are all *except*:**
A. Blood volume increase by 35%
B. SVR ↑ by 5%
C. Normal CVP
D. RV volume increased by 18%

54. **In pheochromocytoma all are seen *except*:**
A. Orthostatic hypotension
B. Clonidine cause catecholamine suppression
C. MEN IIa (may be associated)
D. LV systolic dysfunction

55. **Normal rising carotid pulse can be seen with (AS) in:**
A. Elderly
B. Young
C. Subaortic membrane
D. Inelastic arteries

56. **Ligament of Marshall attaches to:**
A. Coronary sinus
B. Left atrium
C. Pulmonary vein
D. Superior vena cava

57. **Post traumatic patient having cardiac murmur, shows flail tricuspid leaflet on echo, most likely murmur:**
A. Early systolic murmur
B. PSM
C. Continuous murmur
D. Systolic diastolic murmur

58. **58-year-old patient with cleft mitral valve with MR, ECG finding will be:**
A. LAD
B. Right ventricular hypertrophy
C. LBBB
D. WPW type B

59. **ECG finding in LAHB is:**
A. QRS >120 m sec
B. RS in inferior lead with QR in aVL
C. Clockwise rotation
D. qR in inferior lead

60. **In pulmonary embolism all are seen *except*:**
A. ↑ Arterial alveolar gradient
B. Cerebral vasodilatation
C. Normal chest X-ray
D. ↑ minute ventilation

61. **D dimer false is:**
A. High positive predictive value
B. Elisa more sensitive than latex agglutination
C. D dimer >500
D. May be positive in MI

62. **Pericarditis with HIV indicates all *except*:**
A. Poor prognosis
B. HIV-1 may be causative
C. Low CD_4 count
D. Less chance of tamponade

63. **HIV all are true *except*:**
A. DCMP most common
B. Accelerated atherosclerosis
C. Long QT in 1/3 hospitalized patients
D. Pulmonary HTN carries poor prognosis

64. **CRF is defined as:**
A. GFR<60 ml/1.73 m^2 for 3 months
B. GFR<50 ml for 6 months
C. GFR<30 ml/m^2 for 6 months
D. GFR<40 ml/m^2 for 6 months

65. **In renal dysfunction–Drug whose dose need not to be altered:**
A. Atenolol
B. Sotalol
C. Clopidogrel
D. Dofetilide

66. **Digoxin toxicity may present with all *except*:**
A. Paroxysmal atrial tachycardia with varying AV block
B. Mobitz type II
C. Bidirectional VT
D. Regular heart rate in a patient of AF

67. **Bariatric surgery indicated in:**
A. BMI >40
B. BMI >50
C. Diabetes
D. Centripetal obesity

68. **60-year-old female with acute MI presented with cardiac rupture on 4th day. True is:**
A. Less common in hypertensives
B. Rupture is usually in the centre of the necrotic mass
C. More with first MI
D. Right > Left

69. **CAD risk factors: more important in females as compared to males are all *except*:**
A. ↑ LDL cholesterol
B. ↑ TG
C. Smoking
D. DM

70. **All are more common in females than males *except*:**
A. More commonly present with angina
B. Comorbidities are less common
C. Sudden death is less common
D. CABG is associated with more complication

71. **Diabetes and cardiovascular disease:**
A. Optimal HbAc 7.2%
B. 1% decrease to HbAc has 14% ↓ in mortality
C. Only blood sugar level >126 mg/ml is associated with CAD
D. Abdominal aortic aneurysm has consistent and potent relation with DM

72. **Diastolic dysfunction is detected by:**
A. End systolic stress
B. Myocardial dp/dt
C. ↑ Pulmonary blood flow
D. Tau

73. **Anti-parkinsonian drug pergolide withdrawn because of:**
A. MI
B. Valvular regurgitation
C. PPH
D. Constrictive pericarditis

74. **In cardiac tamponade earliest sign is:**
A. RA collapse
B. RV systolic collapse
C. RV diastolic collapse
D. Pulsus paradoxsus

75. **In elderly following are age related changes rather than disease, *except*:**
A. ↑ Pulse pressure
B. LVH
C. ↓ Heart rate variability
D. ↓ Max heart rate

76. **For smoking de-addiction following are used *except*:**
A. Bupropion B. Nicotine gums
C. Cannabinol D. Vareniclline

77. **Which of the following is an odd match?**
A. β receptor – G protein
B. Acetylcholine (Muscarinic G protein)
C. Angiotensin II - cAMP
D. NO -cGMP

78. **Glucose intolerance by all *except*:**
A. ARBs B. Thiazides
C. β blockers D. Nicotinic acid

79. **After cardiac transplant the incidence of following malignancy is increased:**
A. B cell lymphoma
B. Leukemia
C. Rhabdomyosarcoma
D. Mesothelioma

80. **For sildenafil true are all *except*:**
A. PDE 5 stimulator
B. Used in PPH
C. Causes flushing as side effect
D. ↑ cGMP

81. **Most cost effective treatment:**
A. Streptokinase in acute STEMI
B. Gp IIb/IIIa in unstable angina
C. GpIIb/IIIa in primary PCI
D. STK in stroke

82. **HAPE all *except*:**
A. More common in young
B. High altitude people sojourn to low altitude
C. ↑ capillary permeability
D. Sildenafil is used in treatment

83. **Swimming related death is most commonly due to:**
A. Long QT syndrome
B. Brugada
C. Diver's syndrome
D. ARVD

84. **In failing heart which of the following is seen?**
A. Cardiac transient alternans
B. ↓ Cytosolic Ca^{2+}
C. End diastolic wall stress reduced
D. Down regulation of β3 receptor

85. **Myocyte length is longer than normal in:**
A. HOCM
B. Chronic AR
C. AS
D. Thyrotoxicosis

86. **D in ABCD predicting stroke after TIA:**
A. Diabetes B. Duration
C. Delay D. Disability

87. **Operated TOF in childhood, a middle aged female found to have QRS 180 ms with RBBB, cause is:**
A. RV dysfunction B. VT
C. DCMP D. WPW

88. **Mediterranean diet is rich in:**
A. Red wine B. Olive oil
C. Fish oil D. PUFA

89. **Atkins diet initially has:**
A. ↓ Fat ↑protein
B. Low calorie, liquid protein diet
C. ↓ Carbohydrate, normal protein
D. ↓ Carbohydrate, ketosis

90. **Permanent reciprocating functional tachycardia: false is:**
A. May be caused by digoxin
B. Decreases with increasing age
C. Commonly causes tachy cardiomyopathy
D. Most commonly, focus is near the OS of coronary sinus (accessory pathway)

91. **Coronary sinus O_2 saturation:**
A. 35 B. 25
C. 55 D. 45

92. **Secondary prevention trial is:**
A. 4S B. WOSCOPS
C. DASH D. AFCAPS

93. **Takayasusarteritis involves which artery most commonly in India?**
A. Subclavian
B. Renal
C. Innominate
D. Pulmonary artery

94. **Longest refractory period is seen in:**
A. Atrial muscle fibre
B. AV node
C. Purkinje fibre
D. Accessory pathway

95. About RV true are all *except*:
A. RV contracts earlier than LV and continues after LV
B. Moderator band
C. Incomplete RBBB due to RV dilatation
D. In PS, increased afterload of RV

96. True are all *except*:
A. Diastolic BP in upper limb and lower limb are equal
B. Osler's maneuver is used to diagnose pseudo-hypertension
C. SP measurement by sphygmomanometer may not be reliable in shock
D. Phase IV Kortokoff sound – diastolic BP

97. Walk through angina:
A. Ischemic preconditioning
B. Anrep effect
C. Bowditch staircase phenomenon
D. Starling law

98. Acute heart failure, which is not used:
A. Neural endopeptidase
B. Endothelin antagonist
C. Anti TNF α
D. BNP analogue

99. Electrocution all *except*:
A. ↑↑ voltage can cause asystole
B. Low voltage AC current can cause death due to VF
C. Prolonged CPR should not be done if pupils are fixed and dilated
D. Superficial tissue burns cannot indicate deep tissue damage

100. Cyanotic spell all are true *except*:
A. Common in summers
B. May cause stroke
C. May be precipitated by blood transfusion
D. May be seen in VSD in pulmonary atresia

101. In patient with (old MI) with (LVEF 35%) having hemodynamic stable VT treatment of choice:
A. AICD B. Amiodarone
C. β blocker D. EPS

102. If father has CHD max incidence in:
A. Marfan
B. ASD
C. Congenital arotic value stenosis
D. VSD

103. In adult after treatment of CoA false is:
A. HT can be treated
B. Right arm BP > left arm BP always
C. Aortic aneurysm can be seen
D. PGE1 inf used in neonates

104. Cheyne-Stokes respiration all are true *except*:
A. Blunted during REM sleep
B. Min return at the end of apnea
C. Denotes poor prognosis
D. Can occur during awake state

105. Obstructive sleep apnea:
A. AHI
B. Non-invasive saturation
C. Electromyography
D. Heart rate

106. Statin not affected by cytochrome P450:
A. Pravastatin
B. Rosuvastatin
C. Lovastatin
D. Fluvastatin

107. Odd one out:
A. IABP acute AR
B. VSD in MI-device closure
C. MI with MR mitral repair
D. Cardiogenic shock primary PCI

108. High oral bioavailability:
A. Linezolid
B. Propranolol
C. $MgSO_4$
D. Amiodarone

109. Diagnostic marker of MI within 4 hours of onset:
A. CPk MB form
B. Trop I
C. T1/T2 ratio
D. Trop T
E. None of the above

ANSWERS

1	A	2	B	3	B	4	A	5	B	6	B	7	D
8	A	9	A	10	B	11	A	12	C	13	C	14	A
15	A	16	B	17	A	18	B	19	C	20	D	21	B
22	A	23	A	24	D	25	A	26	D	27	B,D	28	D
29	A	30	C	31	A	32	A	33	C	34	A	35	A
36	A	37	C	38	D	39	C	40	D	41	A	42	A
43	D	44	B	45	D	46	B,C	47	B	48	A	49	B
50	C	51	A,B	52	A	53	B	54	B	55	B	56	A
57	A	58	A	59	B	60	A	61	A	62	B	63	A
64	A	65	C	66	D	67	A	68	C	69	A	70	B
71	B	72	D	73	B	74	A,C	75	B	76	C	77	C
78	A	79	A	80	A	81	A	82	B,C	83	A	84	A
85	B	86	B	87	A	88	B,D	89	D	90	A	91	A
92	A	93	B	94	D	95	A	96	D	97	A	98	C
99	C	100	C	101	B	102	A	103	B	104	C	105	A
106	A	107	A	108	A	109	E						

9

AIIMS MAY 2007

1. **Reflex sympathetic dystrophy is seen in all *except*:**
   A. Steroid B. MI
   C. Fracture D. Stroke

2. **ABO incompatible cardiac transplants is done in:**
   A. Never done
   B. Neonates
   C. Identical twins
   D. Women on steroids

3. **Increased amylase in all *except*:**
   A. Strangulated hernia
   B. Perforated PUD
   C. Mallory-Weiss syndrome
   D. Acute cholecystitis

4. **Pathogen for vascular seeding:**
   A. Salmonella
   B. Staphylococcus
   C. Listeria
   D. Streptococcus hemolyticus

5. **DNA adducts in leucocytes are seen in:**
   A. DVT
   B. Sickle cell anaemia
   C. Romano Ward syndrome
   D. Chronic tobacco use

6. **Tolvaptan, all are true *except*:**
   A. V_2 antagonist
   B. Hyponatremia caused by it
   C. Useful in liver cirrhosis
   D. Can be used in renal failure

7. **Hyponatremia is seen in all *except*:**
   A. Diabetes insipidus
   B. Cirrhosis
   C. CHF
   D. Nephrotic syndrome

8. **All cause coagulation deficiency *except*:**
   A. Pregnancy
   B. Cirrhosis
   C. Prolonged heparin
   D. Nephrotic syndrome

9. **In pregnancy all are seen *except*:**
   A. Increased calcium
   B. Increased stroke volume
   C. Increased ESR
   D. Increased creatinine clearance

10. **Drug causing metabolic alkalosis:**
    A. Torsemide
    B. Acetazolamide
    C. Eplerenone
    D. Triamterine

11. **IW, STEMI with ST ↓ in anterior lead, indicate all *except*:**
    A. Increased mechanical complication
    B. Reciprocal electrical changes
    C. PWMI
    D. Anterior wall ischemia

12. **Drugs with decreased mortality in MI:**
    A. Eplerenone B. Digoxin
    C. Milrinone D. Dopamine

13. **Drugs causing AV nodal block:**
    A. Itopride B. Clonidine
    C. Hydralazine D. Erythromycin

14. **Drugs avoided in pregnancy include all *except*:**
    A. INH B. Amiodarone
    C. Valsartan D. Ergotamine

15. **BMPR-2 is seen in:**
    A. PPH B. DVT
    C. MI D. HTN

16. **Maximum mortality is seen in pregnancy with:**
    A. MVA 1.5 cm^2
    B. AVA 1.5 cm^2
    C. Marfan with aortic involvement
    D. Pink TOF

17. **Asymptomatic RBBB on ECG, HV interval should be:**
A. 25
B. 50
C. 85
D. Cannot be determined

18. **Low affinity Hb Kansas is associated with:**
A. Cyanosis **B.** Polycythemia
C. CHF **D.** DVT

19. **Marantic endocarditis, most common cause:**
A. GI adenocarcinoma
B. Multiple myeloma
C. NHL
D. Malignant melanoma

20. **TPI in MI is indicated in:**
A. New onset LBBB with increased PR interval
B. Preexisting LBBB with hypotension
C. IWMI with HR 60
D. Primary AV block requiring beta blocker

21. **Risk factor for increased incidence of ICH with thrombolytics are all *except*:**
A. Obesity
B. Hypertension
C. Ischemic stroke
D. Elderly

22. **For warfarin all are true *except*:**
A. Monitored with anti-Xa level
B. Slow acetylators 1.5 mg may be sufficient
C. Decreased protein C in early period
D. Rifampicin decreases efficacy

23. **Courage trial evaluated PCI vs medical therapy in:**
A. CTO
B. Chronic stable angina
C. LMCA disease
D. Carotid + coronary PCI

24. **Thrombolytics are absolutely C/I in:**
A. 70-year-male with HTN with acute chest pain with new onset diastolic murmur in (L) lower sternal border with ST elevation in inferior leads
B. 40-year diabetic male with recent laser surgery of retina
C. 40-year-female with BP 180/110
D. New onset LBBB with ST ↑ in I, aVL, V_{5-6}

25. **For DCM, all are true *except*:**
A. Decreased dp/dt
B. Decreased aortic dip incissura
C. Decreased PA O_2 saturation
D. Decrease LV relaxation velocity

26. **Drug C/I in cyanotic spell:**
A. ACEI **B.** IV fluids
C. Phenyl ephrine **D.** Methoxamine

27. **Pulmonary embolism is least likely with:**
A. Normal d-dimer levels
B. (N) ABG
C. (N) CXR
D. (N) ECG

28. **ECG in Duchenne's muscular dystrophy all are true *except*:**
A. RAD
B. Right sided accessory pathway
C. Q in I, aVL, V_{5-6}
D. Tall R wave in VI

29. **Coronary sinus saturation:**
A. 30% **B.** 25%
C. 45% **D.** 65%

30. **For cardiogenic shock in acute MI all are true *except*:**
A. Incidence around 7%
B. Medical Rx mortality 50-60%
C. Usually present at admission and rare after hospitalization
D. In minority of cases systemic vascular resistance <1800 dyne/sec

31. **Epidemiology of MI, true are all *except*:**
A. Aggressive reperfusion mortality rate 15% (Trials)
B. Incidence of STEMI decreasing
C. Case fatality rate decreasing
D. Thrombolytics beneficial in elderly

32. **Reperfusion arrhythmia include all *except*:**
A. AIVR
B. AF
C. VF
D. Sinus bradycardia
E. None of the above

33. **p wave alternans is seen with:**
A. Pulmonary embolism
B. PSVT
C. AF
D. Tamponade

34. **Absence of Q wave in STEMI is seen in:**
A. 15% **B.** 25%
C. 35% **D.** 5%

35. **For thrombolytic therapy in STEMI, true are all *except*:**
A. Diabetic > non-diabetic
B. IWMI > AWMI

C. SBP < 100 mmHg > 170 mmHg
D. Younger better than elderly

36. **For MI in females all are true *except*:**
A. With PCI, periprocedural complication 3 times more common
B. Thrombolysis less efficacious in female
C. Increase TG is risk factor for post CABG
D. DM females more mortality

37. **High voltage ECG is seen in:**
A. Pompe's disease
B. Amyloidosis
C. Haemorrhagic pericardial effusion
D. Homocystinuria

38. **1 year old with previously normal history develop ST elevation in precordial leads:**
A. ALCAPA
B. Familial hypercholesterolemia
C. Hyper homocystinemia
D. Myocarditis

39. **Young male 25-year-old with ST elevation in routine ECG, least likely is:**
A. Underdamping
B. Brugada
C. Early repolarisation
D. Persistent juvenile pattern

40. **Artery and venous thrombosis, true are all *except*:**
A. AT III def
B. PNH
C. Polycythemia vera
D. Essential thrombocythemia

41. **MI, least likely to present with:**
A. Pain over trapezous ridge on inspiration
B. Syncope
C. Vomiting
D. Fatigue

42. **Acute MI is least associated with:**
A. Hypoglycemia
B. Decreased vital capacity
C. Increased Hb affinity
D. Increased blood viscosity

43. **Pulmonary embolism all are true *except*:**
A. Hemoptysis indicates massive embolism
B. BNP increased
C. Troponin increased
D. Thrombolytics can be used upto 2 weeks

44. **Septic shock all are true *except*:**
A. Low serum lipids
B. Dohle bodies
C. Decreased SVR
D. Decreased D-dimer

45. **True all *except*:**
A. Sensitivity and specificity are independent of prevalence
B. LRR 0.5 indicates poor test
C. There are no perfect test
D. If prevalence < 10% positivity is less even if test is accurate

46. **Hemoptysis, all are true *except*:**
A. Rigid bronchoscope preferred in massive hemoptysis
B. Coil embolisation effective in Rasmussen aneurysm
C. 30% remain undiagnosed even after extensive investigation
D. Pulmonary parenchymal Kaposi can occur in AIDS

47. **Hyperthyroidism in elderly, least likely present as:**
A. Tremor B. Depression
C. AF D. CHF

48. **In hyperthyroidism with AF true all *except*:**
A. Young patient with AF may not need anticoagulation
B. Digoxin to be given in low dose
C. Non-selective β-blocker preferred
D. Anti-thyroid Rx reverses AF in 2/3 pt at 3 months

49. **Neurocardiogenic syncope, incidence is more than general population in patients with:**
A. AS
B. HOCM
C. Bronchial asthma
D. Carotid hypersensitivity

50. **In syncope all are true *except*:**
A. Neurocardiogenic syncope is associated with afferent from myelinated vagal fibres from LV
B. HR <30 is insufficient to achieve CO even in supine position
C. Micturition syncope is more common in male
D. Can cause syncope by atrial flutter with 1:1 conduction in structurally normal heart

51. **For PPAR all are true *except*:**
A. Is mitochondrial receptor
B. Is transcription factor
C. Modulates hormone metabolism
D. Clofibrate acts on PPAR-α

52. **In a 14-year-male, severe rheumatic MS is least likely to be associated with:**
A. Severe TR B. Severe AS
C. Severe AR D. PR

53. Arterial thoracic outlet syndrome, all are true *except*:
A. Produce weakness in C8 distribution
B. Resection of cervical rib may be needed
C. Digital gangrene can occur
D. Adson's test may be positive

54. Female with MVA= 1.8 m^2, day 2 postpartum develops acute onset of dyspnea, pH 7.2, PO_2 60, $PCO_2$20, cause is:
A. Peripartum CM
B. Pulmonary embolism
C. CHF
D. Hysterical hyperventilation

55. Hypothyroidism true is:
A. ↑ SVR
B. ↓ PVR
C. ↓ MVO_2
D. Normal mixed venous saturation

56. Primary fuel for metabolism of heart at rest:
A. FFA B. Glucose
C. Ketone D. Carnitine

57. CIN prevented by:
A. NAC B. $MgSO_4$
C. Furosemide D. Toxic dye

58. In Noonan's syndrome, all are seen *except*:
A. PV dysplasia B. (N) Stature
C. (N) Karyotype D. HOCM

59. SCD with HOCM is least likely in:
A. Infant B. Noonan's
C. Fredrich's ataxia D. Athletes

60. Maximum exercise with ↓MVO_2, cause:
A. Lung dysfunction
B. Cardiac dysfunction
C. Uncooperative patient
D. Athletes

61. Submaximal exercise in MI, should achieve:
A. 5 METS B. 7 METS
C. 3 MET D. 9 MET

62. TIMI frame count in (N) CAG:
A. 21 B. 41
C. 1 D. Cannot be determined

63. Level of evidence with single large control trial:
A. A B. B
C. C D. O

64. Takotsubo cardiomyopathy true is:
A. Acute emotional stress
B. Anti-neoplastic drugs
C. Cardiac transplant
D. Takayasu arteritis

65. CHF all are true *except*:
A. MVO_2<10 ml indicates poor prognosis
B. Anti-apoptotic drugs shown improved survival
C. 40% of SCD
D. Annual mortality 30-80%

66. In CCF all are true *except*:
A. ↑ BNP
B. ↑ TNF
C. ↑ VC
D. ↓ Pulse pressure

67. Low HDL in all *except*:
A. Tangiers disease
B. Hyperchylomicronemia (FH)
C. Familial hypercholesterolemia (FCH)
D. Familial combined hypertriglyceridemia
E. None of the above

68. For CK-MB and Trop T, true is:
A. Trop T preferred in reinfarction within 1 week
B. CKMB more specific but less sensitive
C. Trop T and I present in both skeletal and cardiac muscles
D. Bedside Trop T can detect upto 5 mg/ml

69. Non-diabetic 40-year-male; with non-specific, ST-T changes epigastric discomfort for 20 min, Trop T negative was given NTG and antacids, all false *except*:
A. Needs observation in emergency
B. Negative Trop T almost shows high possibility of non-CAD diagnosis
C. Needs immediate TMT
D. CT to be done for calcium score

70. Coronary Ca^{2+} best detected by:
A. EBCT B. USG
C. MRI D. ECHO

71. Unilateral diaphragmatic palsy in spontaneously breathing patient best diagnosed by:
A. USG B. Physical exam
C. CXR D. CT angiography

72. Ostial LAD disease can be seen with all *except*:
A. Ankylosis spondylitis
B. Takayasu disease
C. Behcet's disease
D. Prior radiation

73. All are true *except*:
A. LAD can cause IWMI
B. ECG reliably differentiates transmural MI and subendocardiac ischemia
C. CTO can be asymptomatic
D. ECG can be normal in CTO

74. **For congenital CHB true statement are all *except*:**
A. Intermittent (n) conduction can occur
B. Retrograde conduction can occur
C. Epicardial pacing not useful
D. Torsade de pointes and bradycardia can occur

75. **For SLE all are true *except*:**
A. Pericarditis – most common cardiac presentation
B. Libman sac endocarditis less common with APLA
C. MI incidence markedly increase in young female (40 years)
D. Anti RO Ab can cause CHB after 1st trimester

76. **Pericarditis all are true *except*:**
A. Idiopathic – most common cause
B. Pericardial rub usually transient and biphasic
C. Most cases lead to tamponade
D. Uremic pericarditis resolves with hemodialysis

77. **In PCI with S. creat > 4.2 mg/dl drug to be avoided is:**
A. Tirofiban
B. Eptifibatide
C. Abciximab
D. Bivalirudin

78. **On HRT a patient develops MI, what is to be done:**
A. Discontinue HRT
B. Add statins
C. Modify progestin
D. ↓ dose by ↓

79. **For daily fish consumption, all are true *except*:**
A. ↑ VLDL
B. ↓ BP in HTN patients
C. Fishy odour
D. ↑ Anticoagulation efficacy

80. **For AS with LV dysfunction without CHF, all are true *except*:**
A. AVR
B. BAV initially to be tried
C. Gradient ↓ with LV dysfunction
D. CAG preoperatively

81. **Right aortic arch is most common with:**
A. PTA
B. DORV
C. TGA
D. Pulmonary stenosis

82. **For Vitamin E supplementation, true statements are all *except*:**
A. ↑ Hemorrhagic stroke
B. Does not ↓ lung carcinoma
C. ↓ Pancreatic cancer
D. Does not ↓ CV mortality

83. **Equal O_2 saturation in all four chambers is seen with:**
A. TAPVC
B. PS
C. ASD
D. TOF

84. **HOCM true statement is:**
A. Na^+ channel mutation
B. Alcohol ablation of LAD done
C. Brokenborough Braunwald sign present
D. Apical HCM – most common

85. **For uraemia all are true *except*:**
A. Symptomatic uraemia does not occur till Cr Cl < 50 ml/min
B. Single kidney can maintain normal renal function
C. Women have less creatinine clearance compared to men of same weight
D. Digoxin ↓ to half at CrCl <30 ml/min

86. **In MS with large ASD all are true *except*:**
A. Long diastolic rumble at apex
B. PHT
C. Pulmonary plethora
D. Presence of thrill in 3rd ICS indicates associated MS

87. **Pulmonary vasodilators are all *except*:**
A. Endothelin antagonist
B. Sildenafil
C. Neural endopeptidase
D. PGE1

88. **HIV all *except*:**
A. PPH 0.6%
B. Hemodynamically similar to PPH
C. Mostly occur in low CD_4
D. Inflammatory and immunological mechanism

89. **Heat stroke is predisposed by all *except*:**
A. Anti-parkinsonism drugs
B. Anti-cholinergic drugs
C. Diuretics
D. Steroids

90. **In migraine all of the following can be used *except*:**
A. Adenosine antagonist
B. 5HT antagonist
C. PG inhibitor
D. Dopamine antagonist

91. **A young male on herbal drugs presented with bradycardia, ↓BP, ↑K cause is:**
A. Yellow oleander
B. Dhatura
C. Claviceps
D. Nux vomica

92. **In septic shock parameter to be maintained include all *except*:**
A. Urine output > 30 ml/h
B. PCWP 18-22
C. CVP 10-12 CM
D. MAP 60

93. **For biventricular transvenous pacing position of left ventricular lead in:**
A. Posterolateral vein
B. LV through PFO
C. Septal
D. Ant cardiac vein

94. **True statements are all *except*:**
A. PDA always supply AV node
B. SA node supplied by RCA in 60%
C. RCA from right posterior sinus
D. LAD occlusion (CTO) may be asymptomatic and with N ECG

95. **↓ Mortality in STEMI is seen with all *except*:**
A. β blocker 13%
B. Aspirin 22%
C. ACEI 26%
D. Nitrate 18%

96. **Target dose of ACEI are all *except*:**
A. Captopril 50 tds
B. Lisinopril 20 OD
C. Enalapril 10 BD
D. Ranipril 10 BD

97. **NH_3 ammonia in MPI:**
A. Blood flow
B. Metabolism
C. AA metabolism
D. Lipid metabolism

98. **In MI with major depression and LVEF 25% drug which can be used?**
A. Amitriptyline B. Sertraline
C. Trazodone D. Imipramine

99. **DOC for cyclosporine induced HTN:**
A. Diuretic B. ACEI
C. CCB D. β blocker

100. **Broad T wave with ↑ QT:**
A. Hypocalcemia B. Hypothermia
C. Hypomagnesemia D. Hypokalemia

101. **Causes of TDP include all *except*:**
A. Hypocalcemia
B. Flecanide overdose
C. Cisapride
D. SAH

102. **All are ↓ in incidence in thrombolytic era *except:***
A. Primary VF
B. AIVR
C. Pulmonary embolism
D. Dressler's syndrome

103. **Kussmaul's sign is seen in:**
A. Mediastinal lymphoma
B. RVMI
C. Ebstein
D. Pneumothorax

104. **Bad prognostic markers in USA include all *except*:**
A. Not on aspirin
B. Trop T ↑
C. ST-T changes

105. **SIRS is non-infective in all *except*:**
A. Aortic dissection
B. DES
C. Anaphylaxis
D. Post bypass

106. **Proteinuria all are true *except*:**
A. HTN a/w Tamm-Horsfall proteinuria
B. Bence Jones can't be detected by dipstick
C. Coagulation def. due to procoagulants loss in urine
D. Proteinuria can occur in CHF

107. **(N) Echofinding include all *except*:**
A. E > A
B. MV tissue Doppler velocity >8
C. ↑ Pulmonary venous velocity in inspiration
D. PFO in 30% population

108. **Myocyte are produced in vitro by:**
A. Skeletal myoblasts
B. Fetal neuroectoderm cells
C. Hematopoietic stem cells
D. BM mesenchymal stem cells

ANSWERS

1	C	2	A	3	C	4	D	5	D	6	B	7	A
8	A	9	A	10	A	11	A	12	A	13	B	14	A
15	A	16	C	17	A	18	A	19	A	20	A	21	A
22	A	23	B	24	A	25	C	26	A	27	A	28	B
29	A	30	C	31	A	32	E	33	A	34	B	35	B
36	B	37	A	38	A	39	C	40	D	41	A	42	A
43	A	44	D	45	A	46	C	47	B	48	B	49	D
50	A	51	A	52	D	53	A	54	C	55	A	56	A
57	A	58	B	59	C	60	D	61	A	62	A	63	B
64	A	65	B	66	C	67	C	68	A	69	A	70	A
71	C	72	C	73	B	74	C	75	B	76	C	77	B
78	A	79	A	80	B	81	A	82	C	83	A	84	C
85	A	86	A	87	C	88	C	89	A	90	B	91	A
92	B	93	A	94	B	95	D	96	D	97	A	98	B
99	C	100	A	101	B	102	B	103	B	104	A	105	B
106	C	107	C	108	A								

10

AIIMS DECEMBER 2006

1. **Drugs contraindicated in pregnancy are all *except*:**
   A. Spironolactone
   B. Labetalol
   C. Sodium nitroprusside
   D. Enalapril
2. **Non-HDL cholesterol goal in patient of aortic aneurysm with non-obstructive CAD:**
   A. 100 B. 130
   C. 160 D. 190
3. **Thiamine deficiency occurs in all *except*:**
   A. Food faddist
   B. Homocystinuria
   C. Alcohol
   D. Chronic diarrhoea
4. **Cardiac amyloidosis true are all *except*:**
   A. Low voltage ECG
   B. Angina like chest pain
   C. Bronchiectasis
   D. Nifedipine sensitivity
5. **AICD was conceived and designed by:**
   A. Philips B. MirowIsky
   C. Lown D. St. Louis
6. **Most cost effective strategy in non-cardiac surgery in a patient with chronic stable angina:**
   A. Beta blocker B. Statins
   C. Aspirin D. CAG
7. **BNP is metabolized by:**
   A. Chymase
   B. Neural endopeptidase
   C. Phosphodiesterase
   D. Omapatrilat
8. **Coronary artery spasm caused by all *except*:**
   A. Sildenafil
   B. Alcohol
   C. Acetylcholine
   D. Hyperventilation
9. **Pulmonary vasoreactivity assessment can be by all *except*:**
   A. Amlodipine B. Oxygen
   C. Nitric oxide D. Adenosine
10. **Increased pulmonary vascular resistance all *except*:**
    A. Acidosis B. Hyper inflation
    C. Atelectasis D. Anemia
11. **Intrapulmonary right to left shunt occurs in all *except*:**
    A. Atelectasis
    B. Pneumonia
    C. Eisenmenger syndrome
    D. Cirrhosis
12. **Exercise induced sudden cardiac death can occur in all *except*:**
    A. HOCM
    B. Brugada syndrome
    C. Romanowald syndrome
    D. CAD
13. **Drug requiring dose reduction in renal failure:**
    A. Atenolol B. Propranolol
    C. Carvedilol D. Verapamil
14. **AVNRT in newborn treatment include all *except*:**
    A. Diving reflex B. Verapamil
    C. Propranolol D. Adenosine
15. **Potassium channel opener all *except*:**
    A. Minoxidil
    B. Diazoxide
    C. Glibenclamide
    D. Cromakaline
16. **Osler Rendu Weber cath finding are:**
    A. SVC 70 PV 90 aorta 90 saturation
    B. SVC 70 PV 90 aorta 96 saturation
    C. SVC 70 PV 96 aorta 80 saturation
    D. SVC 70 PV 90 aorta 85 saturation

17. **Kawasaki disease are seen in all *except*:**
A. HypergamMaglobulinemia
B. Thrombocytosis
C. Increased ESR
D. Sudden cardiac death

18. **In hypomagnesemia can be seen in all *except*:**
A. Absent tendon reflex
B. Mg < 1 meQ/dL
C. Increased QT interval
D. Chrostek's sign +ve

19. **Pressure half time is 220 then mitral valve area will be:**
A. 1cm^2 B. 0.8 cm^2
C. 1.2 cm^2 D. 2.0 cm^2

20. **Pseudonormalization on ECHO differentiated by:**
A. Pulmonary venous filling pattern
B. Mitral inflow on Doppler
C. JVP
D. Increased LV size with respiration

21. **In asymptomatic AR with normal LV function indication of aortic valve replacement are all *except*:**
A. LVEDD > 75
B. LVED systolic > 55
C. Max MET < 4
D. ST depression increased from 1 mm to 2 mm on TMT

22. **Asymptomatic AS in a 40-year-old male with peak gradient across aortic valve 75 mm with normal LV function, treatment of choice:**
A. TMT to assess symptoms and cardiac reserve
B. CAG
C. Dobutamine echo to assess valvular resistance
D. Balloon aortic valvotomy

23. **50-year-old female with recent onset exertional dyspnea found to have a large ASD at fossa ovalis treatment of choice will be:**
A. Cardiac cath with CAG
B. Echo guided device closure
C. TMT for cardiac evaluation
D. CT angio

24. **SA nodal artery damage occurs in which of the following surgery?**
A. ASD closure
B. CABG on beating heart
C. PDA ligation
D. Closed mitral valvotomy

25. **In a 40-year-old with AMI systolic blood pressure 80 cardiac index 2.1 PCWP 12 initial management will be:**
A. Milrinone
B. Low dose dopamine + dobutamine
C. IABP
D. IV fluids

26. **Prehospital thrombolysis trial was:**
A. ASSENT-2 B. CAPTIM
C. EMERAS D. GISSI-5

27. **True about abciximab are all *except*:**
A. FAB of chimeric monoclonal antibody
B. Thrombocytopenia may occur
C. Aspirin enhances efficacy
D. Cannot be repeated within 7 days

28. **With concealed bypass tract which arrhythmia cannot occur?**
A. Antidromic SVT
B. CHB
C. AVNRT
D. Atrial fibrillation

29. **Which is the most common finding in CAG?**
A. LCX from RCA
B. Sinus node artery from LCX
C. ALCAPA
D. LAD between PA and aorta

30. **All four chambers have same saturation in which of the following condition?**
A. TAPVC
B. TGA
C. Single ventricle
D. Cardiogenic shock

31. **Coronary sinus oxygen saturation is:**
A. 30% B. 40%
C. 50% D. 20%

32. **Staphylococcus bacteremia with prosthetic valve leads to infective endocarditis in:**
A. 10% B. 50%
C. 90% D. 20%

33. **In end stage CHF with NYHA class IV annual mortality is:**
A. 10-20% B. 25-30%
C. 30-35% D. 60-70%

34. **Clubbing occurs in all *except*:**
A. Fungal infective endocarditis
B. Aortic dissection
C. Tricuspid atresia
D. Pulmonary AV fistula

35. **Janeway lesions are commonly associated with:**
A. Strep. bovis IE
B. Staph aureus
C. Libman sack
D. Viridans

36. **Drugs causing hypertension are all *except*:**
A. Levodopa B. NSAIDs
C. Cyclosporin D. Erythropoietin

37. **CYP 3A5 metabolism is affected in liver by all *except*:**
A. Pravastatin B. Atorvastatin
C. Lovastatin D. Simvastatin

38. **On Warfarin INR increases with:**
A. Digoxin B. Aspirin
C. Acetaminophen D. Rifampicin

39. **In digoxin therapy all are true *except*:**
A. Causes infra HIS block in toxicity
B. Indicated in stage 2 heart failure
C. Bidirectional tachycardia can occur
D. Low dose in women

40. **Strept viridans endocarditis can cause all *except*:**
A. ASO positive
B. RA factor positive
C. p-ANCA positive
D. Leucopenia may occur

41. **Aldosterone causes all *except*:**
A. Interstitial fibrosis
B. Edema
C. Magnesium conservation
D. Ventricular hypertrophy

42. **In acute MI, histopathological findings include all *except*:**
A. Coagulation necrosis
B. Myocytolysis
C. Central apoptosis
D. Contraction band necrosis

43. **All are true *except*:**
A. Isolated RVMI in 3-5% autopsy cases
B. LA infarction more common than RA infarction

44. **Which of the following is more common in AWMI as compared to IWMI:**
A. VSD
B. CHB
C. Papillary muscle dysfunction
D. RVMI

45. **All true in AMI *except*:**
A. Short term mortality 30%
B. Half the cases die in 1st half hour
C. Thrombolysis trial – mortality 15-20%
D. Decreased incidence of STEMI in developed countries

46. **In a patient with claudication distance < 100 m (Fontaine's criteria):**
A. IIA B. IIB
C. III D. IV

47. **Most common site of atherosclerotic aneurysm:**
A. Ascending aorta
B. Infra-renal aorta
C. Superior mesenteric aorta
D. Thoracic aorta

48. **Contraindication to thrombolysis are all *except*:**
A. Laser eye surgery < 6 weeks
B. BP difference in arms > 15 mmHg
C. Past history of idiopathic thrombocytopenic purpura
D. CPR > 10 min

49. **In chronic constrictive pericarditis are seen in all *except*:**
A. Pulmonary artery systolic pressure = 50 mmHg
B. BNP > 800 pg/ml
C. Septal bounce
D. Non-specific ST-T changes

50. **In JVP X descent is absent in:**
A. Tricuspid stenosis
B. AF
C. Cardiac tamponade
D. ASD

51. **Ventricular interdependence is seen in all *except*:**
A. Endomyocardial fibrosis
B. Effusive constrictive pericarditis
C. CCP
D. Cardiac tamponade

52. **Echo finding in pulmonary embolism include all *except*:**
A. Isolated RV apical hypokinesia
B. TR
C. Systolic bulging of IVS to LV
D. Thrombus across foramen ovale

53. **Early systolic murmur will be present in all *except*:**
A. Small muscular VSD
B. VSD with severe PAH
C. MR due to chordal rupture
D. MS with functional TR

54. **Early systolic sound is present in all *except*:**
A. Idiopathic dilatation of pulmonary artery
B. Valvular PS
C. Valvular AS
D. Aortic bioprosthesis

55. **Soft S1 is heard in all *except*:**
A. WPW syndrome
B. Flail mitral leaflet
C. LBBB
D. Acute AR

56. Paradoxical split of S2 occurs in:
A. Post operative RBBB
B. Permanent pacemaker
C. Severe MR
D. CCP

57. Continuous murmur may be heard in all *except*:
A. RSOV in LV
B. Coronary AV fistula
C. Aortic pulmonary collaterals
D. Peripheral pulmonary artery stenosis

58. Which of the following is diagnosed better by palpating carotid than peripheral artery?
A. Parvus et tardus
B. Pulsus bisferiens
C. Pulsus alternans
D. Pulsus paradoxus

59. All true *except*:
A. Intraarterial BP correlated best with Korotokoff phase IV
B. Cuff width 40% of arm circumference
C. Narrow cuff also increases diastolic blood pressure
D. Monckeberg's sclerosis causes pseudo HTN

60. Low voltage ECG is seen with all *except*:
A. Addison's B. Obesity
C. Extensive MI D. Anaemia

61. In Addison's disease all are seen *except*:
A. Low renin
B. Low DBP
C. Cardiac atrophy
D. Cortisol <8 μg/dL

62. CHF is associated with all *except*:
A. Hypouricemia
B. Decreased phosphate
C. Decreased Mg
D. Dilutional hyponatremia

63. Left ventricular assist device include all *except*:
A. Contegra B. Novacor
C. Heartmate D. Abiomed

64. Multislice CT is useful in all *except*:
A. Double aortic arch
B. Coronary artery anomaly
C. ARVD
D. CCP

65. Isometric exercise is associated with increase in all *except*:
A. Heart rate
B. Cardiac output
C. SVR (Systemic venous return)
D. Mean arterial pressure

66. Regarding S4 true is:
A. Normal in children
B. Usually present in acute AR
C. Increases with isometric exercise
D. Present in CCP

67. Amyl nitrate inhalation increases all of the following murmurs *except*:
A. HOCM B. TOF
C. AS D. MS

68. For LBBB occurring on exercise, all are true *except*:
A. Permanent LBBB develop in 50% on long term follow up
B. CHB develops in 50% on long term follow up
C. ST depression preceding by LBBB indicates ischemia
D. It may occur or disappear at varying heart rate

69. Drug contraindicated in NYHA class III to IV CHF:
A. Carvediolol
B. Spironolactone
C. Rosiglitazone
D. Metoprolol

70. In neurocardiogenic syncope, least useful test is:
A. Carotid duplex scan
B. Carotid sinus massage
C. HUTT
D. Orthostatic BP monitoring

71. Supravalvular AS is associated with:
A. Coanda effect
B. Increase calcium
C. Pulmonary stenosis
D. Aortic stenosis

72. No reflow phenomenon is decreased in cath by all *except*:
A. Nicorandil B. Adenosine
C. Verapamil D. Metoprolol

73. Neonate with heart failure associated with normal heart size:
A. TGA
B. Obstructive TAPVC
C. Tachycardia induced cardiomyopathy
D. CHB

74. Fetal heart failure occurs in:
A. TR B. HLHS
C. Single ventricle D. TGA

75. In familial PPH, gene involved is:
A. BMPR2 B. Troponin
C. Serotonin D. Endothelin

76. Herceptin cardiotoxicity is mediated by:

A. ERB B 2 B. PPAR α
C. BMPR 2 D. Dopamine 2

77. Cellular mechanism of electrical alternans is mediated by:

A. Ryanodine receptors
B. Norepinephrine
C. Potassium channel
D. Isoprenaline

78. Heavy alcohol intake causes all *except*:

A. Increased LDL
B. Increased triglyceride
C. Sudden cardiac death
D. Decreases CAD

79. Drug eluting stent are better than Bare metal stent in all *except*:

A. Clopidogrel allergy patients
B. Long lesion
C. Diabetes mellitus
D. Restenosis

80. False positive troponin T seen in:

A. CRF
B. Myocarditis
C. Post CABG
D. Pulmonary embolism

81. Cocaine can cause all *except*:

A. Left sided infective endocarditis
B. Decreased QT interval
C. LV dysfunction
D. Aortic dissection

82. Receiver operating curve indicates:

A. Sensitivity vs 1- specificity
B. Specificity vs 1- sensitivity
C. Odds ratio vs confidence interval
D. Sensitivity versus odds ratio

83. Most sensitive test for small to moderate pulmonary embolism:

A. d-dimer B. 12 lead ECG
C. ECHO D. ABG

84. Tendon xanthoma are seen in:

A. Type II B. Type I
C. Type III D. Type IV

85. In a diabetic 50-year-old lady desirable values are all *except*:

A. HDL < 40 B. BP = 120/70
C. LDL <100 D. TG < 150

86. For a 65-year-old man with asymptomatic RBBB on preop evaluation for inguinal hernia. What is to be done?

A. CAG
B. EPS and ablation
C. Routine management
D. Temporary pacing pre-operatively

87. In unstable angina intermediate risks are all *except*:

A. Trop T > 0.01 and < 0.1 ng/ml
B. Rest pain < 20 min
C. Age > 75 years
D. T wave inversion of >0.2 mV

88. Pseudomonas infective endocarditis is seen with:

A. Community acquired pneumonia in elderly
B. Pentazocine IV abuse
C. Patient receiving steroids
D. Post splenectomy

89. Pheochromocytoma is suggested by all *except*:

A. Persistently increased BP
B. Clonidine increased BP
C. Postural hypertension
D. Beta blocker induced coronary spasm

90. DLCO is decreased in all *except*:

A. Goodpasture's syndrome
B. Emphysema
C. PAH
D. ILD

91. Graham Steel murmur may be seen with all *except*:

A. TOF with absent pulmonary valve
B. Recurrent pulmonary embolism
C. MS
D. PDA

92. Most common cause of hypertension in child in India:

A. Takayasu aortoarteritis
B. Fibromuscular dysplasia
C. Fibrointimal dysplasia
D. Atherosclerosis

93. For companion trial all are true *except*:

A. 50% decreased mortality with biventricular pacing
B. QRS > 120 ms
C. LVEF <35%
D. More beneficial in non-ischemic cardiomyopathy

94. True ionotropic effect is:

A. ANREP
B. Windkessel phenomenon
C. Amylnitrate inhalation
D. Lusitrophic effect

95. **P wave inverted in II, III, AVF in all *except*:**
A. Dextrocardia
B. Ectopic atrial tachycardia
C. Coronary sinus rhythm
D. Junctional rhythm

96. **Ezetimibe all are true *except*:**
A. Decreased LDL alongwith statins
B. Decreased plasma level of fat soluble vitamins
C. Increased HDL
D. No effect on triglycerides

97. **Non-cardiogenic pulmonary edema with increased pulmonary capillary Wedge pressure occurs in:**
A. Bilateral renal artery stenosis
B. Narcotic overdose
C. Post CABG
D. ARDS

98. **Prophylactic drug for contrast induced nephropathy:**
A. N-acetyl cysteine
B. Diatrizoite
C. Steroids

99. **All of the following side effects of ACE I are mediated by bradykinin *except:***
A. Ischemic preconditioning
B. Platelet aggregation
C. Angioedema
D. Cough

100. **Regarding heart failure in women all are true *except*:**
A. Diastolic dysfunction is less common
B. More in elderly
C. More commonly misdiagnosed
D. Presents with more disability with equivalent LV dysfunction

101. **LV dysfunction is indicated by all *except*:**
A. EPSS > 10 mm
B. B-bump of mitral valve
C. Decreased end systolic dimension
D. Decreased systolic wall thickening

102. **Relation of LVEDV and LVEDP is:**
A. Curvilinear
B. Straight
C. Inverse
D. Logarithmic

103. **In total situs inversus, most common cardiac finding:**
A. Structurally normal heart
B. TGA
C. AV discordance
D. CHB

104. **Most specific sign of reversible ischemia:**
A. Pseudonormalization of T wave inversion
B. Inversion of U wave
C. ST elevation in Q wave leads
D. Loss of R wave

105. **Causes of pulmonary hypertension include all *except*:**
A. Toxic oil syndrome
B. Scleroderma
C. Methemoglobinemia
D. Cirrhosis

106. **Conduction disturbance are seen in all *except*:**
A. Freidrich ataxia
B. Hemochromatosis
C. Sarcoidosis
D. Myotonic dystrophy

107. **Least risk of CVA in atrial fibrillation in with:**
A. Apatheic hyperthyroidism
B. Mixed mitral valve disease
C. MS
D. HTN

ANSWERS

1	B	2	B	3	B	4	C	5	B	6	A	7	B
8	A	9	A	10	D	11	B	12	B	13	A	14	B
15	C	16	A	17	A	18	A	19	A	20	A	21	D
22	A	23	A	24	A	25	D	26	B	27	D	28	C
29	A	30	A	31	A	32	B	33	D	34	B	35	B
36	A	37	A	38	C	39	A	40	A	41	C	42	C
43	B	44	A	45	C	46	B	47	B	48	A	49	B
50	B	51	A	52	A	53	D	54	D	55	B	56	B
57	A	58	A	59	A	60	D	61	A	62	A	63	C
64	C	65	C	66	B	67	B	68	B	69	C	70	A
71	A	72	D	73	B	74	A	75	A	76	A	77	A
78	D	79	A	80	A	81	B	82	A	83	A	84	A
85	A	86	C	87	C	88	B	89	B	90	A	91	A
92	A	93	A	94	A	95	A	96	D	97	A	98	A
99	B	100	A	101	C	102	A	103	A	104	B	105	C
106	A	107	A										

11

AIIMS MAY 2006

1. **Sudden cardiac death is seen in all *except*:**
   - **A.** Kawasaki disease
   - **B.** LAD from pulmonary artery
   - **C.** LAD from right sinus
   - **D.** Left circumflex from right sinus

2. **Features of hypercalcemia include all *except*:**
   - **A.** Sinus arrest
   - **B.** Short QT
   - **C.** J point elevation
   - **D.** Sino vent conduction

3. **Malignant transformation in pheochromocytoma is characterised by:**
   - **A.** ↑ Dopamine
   - **B.** Hypotension
   - **C.** Epistaxis

4. **Contraction band necrosis all are true *except*:**
   - **A.** Catecholamine induced injury
   - **B.** Ischemic reperfusion injury
   - **C.** YAMA apoptosis injury
   - **D.** Post pump injury

5. **RVMI diagnosed after 48 hours by:**
   - **A.** Echo
   - **B.** Thallium scan
   - **C.** ECG on right side
   - **D.** Radionucleo ventriculography

6. **In amyloidosis true is all *except*:**
   - **A.** Anginal chest pain
   - **B.** Biopsy showing SAA
   - **C.** False +ve thallium
   - **D.** Postural hypertension

7. **6-day-old neonate with shock and impalpable pulses all of the following are possible *except*:**
   - **A.** CoA
   - **B.** Larger VSD
   - **C.** Tachyarrhythmia
   - **D.** HLHS

8. **Fetal intervention is beneficial in:**
   - **A.** Ebstein's anomaly
   - **B.** Absent left pulmonary artery
   - **C.** AS
   - **D.** VSD

9. **In acute AR, all can be absent *except*:**
   - **A.** Diastolic murmur
   - **B.** Duroziez' sign
   - **C.** S_4
   - **D.** Tachycardia

10. **More common in male:**
    - **A.** AV canal **B.** ASD
    - **C.** PDA **D.** D-TGA

11. **Most common presentation of CAD in female:**
    - **A.** Angina **B.** Acute MI
    - **C.** CCF **D.** Sudden death

12. **Graham Steel murmur occurs in all *except*:**
    - **A.** TOF with absent pulmonary valve
    - **B.** PDA with interrupted aortic arch
    - **C.** Pulmonary embolus
    - **D.** MS

13. **Continuous murmur can be seen in all *except*:**
    - **A.** Restrictive ASD with MS
    - **B.** PDA with interrupted aortic arch
    - **C.** Aorto pulmonary window
    - **D.** Supracardiac TAPVC

14. **Pulsus paradoxus in cardiac tamponade is not seen with:**
    - **A.** Positive pressure ventilation
    - **B.** β blockers
    - **C.** Fever
    - **D.** Pulmonary embolism

15. **Dose reduction of anticoagulants required with all *except*:**
    - **A.** Amiodarone **B.** Indomethacin
    - **C.** Phenytoin **D.** Rifampicin

16. **Selective phospodiesterase inhibitors are all *except*:**
A. Sildenafil
B. Tadalafil
C. Aminophylline
D. Dipyridamole

17. **Levosimendan is useful in:**
A. Acute CHF
B. Diabetic CMP
C. PSVT
D. Digoxin toxicity

18. **DAD seen in:**
A. Digoxin toxicity
B. Torsade de pointes
C. Ventricular parasystole
D. AVNRT

19. **Decrease BNP is seen in:**
A. CRF
B. End stage CCF
C. RCMP
D. Senile amyloidosis

20. **Anorectic drug induced PAH, mechanism of action:**
A. 5-HT and potassium channels
B. Neural mechanism
C. cAMP and Na channel
D. NO and CGMP

21. **Female at 2 A:M with 1 minute chest pain, symptoms repeated with syncope, ECG – ST elevation in inferior leads with 2:1 AV block immediate intervention:**
A. NTG
B. Primary PCI
C. Thrombolysis
D. Temporary pacing

22. **More common in inferior wall MI in comparison to anterior wall (MI):**
A. MR
B. VSD
C. Free wall rupture
D. RBBB

23. **Blood supply of anterior papillary muscle:**
A. LAD + left circumflex
B. LAD + right coronary artery
C. PDA
D. RCA

24. **Treatment modality used for PPH *except*:**
A. Sildenafil
B. Heart lung transplantation
C. Inhaled prostaglandins
D. Bosentan

25. **Great cardiac vein accompanies:**
A. LAD B. PDA
C. LCx D. Left MCA

26. **Features of chromosome 22 deletion include all *except*:**
A. Mild mental retardation
B. Ebstein's
C. Thymic hypoplasia
D. Hypocalcemia

27. **Single gene mutation is seen:**
A. Turner's B. Edward
C. Marfan's D. VSD

28. **Drug eluting stents ↓se subacute thrombosis to:**
A. 0.5 B. 0.5-1.0
C. 2-5 D. 10%

29. **Sirolimus all true *except*:**
A. S→G1 block
B. Saccromyces hygroscopicus is the source
C. Twice as effective as paclitaxel
D. I.V. administration causes hyperlipidemia/thrombocytopenia

30. **Drug eluting stents all *except*:**
A. Reduce mortality
B. Used in treatment in stent restenosis
C. Eliminated risk of subacute thrombosis with clopidogrel
D. Decreases chances of reangioplasty

31. **Rx to be used in septic shock:**
A. Vasopressin
B. Nesiritide
C. Trimetazidine

32. **Asplenia is most commonly associated with:**
A. Interrupted IVC B. TAPVC
C. D-TGA D. L-TGA

33. **RV is identified by all *except*:**
A. Moderator band
B. Elliptical shape
C. Coarse trabeculations
D. Septal tricuspid

34. **All true *except*:**
A. Both ventricles from bulbus cordis/ventricle
B. Subpulmonary conus resorbs and subaortic elongates
C. Pulmonary vein arises from first part of LA
D. R and L pulmonary A arises from prox 6th arch

35. **Mitral aortic discontinuity is seen in:**
A. DORV B. TA
C. TOF D. COA with VSD

36. **Man operated 2nd post operation day for colonic carcinoma develops hypotension and restlessness, diagnosis is:**
A. MI
B. Pulmonary embolism
C. Septic shock
D. Wound dehision

37. **Exercise increases VT in all *except*:**
A. Brugada
B. Belhassen tachycardia
C. RVOT-VT
D. HOCM

38. **ARVD diagnosed best with:**
A. MRI B. CT angio
C. PET scan D. ECHO

39. **Most sensitive investigation for ILD:**
A. HRCT B. DLCO
C. PAH by echo D. Chest X-ray

40. **Earliest sign for cardiac tamponade:**
A. Collapse of diastolic RV
B. Pulsus paradoxsus
C. Hypotension
D. Dicrotic pulse

41. **Epicardial fat pad seen between:**
A. Visceral pericardium and myocardium
B. Parietal and sternum
C. Parietal and visceral pericardium

42. **Properties of adenosine 2 receptor are all *except:***
A. Bronchoconstriction
B. Coronary vasodilations
C. ↑ses + TNF - α
D. No reflow phenomenon

43. **AT-I receptor all *except*:**
A. Vasoconstriction
B. Releases NE
C. Releases aldosterone
D. ↑ increases TNF-α

44. **Statins all *except*:**
A. High dose statin reduces acute coronary events
B. 40 mg simvastatin ~ 10 mg of atorvastatin
C. Useful in primary prevention

45. **NO is synthesized from:**
A. Arginine B. Leucine
C. Valine D. Isoleucine

46. **β blocker trial which showed ↑sed mortality cardiogenic shock:**
A. BHAT
B. COMMIT CCS
C. MIAMI
D. ISIS-1

47. **HOPE trial all are wrong *except*:**
A. Low risk
B. Women excluded
C. 5 mg ramipril for 4 years
D. 25% relative risk reduction

48. **ALL HAT trial drug not to be used:**
A. Prazosin B. Doxazosin
C. Minoxidil D. Nifedipine

49. **All are physiological values *except*:**
A. SVR 20 U
B. PVR 2U
C. Cardiac index – 1.6 litre/mm^2
D. MVO_2 7 ml/100 g/min

50. **Most common drug causing dilutional hyponatremia:**
A. Thiazide B. IFN-α
C. ACE-I D. β blocker

51. **Hypertriglyceridemia is caused by all *except*:**
A. β blockers
B. Thiazides
C. ACE-I

52. **Total Ch-260, HDL-40, TG 125, value of LDL:**
A. 195 B. 220
C. 95 D. 100

53. **Chorea is seen in all *except*:**
A. APLA
B. Pregnancy
C. Hypoxia
D. Hyperthyroidism

54. **For rheumatic fever all are true *except*:**
A. Modified Jones criteria not useful in recurrent RF
B. Acute phase reactants normal in chorea
C. Echo added as major criteria
D. Secondary prophylaxis in mild MS with carditis at least 40 years of age

55. **For severity of MR most useful criteria is:**
A. Vena contracta width
B. Jet area method
C. PHT
D. LA dimension

56. **PHT in MS is not useful:**
A. Just after PTMC
B. Associated MR
C. Pregnancy
D. Isolated MS

57. **Lone AF originates from:**
A. Pulmonary vein
B. Coronary sinus

C. Right atrial appendage
D. Left atrial appendage

58. **In CCF which does not improve survival?**
A. Bisoprolol
B. Candesartan
C. Spironolactone
D. Frusemide

59. **Target dose used in trials all *except*:**
A. Carvedilol 25 mg BD
B. Aten 100 mg OD
C. Metoprolol XL 200 mg OD
D. Bisoprolol 5 mg OD

60. **Angiographic catheter all *except*:**
A. Sones B. Judkins
C. Amplatz D. Cournald

61. **GpIIb/IIIa beneficial in all *except*:**
A. USA
B. Thrombolysis in AMI
C. NSTEMI
D. Primary PCI

62. **Aspirin resistance measured by:**
A. Platelet aggregimetry
B. Platelet granular count
C. Total platelet count
D. Occurrence of MI during use

63. **LMWH assay is done by:**
A. Anti XA B. aCT
C. aPTT D. PT

64. **Prehospital fibrinolysis most effective drug:**
A. Urokinase B. Hirudin
C. Tenecteplase D. Alteplase

65. **Restenosis is maximally seen after PCI in stable CAD angina:**
A. LMCA diseases
B. Ostial LAD diseases
C. SVG diseases
D. PDA diseases

66. **High risks USA all *except*:**
A. DM
B. Stable angina
C. Trop T +ve
D. LV dysfunction

67. **Asian Indian CAD all are true *except*:**
A. Hypertriglyceridemia more important than LDL cholesterol
B. APO B/APO A1 is one of most important risk factor
C. Smoking is a risk factor
D. Occurs at younger age

68. **Framingham risk score include all *except*:**
A. HDL
B. LDL
C. Smoking
D. Systolic BP

69. **Complication of sleep apnoea are all *except*:**
A. Seizures
B. Sudden death
C. LV dysfunction
D. PAH

70. **POTS best diagnostic test:**
A. HUTT
B. TMT
C. Autonomic blockade
D. Hyperbaric O_2

71. **Ankle Brachial Index > 0.9 all *except*:**
A. Rest pain
B. Uncomplicated DM
C. Normal
D. Autonomic neuropathy

72. **U wave inversion in TMT:**
A. Prox LAD disease
B. Hypokalemia
C. HOCM

73. **ST changes cannot be used reliable to diagnose CAD in presence of all *except*:**
A. AS
B. LVH
C. Arterial switch operation
D. WPW

74. **VF seen in all *except*:**
A. Malignant neurocardiogenic syncope
B. Malignant hyperthemia
C. WPW
D. IWMI

75. **All seen in HOCM *except*:**
A. Subaortic membrane
B. Concentric LVH
C. RVH
D. Pseudonormalization in Doppler mitral

76. **For CCP, true is:**
A. E>A
B. DT <150 msec
C. Blunting of E wave on tissue Doppler
D. TV Doppler variation in respiration

77. **Single fibre contractility load independent:**
A. V max
B. ↑ Dp/dt (max)
C. LV stroke volume index
D. EF

78. **For adriamycin induced toxicity all are true *except*:**
A. Cumulative dose more important but peak dose is not important
B. Cumulative dose >450 mg/m^2
C. Dexrazone prevents toxicity
D. Toxicity usually appears 3 months after stopping drug but may appear in decades also

79. **Treatment of choice for a sessile rhabdomyoma with AV peak gradient 60 mmHg in a neonate:**
A. Alcohol ablation
B. Surgery
C. Medical management

80. **Asymptomatic female with AS with pressure gradient 60 mmHg 3rd trimester pregnancy, treatment of choice is:**
A. Medical
B. BAV
C. Cesarean with valvotomy
D. Surgical

81. **90% asymptomatic carotid artery stenosis with TVD with LV dysfunction, treatment choice is:**
A. CABG alone
B. CABG now, then endarterectomy
C. Carotid stenting first then CABG
D. CABG+CEA together

82. **Trop T can be false +ve in all *except*:**
A. Ischemic stroke
B. Atrial myxoma
C. Aortic dissection
D. Ruptured aortic aneurysm

83. **In IE with 10 mm vegetation, cardiac stroke occurring is most likely in which of the following involvement?**
A. Mitral valve with staph aureus
B. Aortic valve with strep viridans
C. Tricuspid valve with candida
D. Already treated mitral valve vegetatation with persistent vegetation

84. **↑sed erythropoietin with polycythemia is seen in all *except*:**
A. TOF
B. Polycythemia vera
C. Cerebellar hemangioma
D. Hypoxemia

85. **QT prolongation seen in all *except*:**
A. Toxic myocarditis
B. Myocardial ischemia
C. Normal
D. Sotalol therapy

86. **For cardiac transplantation, most important parameter is:**
A. EF
B. VO_2
C. HLA
D. Weight

87. **Right side aortic arch, least common in:**
A. TOF
B. VSD with Ps
C. Truncus arteriosus
D. Corrected TGA

88. **Failed thrombolysis is indicated by:**
A. T↓ after 4 hours
B. ST resolution >50% at 90 min
C. AI VR
D. VT

89. **Broad complex tachycardia is suggestive of SVT in presence of:**
A. A-V dissociation
B. Fusion beat
C. QRS > 160
D. RSR in V_1 and qRS in V_6

90. **In shock trial, 30 days survival in medically managed patients was:**
A. 56%
B. 44%
C. 41%
D. 76%

91. **ECG normalizes in patients after 1 year of MI in:**
A. 5%
B. 10%
C. 15%
D. 20%

92. **PCI more effective than thrombolysis in all *except*:**
A. Patient present with 1 hour
B. After 3 hours at PCI enabled centre
C. Shock occurs more commonly after PCI than thrombolysis

93. **Takayasus' arteritis commonly involves all *except*:**
A. Pulmonary artery
B. Abdominal aorta
C. MCA
D. Left subclavian artery

94. **Endocarditis is most commonly seen in:**
A. PDA at 5 years
B. Elderly MVP with MR
C. Pregnancy with Ebstein's

95. **Alveolar arterial grad >40 mmHg is seen in:**
A. Chronic mountain sickness
B. GBS polyneuropathy
C. TOF
D. Barbiturate poisoning

96. **Prostacycline causes all *except* (PGE2):**
A. Apnoea
B. Hypotension
C. Hypercalemia
D. Seizure

97. In brain abscess in cyanotic HD all *except*:
A. Fever in 80%
B. MRI for diffuse cerebritis
C. Anti-convulsants for 6 months
D. Endocarditis is not associated with brain abscess

98. Hypersensitive carotid sinus all are true *except*:
A. Common in elderly
B. Sinus pause >3 min
C. Most of the time venipacing is effective
D. Movement of neck causes exacerbation of symptoms

99. Anti-coagulation in AF all *except*:
A. Not used in elderly due to increased risk of haemorrhage
B. INR ~ 1.5 is ineffective
C. Should be given for 3 months after cardioversion
D. Not to be given in lone AF in young

100. Low voltage shock is given in:
A. Ectopic atrial tachycardia
B. Atrial flutter
C. Antidromic reentrant tachycardia
D. Complicated NSVT

101. Balloon atriostomy is done in:
A. Corrected TGA
B. TAPVC
C. Mitral atresia
D. PPH

102. HOCM most common gene involved:
A. Myosin B. Trop I
C. Actin D. Tropomyosin

103. Aortic dissection least likely seen in:
A. Syphilis
B. Homocystinemia
C. CoA
D. Biscup aortic valve

104. Drugs causing cardiovascular disease all *except*:
A. Rofecoxib
B. Cisapride
C. Levodopa
D. Long acting nifedipine

105. Enzyme with shortest life span:
A. Myoglobin
B. SGOT
C. CPK
D. SGPT

106. In resting heart, substrate used for metabolism:
A. Ketones B. Glucose
C. AA D. FAA

107. Syncope seen in all *except*:
A. PE
B. Carotid artery stenosis
C. Internal haemorrhage
D. Cardiac tamponade

108. A person with hyperlipidemia which has highest risk of CAD?
A. Dizygotic twin
B. History of CAD in mother
C. History of CAD in father
D. Both parents

ANSWERS

1	D	2	D	3	A	4	C	5	D	6	B	7	B
8	C	9	D	10	D	11	A	12	A	13	B	14	A
15	C	16	C	17	A	18	A	19	D	20	A	21	B
22	A	23	A	24	B	25	A	26	B	27	C	28	B
29	C	30	A	31	A	32	B	33	B	34	B	35	A
36	B	37	A	38	A	39	A	40	A	41	B	42	C
43	D	44	B	45	A	46	B	47	D	48	B	49	C
50	A	51	C	52	A	53	C	54	C	55	A	56	A
57	A	58	D	59	B	60	D	61	B	62	A	63	A
64	C	65	C	66	B	67	C	68	B	69	A	70	A
71	A	72	A	73	C	74	A	75	A	76	C	77	A
78	D	79	C	80	A	81	B	82	B	83	A	84	B
85	B	86	B	87	D	88	D	89	D	90	B	91	B
92	A	93	C	94	A	95	C	96	C	97	A	98	C
99	C	100	C	101	B	102	A	103	B	104	A	105	A
106	D	107	B	108	D								

12

AIIMS DECEMBER 2005

1. **Least relative risk among current smoker:**
   A. Ca lung
   B. CAD
   C. COPD
   D. PVD
2. **Aptameter is:**
   A. FAS
   B. VEGF
   C. DeCOY
   D. PGEF
3. **CARTO in therapeutic mapping in arrhythmias uses:**
   A. 3 X-ray
   B. 3 D echo
   C. 3 D spectroscopy
   D. 3 D magnetic resonance
4. **Glasgow phenomenon is:**
   A. Increase luminal diameter in early atherosclerosis
   B. Decrease luminal diameter in early atherosclerosis
   C. Increase stiffness in early atherosclerosis
   D. Decrease stiffness in late atherosclerosis
5. **Type A lesion:**
   A. Discrete
   B. Non calcified
   C. Ostial
   D. SVG graft
6. **Mechnical ventilation in COPD true all *except:***
   A. FiO_2: 0.3
   B. I/E ratio 1:1
   C. Tidal volume 10 ml/kg
   D. PCO_2 <45 mmHg
7. **Pulse oximeter not true is:**
   A. Measures PaO_2
   B. Sometime above 90% SaO_2
   C. Cannot be used with methemoglobinemia
   D. Uses Doppler technique
8. **End tidal $PaCO_2$ < 7 suggest all *except*:**
   A. Oesophageal intubation
   B. V/Q mismatch
   C. Spontaneous circulation
   D. Inadequate cardiac compression
9. **Pulses bisferiens best felt at:**
   A. Carotid B. Radial
   C. Brachial D. Femoral
10. **Single S2 is seen in:**
    A. Corrected TGA
    B. Eisenmenger with PDA
    C. TAPVC
    D. PS
11. **Continuous murmur is seen in all *except*:**
    A. Abdominal aneurysm
    B. MS with ASD
    C. RSOV
    D. Peripheral PS
12. **Longest survival in cyanotic heart disease >10 year:**
    A. TOF B. Ebstein
    C. TAPVC D. C-TGA
13. **Migraine is most commonly associated with:**
    A. PPH B. Marfan
    C. PFO D. AS
14. **Not seen in Down's syndrome:**
    A. TGA
    B. Alzheimer's
    C. Tricuspid atresia
    D. Hirschsprung disease
15. **Myocardial biopsy not useful in:**
    A. Acute rheumatic activity
    B. Sarcoidosis
    C. Myocarditis
    D. Amyloidosis

16. **Myocarditis is not caused by:**
A. Hepatitis C
B. Polio
C. Adenovirus
D. HIV

17. **Cardiomyopathy caused by all *except*:**
A. Cisplatin
B. Doxorubicin
C. Cyclophosphamide
D. Herceptin

18. **Myocarditis is caused by:**
A. Captopril
B. Diltiazem
C. Azathioprine
D. Diazepam

19. **Aspirin in female 100 mg/alternate day:**
A. Decrease all cause mortality
B. Decreases breast Ca
C. First MI
D. Decreases stroke

20. **Hyperglycemine caused by all *except*:**
A. Primary aldosteronism
B. Pheochromocytoma
C. Diuretics
D. ACE-I inhibitor

21. **Addison's disease all are features *except*:**
A. Fatigue
B. Weight gain
C. Hypotension
D. Skin pigmentation

22. **Increased BP in standing:**
A. Essential HTN
B. Familial dysautonomia
C. Pheochromocytoma
D. Old age

23. **Not seen in hypothyroidism:**
A. CHB
B. Increase PV resistance
C. Deafness
D. Increase CPK

24. **Amiodarone therapy for 24 hours cause all *except*:**
A. Hypothyroidism
B. TDP
C. Bradycardia
D. Pulmonary toxicity

25. **QT interval increase in all *except*:**
A. Hypothermia
B. Phenytoin
C. TCA
D. Sotalol

26. **In pregnancy all flares *except*:**
A. Ulcerative colitis
B. SLE
C. MVP
D. Rheumatic chorea

27. **All are associated with aorto arteritis *except*:**
A. Crohn's
B. Sarcoidosis
C. Erythema nodosum
D. RPGN
E. None of the above

28. **MS 1.7cm^2 3-month pregnancy treatment of choice:**
A. Spironolactone
B. Beta blocker
C. PTMC
D. MTP
E. BMV in 2nd trimester

29. **Severe MR in pregnancy with normal LV function:**
A. Conservative management
B. Repair
C. Replacement
D. Cesarean at delivery

30. **Balloon dilation is not done in all *except*:**
A. Congenital MS
B. Takayasu
C. Subaortic stenosis
D. Neonatal coarctation

31. **Infective endocarditis (acute cause by all *except*:**
A. Coxiella
B. β-hemolytic streptococcal
C. Staph aureus
D. Listeria

32. **Best treatment for hemoptysis in TOF:**
A. Octreotide
B. Embolism with coil
C. Ligation of collateral
D. Embolisation of pulmonary artery

33. **Prophylaxis not required in all *except* for endocarditis:**
A. Cystoscopy
B. Cesarean
C. Bronchoscopy
D. Tooth extraction

34. **Octreotide used in all *except*:**
A. Mesentric ischemia
B. Vipoma

C. Acromegaly
D. Carcinoid

35. **Flushing with nicotinic acid treatment is:**
A. Aspirin
B. Sedatives
C. Tropical treatment
D. No treatment as it gets relieved within time

36. **BP not readable in infants with:**
A. Oscillometry
B. Flushing technique
C. Doppler
D. Spectroscopy

37. **Ankle edema in elderly caused by all *except*:**
A. Minoxidil
B. Amlodipine
C. Indomethacin
D. Rosuvastatin

38. **TG is not lowered by:**
A. Statin
B. Nicotinic acid
C. Gemfibrozil
D. Ezetimibe

39. **All secondary trials *except:***
A. Woscop B. Lipid
C. 4s D. BPs

40. **Primary trials all *except* for ICD:**
A. MUSTT B. CASH
C. Definite D. CABG patch

41. **Inferior wall MI poor prognosis all *except*:**
A. V1-V3 ST depression
B. Complete heart block
C. RVMI
D. Papillary muscle rupture

42. **Which will require active treatment in MI?**
A. AF B. IV ectopic
C. Vent ectopic D. AIVR

43. **Aflutter joule required for cardioversion:**
A. 25-50 B. 100
C. 15 D. 360

44. **BNP level in acute dyspnea of non-cardiac syndrome:**
A. 90 B. 180
C. 350 D. 500

45. **Normal heart all arrythmias seen *except*:**
A. Flutter
B. Accessory pathway
C. AF
D. PSVT

46. **Adenosine treatment used in all *except*:**
A. AVNRT
B. Other AVRT
C. Anti-dromic AVRT
D. Atrial flutter

47. **Messenger for NO:**
A. c-GMP B. Ca+
C. ADP D. COX

48. **Coronary spasm all seen *except:***
A. Bradycardia
B. Syncope
C. Adenosine induced spasm
D. VF

49. **Most sure sign hypocalcemia suggest by:**
A. Prolonged QU
B. ST elevation
C. Increased PR interval
D. IT wave inversion

50. **Most severity indication of CCP:**
A. Late diastolic collapse
B. Electrical alternans
C. Early diastolic collapse
D. Late systolic collapse

51. **Rx of hyper eosinophilia all *except*:**
A. Imitnib
B. Etanarcept
C. Hydroxy urea
D. IL-2

52. **NCEP ATP-3 metabolic syndrome all *except*:**
A. BP > 130/85
B. Fasting glucose >110
C. Microalbuminuria
D. Raised TG

53. **Definitive diagnosis of metabolic syndrome made by:**
A. BMI>30
B. Wait hip ratio >0.8
C. TG>120
D. HDL>40

54. **Apo B seen in all *except*:**
A. VLDL
B. HDL
C. Chylomicrone
D. VLDL

55. **NSTEMI with significant trop T positive:**
A. Abciximab + medical
B. Abciximab + PCI

C. PCI without abciximab
D. Intergrellin—abciximab—PCI

56. **TLT = PCI in:**
A. < 3 hours B. < 1 hour
C. < 2 hours D. 12 hours

57. **Facilitated thrombolysis true is:**
A. Increased bleeding >75 years
B. Recently used in T bleeding risk
C. Trials have shown benefit
D. Treatment of choice in ST elevation MI

58. **Ximelgatran all *except*:**
A. Oral direct thrombin inhibition
B. No hepatotoxicity
C. No interaction with food
D. No monitoring required

59. **Heparin dose monitored after PCI by:**
A. ACT B. APTT
C. Clot lysis D. PT

60. **90 minutes TIMI3 flow after STK:**
A. 55 B. 35
C. 75 D. 90

61. **PPH gene responsible is:**
A. Serine protease B. Elastase
C. TGF-B D. Arrestin

62. **Athlete all seen *except*:**
A. LVS3
B. Heart rate < 50
C. Mobitz type I
D. Loud P2

63. **Pulmonary vasoconstriction occurs with all *except*:**
A. Arginine
B. Exercise
C. REM
D. Polycythemia

64. **Localized pulmonary edema seen in all *except*:**
A. MS
B. Radiation
C. Pulmonary AV fistula
D. Pulmonary embolism

65. **A1 antitrypsin deficiency all seen *except*:**
A. Atypical emphysema
B. Premature emphysema
C. Bronchiectasis
D. Cirrhosis

66. **Syncope seen in normal health adult:**
A. HR 50 B. BSM <50
C. PCO_2 = 10 D. PO_2 = 60

67. **In normal healthy adult echo can show all *except*:**
A. PR B. AR
C. TR D. MR

68. **Patient having congestive hepatomegaly with marked respiratory flow variation on echo investigation of choice:**
A. CT chest B. TEE
C. MRI D. Chest X-ray

69. **Myocardial viability detected by:**
A. Rest redistribution
B. Exercise SPECT
C. First pass
D. Radionuclide angiography

70. **NH3 in PET estimates:**
A. Coronary flow
B. Fat metabolism
C. Stunned myocardium
D. Anaerobic metabolism

71. **Stent deployment best detected by:**
A. IVUS
B. Contrast CT
C. MRI
D. Pulsatile fluoroscopy

72. **Stress test done by all *except*:**
A. Erjonovine B. Dipyridamole
C. Adenosine D. Dobutamine

73. **All seen in mechanical ventilation in COPD *except*:**
A. Cholelithiasis
B. Hypotension
C. Stress block
D. Non sustained VT

74. **Treatment of vasovagal syncope all *except*:**
A. Disopyramide
B. Biventricular pacing
C. Paroxitine
D. Midodrine

75. **PPI indicated in:**
A. Alternating BBB
B. RBBB
C. Rate related LBBB
D. CBBB

76. **Pacing in AWMI indicated in all *except*:**
A. Transient CHB
B. Bifascicular block without primary block
C. 2:1 AV block after 16 days
D. Alternating BBB with 1:1 conduction

77. **CRT indicated in:**
A. RBBB B. LBBB
C. QRS > 120 msec D. CMB

78. Asymptomatic non-diabetic male for TURP has RBBB pre operative evaluation include:
A. Functional status evaluation
B. Echo
C. Angiography
D. Routine investigations

79. DCMP with severe CHF all not true *except*:
A. Ventriculectomy
B. BT for anemia
C. Amiodarone for prevention of sudden death

80. All true about DCMP *except*:
A. Decreased DP/DT
B. Decreased SVR
C. Poor relaxation
D. Increased EDP

81. Stem cell from bone marrow does not lead to:
A. Astrocyte
B. Endothelium
C. Placenta
D. Pancreas

82. Contrast allergy premedication all *except*:
A. Cimetadine
B. Diphenhydramine
C. Steroids
D. Iodoerone

83. Single and double headed protein:
A. Titin
B. Actin
C. Myosin
D. Troponin

84. Sarcome length does not change in:
A. Isovolumetric relaxation
B. Diastasis
C. Isotonic contraction

85. Rh carditis all are true *except*:
A. Chronic carditis can be seen upto six months
B. Pericarditis does not occur without valvular involvement
C. I/V methyl prednisolone is drug of choice
D. Carditis is early manifestation of severe Rh fever

86. True about Rh fever all are *except*:
A. Erythema nodes seen on fall
B. Subcutaneous nodule suggest carditis
C. Aniskov cell derived from plasma cell
D. Erythema marginatum not seen on face

87. Early closure of mitral valve occur in:
A. Increased PR interval
B. Severe AR
C. MS

88. Severe AS in elderly person is diagnosed by all *except*:
A. Heaving apex
B. Soft S2
C. Carotid upstroke

89. MRI is diagnostic in:
A. ARVD
B. CA myxoma
C. Pericarditis

90. Maximum incidence of acute Rh fever in school children seen:
A. Uttaranchal **B.** Gujarat
C. TN **D.** Others

91. Magnesium can be used in all *except*:
A. Diuretic therapy
B. Migraine
C. Renal failure
D. Pregnancy

92. HOCM all are seen *except*:
A. ASM of mitral valve
B. RV hypertrophy
C. Sub aortic membrane

93. Cox 2 inhibitor all are seen *except*:
A. Decreased GI bleed
B. Decreased non-fatal MI
C. Increased SCD

94. Right axis deviation seen in all *except*:
A. Reversing of left and right arm leads
B. Acute pulmonary embolism
C. Common atrium
D. Dextrocardia

95. In which VSD conduction defects is involved:
A. Outlet VSD
B. Perimembranous VSD
C. Swiss cheese
D. Mid muscular

96. AV duration is affected in all *except*:
A. Age
B. Dextrocardia

97. 2:1 block is affected by all *except*:
A. Exercises
B. Atropine
C. Digoxin
D. Procainamide

98. True about sleep apnea all *except*:
A. Most of them does not have CHF
B. Decrease after LV function improves
C. 10% of CHF patient have sleep apnea
D. CHF patient can have sleep apnea

99. **Affirm trial true is:**
 A. Rate control with oral anti-coagulants
 B. Maze operation
 C. Amiodarone

100. **All are used for smoking de-addiction (withdrawal) all *except*:**
 A. Bupropion
 B. Nicotine
 C. Cimetidine
 D. Cigar smoking

101. **Contrast agent (in echo) used for pulmonary AV fistula:**
 A. Saline agitated
 B. Gadolinium
 C. Adenosine

102. **All draining in coronary sinus *except*:**
 A. Anterior cardiac vein
 B. Great cardiac vein
 C. Small cardiac vein
 D. Middle cardiac vein

103. **RV is identified all *except*:**
 A. Moderator band
 B. Tricuspid valve
 C. Origin of pulmonary artery
 D. Septal attachment of chordae

104. **Prinzmetal's angina cluster:**
 A. After midnight
 B. 6-12 AM
 C. In evening
 D. After awakening

105. **All are standard protocol for MI treatment *except:***
 A. GIK
 B. Clopidogrel
 C. ACE inhibitor
 D. STK

106. **PGE1 in pulmonary atresia causes all *except*:**
 A. Fever
 B. Apnea
 C. HTN
 D. Increased cyanosis

107. **Diabetes mother all *except*:**
 A. Macrosomia
 B. Delayed heavy maturity
 C. Neonatal HTN
 D. Transient HCM

108. **Max wall stress:**
 A. Sub endocardial
 B. Pericardial
 C. Epicardial

ANSWERS

1	B	2	B	3	D	4	A	5	A,B	6	B	7	C
8	D	9	A	10	B	11	A	12	B	13	C	14	A
15	A	16	B	17	A	18	D	19	D	20	D	21	B
22	A	23	A	24	D	25	A	26	C	27		28	B
29	A	30	A	31	A,B	32		33	D	34	A	35	A
36	D	37		38	D	39		40	B	41	B	42	A
43	A	44	A	45	A	46	D	47	A	48	C	49	
50		51		52	C	53	A	54		55	B	56	A
57	C	58	B	59	A	60	A	61	C	62	D	63	A
64	A	65	A	66	A	67	B	68	A	69	A	70	
71	A	72	A	73		74	B	75	A	76		77	C
78	A	79	C	80	B	81	C	82	D	83	C	84	B
85	C	86	A	87	B	88	C	89	A	90	A	91	C
92	C	93	B	94	C	95	B	96		97		98	
99	A	100	D	101		102	A	103	C	104	A	105	A
106	D	107	C	108	A								

13

AIIMS MAY 2005

1. **Rate >150, sudden onset cause:**
   A. Sinus tachycardia
   B. PSVT
   C. AF block
   D. VT
2. **Hairless pubic and axillary, cardiomyopathy, heart block:**
   A. Hemochromatosis
   B. Addison's
   C. Kearnssayre
   D. Klinefelter
3. **Drugs that worsen angina are all *except*:**
   A. T3
   B. Sumatriptan
   C. Oxyphedrine
   D. Dipyridamole
4. **Adverse prognosis in TMT all *except*:**
   A. <6 min
   B. Hypotension during recovery
   C. ST elevation
   D. Symptomatic VT
5. **In TMT all *except*:**
   A. SVT are normal
   B. VPC which disappear during exercise suggest CAD unlikely
   C. Post MI VPC have bad future prognosis
   D. PVC only during stress indicates ischemia
6. **TMT ST ↓ occurs without CAD in all *except*:**
   A. AS
   B. LVH
   C. WPW
   D. Physical deconditioning
7. **TMT with WPW all *except*:**
   A. Disappearance of delta wave suggest antegrade short ERP
   B. PSVT common
8. **20 years male with CAD likely to have:**
   A. Tendon xanthoma
   B. Tubero eruptive
   C. Planar
   D. Eruptive
9. **Apo B is not present in:**
   A. Chylomicrons **B.** VLDL
   C. LDL **D.** HDL
10. **Morphology like HOCM all *except*:**
    A. Amyloidosis
    B. Hyperparathyroid
    C. Ducehnne's
    D. Noonan
11. **Pain with LBBB in 1st hour most appropriate:**
    A. Thrombolyse with tPA full dose
    B. Primary PTCA to centre at distance of 1 hour
    C. Trop T confirmation
    D. Gp IIb/IIIa + ½ tPA + PTCA
12. **Drug of choice for cyclosporine induced HTN:**
    A. Beta blockers **B.** CCB
    C. Diuretic **D.** ACE
13. **Not used in pregnancy all *except*:**
    A. ACE
    B. ARB
    C. Propylthiouracil
    D. Aldosterone antagonist
14. **HTN + metabolic alkalosis + hypokalemia seen in all *except*:**
    A. Cushing's
    B. Conn's
    C. RTA type IV
    D. Liquorice ingestion
15. **Seen in pregnancy all *except*:**
    A. Left sided straightening of border
    B. Pulmonary basal rales
    C. ↑ R/S in V_1-V_2
    D. S2 soft

16. **Persistent fetal circulation all *except*:**
A. Differential cyanosis
B. Metabolic alkalosis
C. Normal shaped heart
D. PHT

17. **Dopanine D_1 diagonist:**
A. Dobutamine
B. Sumatriptan
C. Bromocriptine
D. Fenoldopam

18. **Pulmonary artery stenosis seen in all *except*:**
A. Down B. Rubella
C. Alaigille D. William

19. **Coronary artery spasm by all *except*:**
A. Ach (Acetyl choline)
B. Ergonovine
C. Alcohol
D. Serotonin

20. **In plaque rupture all seen *except*:**
A. ↑ 5-HT
B. ↓ Metalloproteinase
C. ↓ NO
D. ↑ TXA_2

21. **In fountain classification <200 m claudication class:**
A. I B. IIa
C. IIb D. III

22. **TIMI risk factor '3' is for STEMI given to:**
A. Age 65-74 B. HR > 100
C. SBP<100 D. Killip III-IV

23. **Act on thrombin through antithrombin:**
A. Agratroban
B. Fondaparinaux
C. Enoxaparin
D. Bivaluridin

24. **Which of following not give to infant with PSVT?**
A. Ice pack over face
B. Adenosine
C. Verapamil
D. Digoxin

25. **MVP associated with all *except*:**
A. Kyphoscoliosis
B. Ostium primum
C. Left sided bypass tract (accessory pathway)
D. Marfan

26. **Square root sign in all *except*:**
A. CHF
B. MR
C. Autonomic neuropathy
D. ASD

27. **Flash pulmonary edema with HTN seen in:**
A. RAS B. CoA
C. PIH D. Conn's

28. **Pulmonary embolism all true *except*:**
A. 50-60% No DVT
B. Q wave 2,3 aVF
C. RV hypokinesia except apex
D. Normal D-dimer rules out diagnosis of PE

29. **In RCMP all *except*:**
A. PA > 50
B. RVEDP < 1/3 RVSP
C. LV and RV filling pressures difference less than 5 mm
D. Square root sign

30. **Reverse pulsus paradoxus seen in:**
A. HOCM
B. Absent pericardium
C. RVMI

31. **HLHS with collapse treatment:**
A. PGE1
B. Transplant
C. Norwood
D. Percutaneous aortic valvotomy

32. **BMV not done in:**
A. With mild MR
B. Mild AR
C. AF
D. Congenital MS

33. **PHT is useful all *except*:**
A. Post PTMC
B. Valid in isolated MS
C. Not valid in MR/AR
D. Not valid in HTN

34. **Senile amyloidosis due to:**
A. Transthyretin
B. Calcitonin
C. Prealbumin
D. ANP

35. **LA myxoma systemic symptoms are due to:**
A. IL-6
B. IFN-α

36. **Amiodarone induced thyrotoxicosis all *except*:**
A. Papillary CA
B. Thyroiditis
C. Jod Basedow
D. Autoimmune

37. **Early systolic murmur in all *except*:**
A. IE
B. Severe MR due to MI
C. Small VSD
D. Mild rheumatic MR

38. Cannot diagnose by fetal echo in second trimester:
A. Small VSD B. Ebstein
C. CHB D. AS

39. Risk of restenosis maximum after PTCA:
A. USA
B. Venous graft
C. Stent like result of balloon PTCA
D. Primary PTCA

40. Cyanotic spell with PS all *except*:
A. ASD B. VSD
C. TGA D. Single ventricle

41. Single S2 all *except*:
A. TOF B. Eisenmenger
C. ASD repair D. TA

42. Hibernation myocardium detect by all *except*:
A. High dose dobutamine echo
B. SPECT
C. PET
D. Second dose thallium

43. After thrombolysis most common cause of death:
A. Cardiogenic shock
B. Reperfusion arrhythmia
C. CVA
D. Ventricular rupture

44. Thrombolysis absolute contraindication all *except*:
A. Ischemia CVA < 6 months
B. Closed head trauma < 3 months
C. AV malformation
D. Aortic dissection

45. PCI effect of heparin assessed by:
A. APTT
B. Clot lysis time
C. ACT
D. BT

46. In aortic dissection symptoms all *except*:
A. Syncope
B. Paraplegia
C. Right pleural effusion
D. CVA

47. Hepatojugular reflux seen in all *except*:
A. ↑ PCWP B. ↓ afterload
C. TR D. RVMI

48. Infection common after splenectomy *except*:
A. Pneumococci
B. H influenzae
C. Babesiosis
D. Infectious mononucleosis

49. Multislice CT angiography can detect all *except*:
A. Anomalous coronary artery
B. Stent stenosis
C. Main left coronary
D. SVG patency

50. Takayasu disease associated with all *except*:
A. Crohn's disease
B. UC
C. RA
D. PPH

51. Cyanosis with haemoptysis is seen in all *except*:
A. TOF
B. Truncus arteriosus
C. Schimitar syndrome
D. Osler Weber Rendu syndrome

52. In cath data all are true *except*:
A. A>V in LA pressure tracing

53. Causes of MR in infant all *except*:
A. ALCAPA
B. Endocardial Cushing defect
C. Tricuspid atresia
D. Endomyocardial fibroelastosis

54. Ductus arteriosus develops from:
A. Distal 6th arch B. 4th arch
C. 1st arch D. 3rd arch

55. Pulmonary artery develops from:
A. Proximal 6th arch
B. 3rd arch
C. 4th arch
D. Distal 6th arch

56. NTG causes all *except*:
A. Hypotension with bradycardia
B. ↑ SGOT
C. Methemoglobinemia
D. Mild PO_2↓

57. Migraine associated with all *except*:
A. Temporary brain stem ischemia
B. Syncope
C. Prinzmetal angina
D. Pulmonary HTN (PPH)

58. Severity of MR associated with all *except*:
A. Pulmonary venous flow reversal
B. Regurgitation volume >40 ml
C. Jet area in LA >50%
D. Vena contracta > 6 mm

59. All true of acute RVM I *except*:
A. Improved by IABP
B. Hypoxemia
C. Persistent ST elevation in V_4R
D. Pulsus paradoxus

60. ↑ PAP (20 mmHg) on inspiration and attenuated γ descent:
A. Cardiac tamponade
B. MS
C. CHF
D. Pulmonary embolism

61. ARVD all *except*:
A. Thinning of RV on echo
B. Left myocarditis in biopsy
C. LBBB morphology in VT
D. Familial

62. Infective endocarditis all *except*:
A. MCD
B. RPGN
C. MPGN
D. Focal segmental GN

63. Major criteria of Framingham:
A. Exertional dyspnea
B. Pedal edema
C. X-ray cardiomegaly
D. Tachycardia >120

64. Late ECG changes in severe hypokalemia:
A. ↑ QU interval B. ↑ PR
C. ↓ T D. ST ↓

65. Protein losing enteropathy is seen in all *except*:
A. Constrictive pericarditis
B. After Fontan operation
C. Cardiac transplantation
D. Menetrier's disease

66. RV is a systemic pump in all *except*:
A. CTGA B. TGA
C. Baffle D. Arterial switch

67. Characteristic of VT all *except*:
A. Capture beat
B. VA dissociation 2:1
C. QRS >120 ms

68. Holiday heart syndrome all *except*:
A. AF B. AFL
C. CHB D. VPC

69. Free wall rupture all *except*:
A. Most common in 1-4 days
B. With previous MI
C. With HTN
D. Thrombolysis increase the risk

70. ST ↑ in V_1 all *except*:
A. Brugada B. LBBB
C. ↑ Ca^{2+} D. Post wall MI

71. Gene therapy in all *except*:
A. HOCM
B. PVD
C. Ischemic CMP

72. Drug in metabolic syndrome:
A. Acarbose B. Pioglitazone
C. Nateglinide D. Aspirin

73. >10 mmHg diff in both arm all *except*:
A. Supravalvular AS
B. PVD
C. Takayasu
D. Modified BT shunt

74. Maximum cardiac risk in:
A. Hip surgery
B. Iliofemoral bypass
C. Hemicolectomy
D. Radical mastectomy

75. Prophylaxis for IE required in:
A. Caesarean
B. TURP
C. Coronary angiography
D. TEE
E. None

76. Normal in a Marathon runner (athlete) all *except*:
A. LVS3
B. Mild MDM at LLSB
C. Grade II aortic ejection systolic
D. HR 55/min

77. Early in prosthetic valve IE leading to myocardial and cerebral abscess:
A. Candida
B. HACEK
C. Pseudomonas
D. Staphaureus

78. Organism causing cerebral abscess in cyanotic child:
A. Strepto spp
B. Staphaureus
C. Pseudomonas
D. Neisseria

79. Angiography in MI showing hemodynamically significant CAD:
A. >75% occlusion diameter (of all 3 vessel)
B. >50% stenotic area
C. Associated with acute MI
D. >90% ischemia defect

80. Edema by all *except*:
A. Minoxidil B. Pioglitazone
C. Lovastatin D. NSAID

81. **More common in inferior wall MI than anterior wall MI all *except*:**
A. Idioventricular rhythm
B. Papillary rupture
C. Mobitz type II block
D. Vomiting

82. **HOCM all *except*:**
A. Apical good prognosis
B. Mutation of MHC
C. Septal alcohol ablation relieve symptom
D. Post PVC potentiation of murmur

83. **Drug of 1st choice for prophylaxis in portal hypertension:**
A. Beta blocker
B. Nitrate
C. Vasopressin
D. Somatostatin

84. **APLA syndrome all *except*:**
A. ↑ PTT
B. 50% SLE
C. Recurrent arterial thrombosis
D. Thrombocytopenia

85. **In non ketotic hyperosmolar coma all *except*:**
A. Vomiting with abdominal pain
B. Osmolality 350
C. Normal phosphate
D. Normal anion gap

86. **Acquired tosade de pointes initial drug:**
A. Beta blocker
B. Mg^{2+}
C. CA^2 gluconate

87. **In HF all *except*:**
A. ↑ B_1 receptor
B. ↑ basal Ca^{2+}
C. RMP less negative
D. Decreased AT Pase

88. **H wave in JVP all *except*:**
A. Isovolumetric relaxation
B. Diastosis

89. **O_2 consumption in normal adult during exercise depends upon:**
A. Hb
B. Cardiac output
C. Total lung capacity
D. Skeletal muscle fitness

90. **INR in prosthetic mitral valve:**
A. 1.5-2.5
B. 2.5-3.5
C. >3.5
D. >3

91. **On HRT therapy woman develop MI what to do?**
A. Stop HRT
B. Start after one year
C. Continue same dose
D. Shift to low dose progesterone

92. **Choice of bioprosthesis over mechanical value all *except*:**
A. Patient choice
B. CRF on dialysis
C. Life expectancy less
D. Pregnancy expected

93. **Indication of cardiac transplant all *except*:**
A. Low EF
B. Recurrent symptomatic VT
C. Killip 3-4 not amenable to PTCA/CABG

94. **CHF with sleep apnea treatment of choice:**
A. Weight reduction
B. Uveopalatopharngealplasty
C. Nasal CPAP
D. Ambulatory oxygen therapy

95. **Adriamycin toxicity all *except*:**
A. Years after drug stoppage possible
B. Once occurred worse prognosis than DCMP
C. ACE contraindicated
D. Dexrazoxane can be used to ↓ toxicity

96. **In ageing all seen *except*:**
A. ↓ CO in stress
B. ↑ Sugar in acute stress
C. ↑ S. creatinine
D. ↓ TLC

97. **Billow pulmonary valve worst likely in:**
A. MS
B. TS
C. PS
D. AR

98. **True for $MgSO_4$ all *except*:**
A. For seizure act through D1 receptor
B. No benefit in MI
C. Useful in Torsade de pointes
D. Aldosterone ↑ Mg^{2+} level

99. **Classic PAN all *except*:**
A. P-ANCA +ve
B. CHF
C. Eosinophilic granuloma
D. Testicular pain

100. **Peripheral pulse palpable with gangrene:**
A. Abdominal aneurysm
B. Diabetic
C. Beurger of Toe
D. PAD

101. All are true *except*:

A. Lactate level reliable in diagnosis of ischemia
B. Myocardial bridges in normal person
C. Dipyridamole induce ischemia reversed by adenosine
D. LVEDP ↑ before ST depression

102. Warfarin effect ↓ by all *except*:

A. Vitamin K oral intake
B. Rifampin
C. Amiodarone
D. Phenobarbitone

103. True of hypothyroidism all *except*:

A. Normal HR response on exercise
B. Large pericardial effusion frequently causes tamponade
C. Pulmonary edema less occur

104. Infradiaphragmatic TAPVC all *except*:

A. Ground glass X-ray
B. Normal heart
C. Split S2
D. TR velocity >2 m/sec

ANSWERS

1	A	2	A	3	D	4	B	5	D	6	C	7	
8	A	9	D	10	B	11	A	12	B	13	C	14	C
15	D	16	B	17	D	18	A	19	D	20	B	21	C
22	C	23	C	24	C	25	B	26	B	27	A	28	B
29	C	30	A	31	A	32	D	33	A	34	A,D	35	A
36	A	37	A	38	A	39	B	40	A	41	C	42	A
43	A	44	A	45	C	46	C	47	B	48	D	49	B
50	D	51	C	52	A	53	C	54	A	55	A	56	B
57	D	58	B,D	59	A,C	60	A	61	B	62	A	63	C
64	D	65	C	66	D	67	C	68	C	69	B	70	D
71	A	72	B	73	D	74	B	75	E	76	B	77	D
78	A	79	A	80	C	81	A,C	82	D	83	A	84	B
85	B	86	C	87	D	88	A	89	B	90	D	91	A
92	B	93	A	94	C	95	C	96	C	97		98	D
99	A,C	100	A	101	C	102	C	103	B	104	C		

14

AIIMS DECEMBER 2004

1. **Right anterior loop (instead of left anterior) loop leads to:**
   A. DTGA
   B. L-TGA
   C. Ebstein's anomaly
   D. PAPVC
2. **Least nephrotoxic:**
   A. Iohexal
   B. Iodixinol
   C. Urograffin
   D. Iopa
3. **Giant cell arteritis all *except:***
   A. Jaw claudication
   B. Elderly more
   C. Arch involvement
   D. Blindness
4. **In ASD 2nd ICS thrill not seen:**
   A. ASD with MS
   B. ASD with MR
   C. ASD with PS
   D. ASD with Eisenmenger
5. **28 years female severe MR → with LVS-60 ml, treatment:**
   A. MVR
   B. MV repair
   C. ACE inhibitor
6. **Pregnancy all cannot be given *except*:**
   A. Labetalol B. Spironolactone
   C. Captopril D. STK
7. **HTN crisis with hematuria with renal insufficiency drug of choice:**
   A. SNP
   B. Methyl dopa
   C. Fenoldopam
   D. Stencler
8. **Oral anti-coagulant dose ↓se required in:**
   A. Amiodarone
   B. Thyroxin
   C. Digoxin
   D. Rifampicin
9. **Digoxin toxicity by all *except:***
   A. Dilzem
   B. High dose diuretics
   C. Amiodarone
   D. Propranolol
10. **Nitrates 1st used in angina by:**
    A. Burnion
    B. Ludwig
    C. Davis
11. **Myocardial resyncronization trial:**
    A. Companion
    B. Madit-2
    C. Cast
    D. Definite
12. **Conduction defect exclusively seen in:**
    A. Fredriech's
    B. DMD
    C. Myotonic dystropy
    D. Familial periodic paralysis
13. **CCP all *except:***
    A. ↑ PCWP–CVP ↑PADP ↑RVDP
    B. Near normal COP
    C. Septal interdependence
    D. Abnormal tissue Doppler study
14. **Neonatal HF not seen:**
    A. ↑ JVP
    B. Cardiomegaly
    C. Hepatomegaly
    D. Respiratory distress

15. **PA banding in all *except:***
   A. Sinus cheese VSD
   B. Ebstein's without PS
   C. Univentricular heart without PS
   D. Tricuspid atresia with PAH

16. **Cardiac transplantation in neonate all *except:***
   A. DCMP
   B. Ebstein's anomaly with severe PVD
   C. HLHS
   D. Multiple VSD

17. **Small defect need not to be closed:**
   A. PDA
   B. VSD
   C. A-P window
   D. Truncus arteriosus

18. **Which of the following cannot be diagnosed by fetal echo?**
   A. C-CHB
   B. Ebstein's
   C. COA

19. **Fetal echo all *except*:**
   A. AVSD
   B. Diaphragmatic hernia
   C. Small VSD

20. **PSVT neonate all *except:***
   A. AVNRT is rare
   B. Verapamil is useful for conversion to NSR
   C. All seen in normal heart
   D. S. tachy up 220 min is normal (200)

21. **Bicuspid AV all *except:***
   A. Most common CHD
   B. Markedly dilated ascending aorta seen
   C. IE prophylaxis necessary
   D. AR can develop

22. **Least common coronary anomaly:**
   A. RCA from LCx
   B. LCx from RCA
   C. Left from non-coronary sinus
   D. Conus from separate ostium

23. **HOCM:**
   A. NSVT—absence good prognosis
   B. Elderly onset—may develop SCD
   C. Elderly syncope more severe than child
   D. Asymptomic can do sporting activity

24. **Monomorphic VT in all *except:***
   A. ACS
   B. DCMP
   C. HOCM
   D. Vent. aneurysm

25. **Normal value all *except:***
   A. TPVR = 150-250
   B. CI = 1.8 to 4.2
   C. A-VO_2 = 30-48
   D. LVEDV = 60-90 ml/m^2

26. **CABG useful in all *except:***
   A. Px LAD
   B. DVD with LCx and RCA
   C. LMCA
   D. TVD with LV dysfunction

27. **Steep Y descent all *except:***
   A. Cardiac tamponade
   B. CCP
   C. CHF
   D. TR

28. **Hibernating myocardium diagnosed by:**
   A. Dobutamine echo
   B. TC-Pyrophospate scan
   C. TMT with adenosine
   D. Contrast echo

29. **All drugs have calcium mediated effect *except*:**
   A. Milrinone
   B. Digoxin
   C. Adrenaline
   D. Nicorandil

30. **HTN in children all *except:***
   A. Age
   B. Height
   C. Weight
   D. Race

31. **H-J reflux correlates with:**
   A. COP
   B. PCWP
   C. PASP
   D. Blood volume

32. **Systolic HTN in elderly:**
   A. Correlates with CV mobidity
   B. β blocker 1st choice
   C. ACE I effective

33. **Toe gangrene with palpable pulse:**
   A. DM
   B. Bergurs
   C. AO aneurysm
   D. Raynaud's

34. **Thrombus at LV apex all *except*:**
   A. STK has ↓ed incidence
   B. Lifelong coagulation
   C. May develop in logilower
   D. Aspirin should be added

35. **RV dyskinesia in RV free wall and base with sparing apex:**
A. PPH
B. PTE
C. RVMI
D. RVD

36. **Typical of large PTE all *except*:**
A. > 50% involved
B. Pulmonary infarction
C. Syncope
D. RV kinesia

37. **Mitral annular calcification all *except*:**
A. Seen in elderly female
B. Newborn seen in Marfan's
C. Associated with AS
D. Associated with MR

38. **LQTS all *except*:**
A. LQT_3 provoked by exercise
B. Competitive sports contraindicated
C. Stress can ↑QT
D. 10% due to sudden death

39. **LQT–treatment not given are all *except*:**
A. I.V. isoprenaline
B. β blockers
C. Pacing
D. Correct electrolytes

40. **Amiodarone in primary resistant VF or pulseless VT:**
A. 300 mg IV over 5 min
B. 300 mg IV push
C. 150 mg slow over 1 min
D. 150 mg IV push

41. **AICD best in:**
A. Brugada with history of VF
B. Child with LQT
C. MI with low EF with NSVT with no inducible VT
D. MI normal EF with prim. VF at MI

42. **Prognosis in acute MI affected by:**
A. RBBB
B. NSVT
C. AIVR
D. Prim VF

43. **Lovastatin induced myopathy exaggerated by all *except*:**
A. Paracetamol
B. Ketoconazole
C. Cyclosporine
D. Erythromycin

44. **Dysynchrony in vent. contraction seen:**
A. LBBB with HF
B. Concealed bypass
C. Junctional tachycardia

45. **Not included in Jones criteria:**
A. Polyarthritis
B. Subcutaneous nodules
C. ↑ ASO
D. Echo diagnosed carditis

46. **Sodium channel blocker all *except:***
A. Lidocaine
B. Phenytoin
C. Manganese
D. Flecanide

47. **VEGF antagonised by:**
A. Von Hippel Lindau protein
B. IL
C. FGF
D. TNF-α

48. **Ductus is present in all *except*:**
A. TOF with absent PV
B. Aortic atresia
C. PA with intact IVS
D. PA with VSD

49. **Ductus develops from:**
A. 3rd
B. 4th
C. 5th
D. 6th AA

50. **Cyanotic spell in TOF precipitated by all *except:***
A. Winter
B. Anaemia
C. Digoxin
D. SVT

51. **Chorea all *except:***
A. 20% develop mitral stenosis in 20 years
B. Associated in 80% of acute rheumatice fever
C. Secondary prophylaxis required
D. Hemichorea can occur

52. **Cardiac depressed in all *except:***
A. Hyponatremia
B. Hypophosphatemia
C. PJRT
D. Selenium deficiency

53. **Down's syndrome all *except:***
A. TGA
B. Hypothyroid
C. Duodenal atresia
D. AD

54. **Dicrotic seen in all *except:***
A. CHF
B. Fever
C. Hypovolemia
D. Cardiac tamponade

55. **Changes in pulse as goes pripheral all *except:***
A. Diastolic BP ↑
B. Dicrotic wave more prominent
C. Upstroke steep with ↑ amplitude
D. Dicrotic moves downward

56. **LVEDP minimally raised in all *except:***
A. Angina
B. Chronic MR
C. CCP
D. Acute AR

57. **Cilostazole all *except:***
A. PDE III inhibitor
B. ↓ HDL
C. ↑ claudication distance
D. ↓ platelet count

58. **Orthostatic hypotension—most effective drug:**
A. Indomethacin
B. Clonidine
C. Midodrine
D. Prednisolone

59. **pH-7.2 HCO_3 10, PCO_2 20, PO_2 87:**
A. Ethylene glycol poisoning
B. Hyperventilation
C. High altitude
D. Pulmonary edema

60. **Cardiac amyloidosis all *except:***
A. Primary amyloidosis death < 1 year
B. ANP deposits in atria in atrial amyloidosis
C. Stem cell useful familial amyloidosis
D. Supportive therapy in SSA

61. **Coronary artery spasm all *except:***
A. Adrenaline
B. 5-FU
C. Ergot
D. Cocaine

62. **Metabolic syndrome all *except:***
A. Abdominal obesity
B. Insulin resistance
C. ↑ TG
D. ↑ LDL

63. **Metabolic regulator of coronary vessels:**
A. Adenosine
B. Prostaglandins
C. CO_2
D. NO

64. **Saphenous vein graft PTA all *except:***
A. GP IIb IIIa ↓ distal embolism
B. Distal protection device reduces infarction
C. Periprocedural infarction ↑
D. BMS are preferred over DES in SVG PTCA

65. **Electrocution all *except:***
A. Death due to apnea
B. Fixed dilated pupil indicate irreversible ischemia
C. EKG simulate hyperkalemia
D. Causes AMI

66. **EAD by:**
A. Sotalol
B. Hyperkalemia
C. β block
D. Digoxin

67. **CAG all *except:***
A. Can be done transradial
B. Contraindicated in acute MI
C. RCA injection may cause bradycardia and asystole
D. Nonionic dye reduces renal complication

68. **Sertaline causes:**
A. Bradycardia
B. Hypotension
C. Long QT
D. VPC

69. **Brain abscess all *except*—in cyanotic CHD:**
A. ↑ by (Fe ↓) iron deficiency
B. ↑ by polycythemia
C. Posterior fossa
D. Caused by anaerobic streptococci

70. **Rheumatic carditis all *except:***
A. Isolated chorea
B. Carry Coomb's murmur
C. Subcutaneous nodules
D. Erythema marginatum

71. **TPI before surgery all *except*:**
A. Asymptomatic CHB
B. Intermitted trifasicular block
C. RBBB + CAD
D. SSS with long pauses

72. **MR severity by Doppler all *except:***
A. PHT
B. PISA
C. Jet area
D. Width of jet

73. **Drug withdrawn from market due to cardiac side effect:**
A. Cerivastation
B. Rofecoxib
C. Nimuslide
D. Troglitazone

74. Sarcoidosis all *except:*
- **A.** Pericarditis
- **B.** PHT
- **C.** High degree AV block
- **D.** Causes AR

75. Pericarditis most common cause—all *except:*
- **A.** Idiopathic
- **B.** Cox A virus
- **C.** TB
- **D.** Post MI

76. TLT all *except:*
- **A.** Urokinase does not cause anaphylaxis
- **B.** Intracranial bleed in 10%
- **C.** PVD can be given after 2 weeks
- **D.** PTE treatment can be given 3-4 days

77. PVD relative risk - max with:
- **A.** HTN
- **B.** Smoking
- **C.** DM
- **D.** Hypercholestenolemia

78. Atherosclerotic RSA all *except:*
- **A.** DM
- **B.** Smoking
- **C.** PVD
- **D.** Bilateral small kidney

79. Alcoholic CMP all *except:*
- **A.** Usually resembles idiopathic CMP
- **B.** Does not occur in absence of nutritional deficiency
- **C.** Usually not associated with hepatic disease
- **D.** Heavy consumption > 20 years

80. True about DES all *except:*
- **A.** Restenosis < 5-7%
- **B.** Steroid and heparin coated did not effect restenosis
- **C.** Restenosis ↑ in DM
- **D.** Not preferred in Px LAD lesion

81. Critical limb ischemia all *except:*
- **A.** Parasthesia
- **B.** ABI 0.6-0.8
- **C.** Dependent edema
- **D.** Rest pain

82. Hydatid cystic all *except:*
- **A.** Never calcified
- **B.** Surgery conducted in asymptomatic
- **C.** Echo investigation of choice
- **D.** Cause pulmonary embolism

83. Not used in persistent PPH of newborn:
- **A.** High frequency ventilation
- **B.** Controlled cryoventilation
- **C.** Surgery
- **D.** Sildenafil

84. PPH all *except:*
- **A.** Nifedipine used in all patients
- **B.** IV PG prolongs survival
- **C.** BMPR2-mutation associated

85. Carotid artery stenosis all *except:*
- **A.** Unilateral CAS cannot cause syncope
- **B.** Surgeons with periop stroke rate of 10-20% should do surgery in carotid art stenosis
- **C.** Person ↓going CABG should have surgery for severe asymptomatic carotid stenosis

86. β blockers in heart failure—all *except:*
- **A.** β_1 downregulation > β_2
- **B.** ββ more effective in III-IV than ACE I
- **C.** Mild to moderate HF mortality 5-15%

87. IABP least effective in:
- **A.** DCMP
- **B.** Unstable angina
- **C.** High risk PTCA
- **D.** Post CABG LVD

88. RVMI–ECG s/o Px RCA occlusion in V4R:
- **A.** ST ↑ 1 mm with ↑ T
- **B.** ST N with ↑T
- **C.** ST ↓ 1 mm with T ↓
- **D.** CHF

89. Cardioplegia commonly used in open heart surgery is:
- **A.** Hypothermia
- **B.** Ach
- **C.** Hyperkalemia
- **D.** Mechanical

90. ARVD all *except:*
- **A.** RBBB on ECG
- **B.** VT with LBBB
- **C.** RV dilatation
- **D.** Fatty infiltration in atrial septum

91. HYTI episode occurs in all *except:*
- **A.** Vasovagal
- **B.** Emotion
- **C.** Cough
- **D.** Micturition

92. Hypophosphatemia seen in all *except:*
- **A.** Alcoholic
- **B.** Hyperalimentation
- **C.** DKA recovery
- **D.** Respiratory acidosis

93. HIV pericardial effusion all *except:*
A. Low blood CD-4 count
B. Spontanous resolution in 20%
C. Mild effusion
D. Etiology not known in most

94. Warfarin all *except:*
A. Bolus dose should not be given
B. INR 2-3 in MVR
C. Emergency reversed by FFP
D. Cause skin necrosis

95. CAD in female true in:
A. HRT not effective
B. 2nd most common cause of death
C. LDL

96. Device closure not done in:
A. PDA—6 mm
B. Muscular VSD
C. A-P defect
D. Coronary A-V fistula

97. Spontaneous closure in neonates occurs in small:
A. PDA
B. VSD
C. ECD
D. AS

98. Eisenmenger syndrome occurs in all *except:*
A. Congenital MS
B. TGA
C. Ebstein's
D. Truncus

99. Chromosomal anomaly in Truncus asteriosus:
A. 22q
B. Trisomy 13
C. XO
D. Trisomy 2 deletion

100. Transfatty acid, rich source is:
A. French fries
B. Coconut oil
C. Olive oil
D. Milk

101. Elevated trop. T levels all *except:*
A. Advanced HF
B. Exercise
C. PTE
D. NSTEMI

102. Risk of restenosis after intervention all *except:*
A. Small vessel
B. Ostial
C. Long lesion
D. Primary PTCA

103. Asymptomatic severe AS:
A. PTA in peak gradient > 60 mm in children
B. Surgery not indicated
C. ↑cholesterol is a risk factor

104. Tricuspid atresia all *except:*
A. LAD
B. Glenn done at 1 month
C. Restrictive ASD balloon septostomy
D. Can present with typical cyanotic spell

ANSWERS

1	B	2	B	3	B	4	D	5	B	6	C	7	C
8	A	9	D	10	A	11	A	12	C	13	D	14	A
15	B	16	D	17	B	18	C	19	C	20	B	21	C
22	C	23	A	24	A	25	B	26	B	27	A	28	A
29	D	30	D	31	B	32	A	33	C	34	B	35	B
36	B	37	C	38	A	39	B	40	B	41	A	42	A
43	A	44	A	45	D	46	C	47	A	48	A	49	D
50	A	51	B	52	A	53	A	54	A,B,C	55	A	56	D
57	C	58	C	59	A	60	C	61	A	62	D	63	
64	D	65	B	66	A	67	B	68	A	69	C	70	A
71	A	72	A	73	B	74	D	75	A	76	D	77	B
78	D	79	B	80	D	81	B	82	A	83	A	84	A
85	B	86	B	87	A	88	A	89	C	90	D	91	D
92	D	93	B	94	B	95	B	96	C	97	B	98	A
99	A	100	A	101	B	102	B	103	A	104	B		

15

BHU 2010

1. **SLE criteria are all *except*:**
   A. ANA
   B. APLA
   C. Elevated AST/ALS
2. **Cyclophosphamide true is:**
   A. 500 mg monthly for 6 months
   B. 500 mg monthly × 6 weeks
   C. 1000 mg daily for 6 weeks
   D. 500 mg daily for 6 months
3. **RA in rheumatic arthritis:**
   A. Has high predictive value
   B. 75% cares +ve, can be used for screening
   C. Can be used as screening test
4. **HLA - association in Type - I DM:**
   A. HLA – DRB * 404
   B. HLA – DRB
   C. HLA – DR3
   D. DR4
5. **Hyperthermia seen in all *except*:**
   A. Enteric fever
   B. Fluoxetine
   C. Thyrotoxicosis
   D. Phenothiazine
6. **Abnormal organization of cells:**
   A. Dysplasia
   B. Disruption
   C. Malformation
   D. Deformation
7. **HPU all *except*:**
   A. Increase rate
   B. Permissive hypercapnia
   C. Increase pressure in airways
8. **ARDS Rx all *except*:**
   A. Corticosteroids
   B. Decrease LAP
   C. Surfactant
   D. Low tidal volume
9. **L. donovani infection finding most common:**
   A. Asymptomatic
   B. Splenomegaly
10. **Auto immune hepatitis all true *except*:**
    A. Amenorrhoea
    B. Hypogammaglobulinemia
    C. Thyroiditis
11. **Most common immuno deficiency:**
    A. IgA deficiency
    B. CVID
    C. SCID
12. **PPH all *except*:**
    A. Prostaglandin 12
    B. Indomethacin
    C. Sildenafil
13. **Absent pain and temperature on one side/loss of proprioception low of motor:**
    A. Brown-Sequard syndrome
    B. Harlequine sensory loss
14. **Treatment of uncomplicated P. vivax:**
    A. Chioroquines B. Proguanil
    C. Qunidine D. Mefloquine
15. **NCC not a minor criteria is:**
    A. + cigar shaped
    B. Antibodies in CSF
    C. Antibodies ELISA (Serum)
    D. MRI finding suggestive of NCC
16. **Category A – Bioterrorism:**
    A. Smallpox
    B. Anthrax
    C. Brucellosis
17. **Case of viral infection:**
    A. Adult T-cell leukemia
    B. Burkitt's lymphoma B
    C. Hairy cell leukemia
    D. Mycosis fungoides

18. Patient on follow up of methotrexate treatment investigation done:
A. Hemogram + urine
B. Hemogram + liver enzymes
C. Urine
D. Hemogram

19. Nazar criteria all *except*:
A. Albumin B. Bilirubin
C. AST D. PT

20. Dejjerine-Sotto syndrome all *except*:
A. Ant. cranial artery involvement
B. Pain in opposite side

21. Apoptosis all *except*:
A. CD95 is required
B. Inflammation is seen
C. DNA cleavage

22. CEP:
A. HMB synthase
B. URO synthetase
C. ALA dehydratase

23. HIV CD4 +se toxoplasma seen at:
A. > 350 B. < 350
C. < 100 D. < 50

24. Acute pancreatitis all *except*:
A. Hemochromatosis
B. Hypercalcemia
C. PTH adenoma
D. Cushing's syndrome

25. PR interval alternans:
A. Dual A-V node pathway
B. AVRT
C. Pulmonary embolism

26. Pacemaker in sinus node dysfunction with normal AV node:
A. AAI
B. VVI
C. DDD

27. Brugada with VT mechanism:
A. Phase 0 B. Phase 1
C. Phase 2 D. Phase 4

28. Carotid sinus hypersensitivity:
A. Sinus pause > 3 sec or SBP decrease 50
B. Sinus pause > 3 sec and SBP decrease 50
C. Sinus pause > 5 sec and SBP decrease 30
D. Sinus pause > 5 sec or SBP decrease 30

29. Myocardial cell specific gravity:
A. 1.02 B. 1.04
C. 1.06 D. 1.08

30. Dose decrease in renal failure:
A. Verapamil B. Metoprolol
C. Atenolol D. Carvedilol

31. Worst prognosis in pulmonary A HTN:
A. Idiopathic
B. Eisenmenger's
C. Anorexdyenic
D. With connective tissue disorder

32. MRI C/I in all *except*:
A. Electronic pump infusion
B. Cochlear implant
C. Neurovascular clips
D. Prosthetic implants

33. II, III, aVF and V4R ST election B.P. = 90/60, shouldn't be done:
A. IV fluids B. STK
C. NTG D. Dopamine

34. LMCA stenosis DX by:
A. aVR elevation >V1
B. aVR elevation <V1
C. ST depression in II, III, aVF, I, aVL, V3V4
D. ST elevation in V1-V3

35. LCX ECG changes:
A. V1 ST elevation with T inversion
B. V1 ST elevation with T upright
C. V1 isoelectric with T upright
D. V1 ST depression, T wave inversion

36. Primary angio v/s thrombolysis is beneficial in:
A. Hypertensive 80 years non obese
B. Hypertensive 80 years obese
C. Non-hypertensive 80 years obese
D. Non-hypertensive 80 years thin limb

37. Mechanism of action of fibrates through inhibition of:
A. PPAR-(alpha)
B. PPAR-(gamma)
C. HMGCoA

38. Max risk of CAD by which ratio?
A. TC : HDL
B. LDL : HDL
C. Apo B 100 : HDL
D. Apo B : Apo A1

39. Life saved by thrombolis is STEMI per 100 is:
A. 7 B. 14
C. 21 D. 2

40. Most effective in decreasing cardiac mortality in MI:
A. Beta blocker B. Aspirin
C. ACE I D. NTG

41. Which diuretic decrease mortality in STEMI?
A. Frusemide
B. Spironolactone
C. Indapamide

42. CAD in female true all *except*:
A. Angina more in female
B. CHF more in female
C. VF and SCD less
D. Comorbidities less

43. MI with cardiogenic shock true all *except*:
A. Early revascularization decrease 30 days mortality in >75 years
B. Decrease 6 months mortality
C. No benefit with revascularization

44. On TMT more likelihood of multi-vessel and bad prognosis CAD all *except*:
A. SBP failure to increase 120 or decrease 10
B. ST depression (excluding aVR)
C. Exercise < 7 METs
D. ST elevation in all leads in except aVR

45. On TMT good (best) predictor of survival:
A. SBP × HR >24000
B. MET > 13
C. –nce of ST depression

46. Mitral value used with pressure half time 540 ms:
A. 0.6 B. 0.7
C. 0.8 D. 0.9

47. Pulmonary flow velocity 120 cm/sec and acceleration time 60 sec what is PASP?
A. 40 B. 50
C. 60 D. 70

48. Pulmonary HTN is defined by pulmonary artery pressure:
A. 25 B. 30
C. 20 D. 40

49. Migratory arthritis in rheumatic fever all *except*:
A. Mostly involve small joints
B. HIP rarely involvement
C. NSAIDs and salicylates after confirmation
D. Last for few weeks

50. During valsalva if Korotkoff's sounds in all phases:
A. Decrease EF
B. Increase afterload
C. Increase filling pressure

51. Korotkoff's sound in which phase of valsalva is normal?
A. I and IV B. I and III
C. III and IV D. All phases →I/IV

52. BAV fusion most common between:
A. Right and non coronary cusp
B. Left and non coronary cusp
C. Right and left coronary cusp
D. None

53. ECG in CCP all *except*:
A. Low voltage common
B. AF 5-10% T
C. ST/T changes are seen most commonly
D. 50% ECG normal

54. Maximum effective orifice area in which condition of mitral valve?
A. Bileaflet B. Heterograft
C. Ball cage

55. Investigation of choice for acute viral pericarditis:
A. ECG B. ECHO
C. CT D. MRI

56. Valvular AS is diagnosed by:
A. Clinical examination
B. ECG
C. History

57. In CHF all decrease long term mortality *except*:
A. Digoxin
B. ACEI
C. Hydralazine + nitrate
D. Beta blocker

58. Which is not a vascular phenomenon?
A. Roth spot
B. Janeway lesion
C. Mycotic aneurysm
D. Septic pulmonary infarct

59. In CCP LV pressure volume curve:
A. Rightward B. Leftward
C. Upward D. Downward

60. Mitral annular calcification seen in all *except*:
A. HOCM
B. Juvenile MS
C. Hyperparathyroidism

61. Severe MR true are all *except*:
A. Axillary radiation of murmur
B. Flow murmur of mitral valve
C. Loudness (intensity IV or more)
D. Cardiomegaly

62. Most common type of ECD in Down's:
A. Type A B. Type B
C. Type C D. None

63. Highest risk of congenital malformation in baby with mother of:
A. Marfan's B. ASD
C. VSD D. TOF

64. Most common coronary anomaly in TGA:
A. Single left anterior descending
B. Single RCA
C. LCX from RCA

65. Inverted IVC seen in:
A. Asplenta
B. Polysplenia
C. Down's syndrome
D. All

66. True about by congenital absence of pericardium is all *except*:
A. Left side more common
B. Pericardiectomy TOC
C. LBBB seen

67. In HOCM, LV pressure volume shift:
A. Leftwards up
B. Rightwards up
C. Upwards left
D. Downward right

68. In situs solitus with dextroversion most common:
A. D-TGA **B.** C-TGA
C. TAPVC **D.** TOF

69. Increase pulmonary blood flow in all *except*:
A. Tr. atresia
B. HLHS
C. TGA
D. Device malformation

70. AF with highest risk of embolism with previous IE:
A. AF with previous history of previous embolism
B. AF with DVT 1 month
C. AF with prosthetic valve 1 month
D. AF recent onset

71. Class I indication for Holter monitoring (ambulatory):
A. Routine post MI
B. Silent ischemia
C. Malfunction pacemaker
D. Vasovagal syncope

72. True about angiosarcoma is all *except*:
A. Cardiotransplantation Rx of TOC
B. RA is most common site
C. Cardiac sarcoma in adults is most common primary tumor
D. Familial occurrence rare

73. POTS all true *except*:
A. NE > 300
B. SBP transiently decrease by 20
C. Tachycardia > 30 b/min
D. Severe orthostatic symp

74. HTN goal JNC - 7 in HTN + CRF:
A. 140 and 90 **B.** 130 and 80
C. 120 and 80 **D.** 130 and 85

75. Which not lead to RCMP?
A. Gaucher's
B. Fabry
C. Hemochromatosis disorder
D. Glycogen storage

76. Fabry's disease true all *except*:
A. Cerebroside accumulation
B. Minimal symptomatic
C. Normal epicardial coronaries
D. MI can occur

77. Indication of IABP all *except*:
A. AR
B. Cardiogenic shock
C. CABG
D. PCI

78. Coronary blood flow:
A. 8-10 ml/min **B.** 7-1 ml/min
C. 2-3 ml/min **D.** 5-6 ml/min

79. 2 months old with ESM with cyanosis with decrease pulmonary vascularity with LAD diagnosis is:
A. Ebstein **B.** Tricuspid atresia
C. TOF **D.** TGA

ANSWERS

1	C	2	A	3	B	4	C	5	A	6	A	7	C
8	A	9	B	10	B	11	A	12	B	13	A	14	A
15	C	16	A,B	17		18	B	19	A	20	A	21	B
22	B	23	C	24	D	25	A	26	A	27	C	28	B
29	C	30	C	31	B	32	D	33	C	34	A	35	D
36	B	37	A	38	A	39	D	40	B	41	B	42	D
43	B	44	C	45	B	46	A	47		48	A	49	A
50	C	51	A	52	C	53	D	54	A	55	D	56	A
57	A	58	A	59	B	60	A	61	C	62	A	63	A
64	C	65	B	66	C	67	A	68	B	69	A	70	A
71	C	72	A	73	A	74	B	75	A	76	A	77	A
78	A	79	B										

16

BHU 2009

1. **Lipoprotein H+ all *except*:**
   A. Halts the progress of atherosclerosis
   B. Step IAHA diet <30% of fat
   C. Preg → diet
   D. Post CABG dietary modification
2. **Clopidogrel resistance all *except*:**
   A. P_2 X $_{12}$ receptor
   B. Cy P_{3a} polymorphism
   C. Decrease ADP
   D. Alter platelet action
3. **Ramsay Hunt most characteristic:**
   A. Blister on pinna
   B. Infranuclear VII
   C. Lots of taste in ant 2/3 of tongue
   D. Bell's phenomena
4. **About atheroembolism all are true *except*:**
   A. Catheter
   B. Livido reticularis
   C. Retinal art → Chol. crystal
5. **Absolute contraindiction to exercise plan:**
   A. DM
   B. DCM
   C. IHD
   D. No pace advance AV block
6. **Asefun. hyper all *except*:**
   A. Infant < 6 m
   B. PS
   C. ΛWMI
   D. Hyperthyroidism
7. **Obesity all *except*:**
   A. Decrease CO
   B. Eccentric hypertrophy
8. **DM with increase TGC treatment goal is:**
   A. 100 B. 150
   C. 200 D. 125
9. **Thalium sensitivity and specificity for CAD:**
   A. 90-90 B. 95-95
   C. 90-70 D. 80-50
10. **Fondaparinaux – all *except*:**
    A. Decrease platelet function
    B. Pentasaccharide
    C. Through anti-thrombin Xa
11. **Atrial infarction all *except*:**
    A. More in RA
    B. < 20%
    C. Atrial arrhyth uncommon
    D. Atrial rupture can occur
12. **Prinzmetal angina all *except*:**
    A. 2/3 associated with stenosis
    B. RCA → normal coronary angio
    C. Ach → sensitive sp in inducing spasm
    D. ST increase in TMT
13. **Most common cause of pulmonary oedema after IWMI:**
    A. Papillary muscle dys
    B. IVS rupture
14. **Myocardial contractility best by:**
    A. LV end syst. pulm. volume in Dp/df
    B. Circumferential myocardial shortening
15. **Reperfusion all *except*:**
    A. AIVR
    B. Normal BP
    C. Decrease chest pain
16. **Reperfusion injury all *except*:**
    A. Accelerated necrosis
    B. Hemorrhage
    C. No reflow phenomena
    D. Carcinoma increase
17. **Cardiogenic shock true all *except*:**
    A. SBP <90
    B. PCWP <18

C. Cardiac index 2.2
D. Hypoperfusion

18. **Cardiac tamponade all *except*:**
A. Occur intrapericardial and RV diastole pr. equal
B. Severe tamponade → bradycardia
C. Initial increase stroke volume due to equal diastolic
D. Hypovol → difficult to diagnose

19. **All increase murmur in HCM *except*:**
A. Standing
B. Amyl nitrate

20. **CHF JV valsalva:**
A. 1 and 4 blunt
B. 2 and 4
C. 1 and 9

21. **AVR in AS:**
A. Mean >50
B. Peak to peak >50
C. Comp. sport peak to peak – 30-50
D. Area – 0.7-0.9 m/BSA

22. **Prosth valve. surgery its indication:**
A. Fungal
B. HF
C. Veg
D. Echo
E. Conduction block

23. **Oral cyanosis + asymptomatic with SaO_2 – 100%:**
A. Alveolar decrease affinity Hb %
B. Alveolar ventilation ventil decrease
C. Decrease diffusion

24. **Combined perip + central cyanosis without dyspnoea:**
A. Methen
B. Cyanide
C. CO

25. **Cardiac dyspnoea all *except*:**
A. Decrease FRC
B. Decrease VC
C. Decrease diff. capacity
D. Decrease compliance

26. **Isovolumic phase all *except*:**
A. Vmax
B. Vpm
C. Max Dp/D_t
D. Mean Vcf

27. **CHF:**
A. α 2 receptor normal α 1 increase
B. α 2 decrease α1 decrease
C. G protein α 1 decrease α 2 decrease

28. **Increase pulmonary blood flow + cyanosis:**
A. Ebstein
B. TAPVC
C. TA

29. **All tolerated in pregnancy – *except*:**
A. Marfan
B. ASD
C. USD
D. CoA

30. **TOF all *except*:**
A. VSD distal to RVOT obs in some
B. 4 criteria
C. Pseudo trembles TOF

31. **Most common coronary art anomaly:**
A. AV fistu
B. ALCAPA
C. LCX from RCA
D. LCA from right sinus

32. **Myxoma all *except*:**
A. 50% of cardiac tumor
B. Recurrence 20%
C. Right → malignancy

33. **Eisenmenger all *except*:**
A. Familial disposition → small stent
B. Worse prog with cong than PPH
C. All may not have cyanosis at rest

34. **Stridor + Dyspnoea:**
A. Doub arch
B. Left aortic arch + aberrant right subclavian
C. Right aortic arch + aberrant left subclavian
D. Right aortic arch with mirror image

35. **VDD all *except*:**
A. AV syndrome
B. Atrial pacing at slow rate
C. Both chamber sensed

36. **Class I indi for PPM – all *except*:**
A. Mobitz I
B. Neurocardio + Bradycardia with HUTT

37. **Antiarrhythmia all *except*:**
A. IA decrease Vmax increase APD
B. IB increase Vmax increase APD
C. IC decrease Vmax increase APD
D. III increase repolarisation

38. **WPW all *except*:**
A. PP
B. 120 ms
C. Delta + wide QRS

39. **True:**
A. Atropine + CSM → decrease both
B. Atropine increase + CSM decrease

40. **Max cond. velocity:**
A. SAN
B. AVN
C. Purkin
D. Ventricle

41. **Pseudoseizure vs seizure:**
A. Increase prolactin
B. Increase lactate
C. Decrease glucose
D. Increase IGF

42. **Mosan Likar modification:**
A. LAD
B. Q in aVL
C. Q in inf. lead
D. Decrease in inf. lead

43. **Purkinje fibre – True:**
A. Less resistant to ischemia
B. Inner 2/3 of endocardium
C. More in papillary muscle tip
D. More rapid repolarisation time

44. **CREST:**
A. PSS
B. PAN
C. SLE

45. **AF with renal failure safe the DOC is:**
A. Defetilide
B. Sotalol
C. Flaccaine
D. Propafenon

46. **EAD:**
A. Increase by CCB
B. Decrease by catecholamine
C. Increase by long cycle

47. **Chronic anaemia all *except*:**
A. O_2 diss. curve to left
B. Decrease after load

48. **Pain in interscapular + coldness right hand:**
A. Type I A diss.
B. Type 2
C. Takayasu

49. **Met. synd all *except*:**
A. Increase HDL
B. LDL
C. TG

50. **Familial increase TG all *except*:**
A. AD
B. Acute pancreatitis
C. Increase by alcohol
D. Increase atherosclerosis

51. **Syndrome X all *except*:**
A. Good prognosis
B. With LBBB worse prog.
C. 20% TMT +ve
D. Generally typical angina

52. **Pulmonary AV fistula associated with:**
A. Osler - Weber redu. syndrome

53. **Radiation induced cardiac all *except*:**
A. Valvular stenosis
B. CAD
C. Pericarditis

54. **Non-cardiac surgery in >40-year-old male increase risk *except*:**
A. Class II CSA
B. S_3
C. AMI < 3 m
D. VPC > 5/min in preop ECG

55. **Type II hyperlipidemia all *except*:**
A. Tendon xenthoma
B. Corneal arcus
C. Increase atherosclerosis
D. Pancreatitis

56. **Warfarin increase:**
A. Phenobarb
B. Allopurinol
C. Rifampicin
D. Sucralfate

57. **Use of IABP:**
A. Stabilization of cardiac shock patient during angioplasty
B. AR and aortic disease
C. Refractory HTN

58. **BCR - ABL gene is seen in:**
A. CML
B. ALL
C. AML
D. Follicular lymphoma

59. **Significant hematuria (single HPF):**
A. 3 – 100
B. 5 – 50
C. 10 – 100
D. 20 – 100

60. **Antibiotic:**
A. Anthrux
B. Botulism
C. Echo

61. **Pulmonary oedema all *except*:**
A. Increase PAP
B. Increase oncotic pressure
C. Pulmonary venous pressure increase

62. **Decrease complement level seen in all *except*:**
A. Acute PSGN
B. Anti GBM disease
C. Mesangioproliferative type II
D. Lupus nephritis

63. **Lung rarely involved in:**
A. PAN
B. PSS
C. SLE

64. **Cyt P_{450} inhibitory effect on:**
A. Pento prazole
B. Esomeprazole
C. Omeprazole
D. Rabiprazole

65. **P_{53} true:**
A. Decrease apoptosis
B. Prevents entering cells in S phase
C. 1st event is inactivation in colonic carcinoma

66. **SIRS all *except*:**
A. Polytrauma
B. Sepsis
C. Immune mediated origin
D. Cytokine infusion

67. **Anti-retroviral – nephrocalcinosis is seen in:**
A. Indinavir
B. Saquinavir
C. Retonavir
D. Tenofovir

68. **IE most common renal manifestation is:**
A. Interstitial B. Crescentric
C. Membranous D. FSGS

69. **TNF-α true:**
A. Cachexia
B. Weight gain

70. **Human genome no. of genes are:**
A. 30-4000 B. 10-20,000
C. 20-3000 D. 50-60

71. **High anion gap all *except*:**
A. Diarrhoea B. Renal failure
C. Ethylene D. Methanol

72. **I_{131} antidote:**
A. KOH B. K1
C. Ca DTPA D. Zn DTPA

73. **Desquamative interpruritis all *except*:**
A. Common in 2nd decade
B. Exclusive in smoker
C. Haziness in chest X-ray and CT
D. Increase macrophage in alveolar space

74. **APC:**
A. Dendritic cell B. Monocyte

75. **Laptin true:**
A. Hypothalium
B. Increase appetite
C. Decrease appetite
D. Decrease in obese

76. **Lacrimation + miosis + blurring of vision:**
A. Nerve gas
B. Phosgene
C. N. mustan

77. **Parvovirus B_{19}:**
A. Erythema infarction
B. Persistent anaemia

78. **Hepatitis C:**
A. 90% in hemophilia
B. DNA virus
C. Rare chronic liver disease

17

CMC VELLORE 2008

1. **Down's syndrome not seen:**
   A. TOF
   B. TGA
   C. High risk hematological malignancy
   D. Hypotension risk

2. **Rubella not seen:**
   A. VSD B. PDA
   C. TOF D. PAS

3. **CHD most common in male all *except*:**
   A. ASD
   B. TGA

4. **CHD common in females all *except*:**
   A. Truncus arteriosus
   B. ASD
   C. PDA
   D. Eisenmenger

5. **Eisenmenger not true is:**
   A. Cyanosis
   B. Pulmonary hypotension is not reversible
   C. Pregnancy mortality > 50%

6. **DORV with subaortic VSD all *except*:**
   A. Mitral aortic discontinuity
   B. Aortic override > 50%
   C. Aortic pulmonary value at same level

7. **X-ray left heart border formed by:**
   A. Pulmonary art — aorta — LA — LV
   B. Pulmonary art — aorta — LA app — LV
   C. Aorta — PA — LA app— LV
   D. Aorta — PA — LA — LV

8. **Straight left heart border:**
   A. MS B. LBBB
   C. RA dilatation D. Ebstein

9. **Surgery in ASD to avoid late onset AF:**
   A. < 5 years B. < 25 years
   C. 40 years D. < 50 years

10. **Const. pericardiotomy (CCP) true is:**
    A. Surgical pericardiotomy is universally/commonly curative
    B. Cardiomegaly is seen
    C. AF is common
    D. Peripheral edema is more than ascites and hepatomegaly

11. **Acute pulmonary edema all *except*:**
    A. Cyanosis
    B. RH failure absent
    C. Morphine is given
    D. Diuretics beneficial

12. **Kussmaul is not seen:**
    A. CCP
    B. Cardiac tamponade
    C. RVMI

13. **Cardiac tamponade all *except*:**
    A. Bradycardia B. Hypotension
    C. JVP D. Kussmaul

14. **True is:**
    A. Pulsus alternans is not seen in HF
    B. Pulsus alternans is due to calcium
    C. Pulsus parvus et tardus seen in 4R

15. **Murmur pitch true is:**
    A. Early systolic is heard with diaphragm
    B. Mid diastolic is heard with : Bell
    C. Opening snap is best heard diaphragm
    D. S_3 and S_4 is high rich pitched sound

16. **NTG true is:**
    A. ↓ses both preload and afterload
    B. ↓ses pulmonary congestion in HF

17. **Drugs acting on 4V node all *except*:**
    A. Adenosine
    B. β-blocker
    C. Diltiazem
    D. Lidocaine

18. **Valsalva:**
 A. N. pattern of valsalva is sinusoidal
 B. IVth phase overshoot is common in HF
 C. IInd phase-inc. HR

19. **Paradoxical S_2 split:**
 A. Pacemaker
 B. RBBB
 C. HOCM
 D. Mild AS

20. **S_1 LOUD seen in all *except*:**
 A. MS
 B. LBBB
 C. LA myxoma

21. **Tall R in V1:**
 A. Normal variant
 B. WPW-B
 C. Post-wall MI

22. **True in Brugada:**
 A. RBBB with ST ↑
 B. QT prolongation
 C. Induced by transvenous pacing
 D. Structural abnormal heart

23. **Acute pancreatitis all *except*:**
 A. Transient myocarditis leads to ↑ set card. enz
 B. Friction rub is seen
 C. Pain in chest on deep breath
 D. Global ST ↑ in all 12 leads

24. **TMT high risk all *except*:**
 A. ST dec > 2 mm in > 5 lead ≤ 5 min
 B. Abnormally high BP
 C. Angina at any stage
 D. Arrhythmias present

25. **TMT high risk:**
 A. ST 4 > 2 mn in > 5 lead
 B. Angina at any stage

26. **MET:**
 A. 3.5 **B.** 2.5
 C. 2.0 **D.** 1.5

27. **AVNRT true all *except*:**
 A. Ablation is success in most cases
 B. Associated with structurally abnormal heart
 C. Involves AV node and right atrium for reentry

28. **True/False:**
 A. Lead I → R arm negative – L arm +
 B. Lead I → R arm + , L arm –
 C. aVl → L arm +, sum of all 3 leads –

29. **True/False:**
 A. Wilson terminal formed by sum of all 3 leads with 5000

30. **↓se mortality in HF true:**
 A. β-blocker (carvedilol)
 B. Spironolactone
 C. Diuretics
 D. Digoxin

31. **Contraindication in pregnancy:**
 A. Labetalol
 B. Aliskiren
 C. Hydralazine
 D. Clonidine
 E. Long acting nifedipine

32. **Cardiac arrest asystole all true *except*:**
 A. Atropine can be given
 B. Adrenaline is useful
 C. CPR to be done
 D. Defibrillation not required if monitor shows flat line

33. **MRI all true/*except*:**
 A. Contrast agent not required/used
 B. Valvular flow velocities can be calculated quantitatively
 C. Viability can be seen
 D. RV surface can be easily visualized
 E. Coronary artery can be visualised

34. **RAS can be predicted by (1,3) (2,4) (4) all:**
 A. Associated with multivessel coronary disease
 B. Associated with PAD
 C. Age of onset of hypotension 30 – 55 years
 D. Renal dysfunction

35. **BNP is raised:**
 A. ↑ in female
 B. NYH Δ st I
 C. HF/pulmonary edema < 1 hour

36. **Most common site of aneurysm:**
 A. Infrarenal aortic
 B. Ascending thoracicaorta
 C. Suprarenal abdominal aorta
 D. Descending thoracic aorta

37. **All true *except*:**
 A. PDA lies in Post/Inf. interventricular groove
 B. L dominance is more than R

38. **All true *except*:**
 A. ↓sed heart rate is due to ↓sed sympathetic
 B. β1 muscarinic receptors supply AV node

39. **JVP all true *except*:**
 A. Cath. tip is put in upper part of RA
 B. JVP raised or decreased can be assed by ext. jugular venous
 C. Level is assessed at MAC (mid axillary line)
 D. Louis Angle > 5 cm is ab. N

E. Jugular venous catheter measures 6 – 8 cm more than measured by JVP and Louis Angle

40. HUTT all *except*:
A. Head is tilted at neck in super position upto 70°
B. Profound bradycardia
C. Hypothermia

41. Transplanted heart all *except*:
A. Lymphoproliferative malignancy caused by Epstein-Barr virus is most common
B. Atherosclerosis is ↑sed
C. Opportunistic inf. more than nosocomial after initial hospitalization
D. Angina is uncommon

42. VT suggested by all *except*:
A. AV dissociation
B. Fusion beats / capture beats
C. Severe LAD
D. QRS 120–140 ms
E. R to Nadir of S > 60 ms

43. VT True/False:
A. Fusion beat-T
B. Associated with MI-T
C. Q to Nadir of S > 60 n

44. Drug causing acute pancreatitis:
A. Deflazacort
B. Methysergide
C. Emetine
D. Mycophenolate mofetil

45. Cyt P40 True/False:
A. Pravastatin B. Rosuvastatin
C. Simvastatin-T D. Atorvastatin-T

46. True treatment in USA 1329:
A. Abciximab used in conservative management
B. Clopidogrel
C. Aspirin
D. Enoxaparin
E. Tirofiban before PCI

47. Prehospital thrombolysis by IV bolus best:
A. Alteplase B. Reteplase
C. TNK D. STK

48. All false *except*:
A. 90 min patency is equal in all
B. STK has highest 90 min patency
C. TNK – tpA has highest 90 min patency

49. True:
A. Diabetic patients in India = 3.1 million
B. CVD patients in India by 2010 > 60% by whole world
C. Insulin resistance in Indians is more than western people
D. CVD mortality more in urban India
E. CVD mortality max in > 70 years in India

50. Eisenmenger:
A. Differential cyanosis in lower limbs if PDA present
B. VSD with AR does not cause Eisenmenger

51. VSD True/False:
A. Membranous and muscular VSD most common-T
B. Large VSD → ↑sed murmur
C. Perimembranous VSD associated with aortic regurgitation

52. ASD all true *except*:
A. Operate only if > 1.5 : 1
B. Female twice as common than male
C. Systolic murmur at pulmonary area
D. Diastolic murmur loudest at apex

53. Device closure done in all *except*:
A. 1° ASD
B. PDA
C. Coronary artery fistula
D. Membranous VSD

54. DCMP true:
A. Interstitial fibrosis seen
B. Thickening of walls +

55. Hollen Hurst plaques:
A. Thromboembolic plaque
B. High lipid plague

56. Stable plague:
A. SM cells
B. Calcification
C. Thick fibrous cap
D. High lipid content

57. I.E. True/False:
A. Blood sample for culture taken aseptically
B. From two different sites
C. Better when fever is present
D. Intra arterial line will yield better results

58. Long duration AF which improves on maneuvers and drugs:
A. Prolonged AF B. Lone AF
C. Persistent AF D. Paroxysmal AF

59. ↑HR ↑ses with contractility:
A. Bowditch
B. Anrep

60. Angiogenesis defined as:
A. Sprouting from collateral
B. Opening of pre existent vessels

61. Early systolic murmur in all *except*:
A. Acute MR
B. TR with ↑ PA press
C. Small VSD

62. **Patient with HR 175/min, visible P wave with QRs after each P wave:**
A. AVNRT B. AVRT
C. Sinus tachycardia D. Atrial tachycardia

63. **If PR interval is shorter than RP interval then answer is:**
A. AVNRT
B. AVRT
C. Sinus tachycardia
D. Atrial tachycardia
E. Atrial flutter

64. **What drug to be given all *except*, patient asymptomatic?**
A. Adenosine
B. DC shock
C. Beta-blocker
D. DC cardioversion

65. **Patient asymptomatic with tachycardia, carotid massage, fails, next to do:**
A. Adenosine
B. DC shock
C. β-blocker
D. Verapamil diltiazem

66. **Early mortality in PCI, true:**
A. Female
B. Renal dysfunction
C. DM
D. Lung diseases

67. **Aortic dissection true:**
A. Pain between shoulder blades
B. Asymmetrical pulses
C. Can lead to renal dysfunction
D. Can be associated with AR

68. **Free wall rupture false:**
A. After previous MI
B. Hypotension
C. Elderly
D. Female

69. **CAD right true all *except*:**
A. Generally describes as heaviness
B. May present as breathlessness
C. May occur on lying down
D. Relieved by mitral
E. Improves in 5 minutes

70. **MS false:**
A. Severe MS < 1.0 cm^2/m^2
B. AF can cause sudden pulmonary edema
C. PAH improves MS symptoms
D. Symptoms don't appear unless MVA > 2.0 cm

71. **Cyanotic spells all *except*:**
A. Does not occur in < 2 years of age
B. Occurs with crying/feeding
C. During spell murmur absent
D. Adrenergic stimulation causes obstruction

72. **RSOV all true *except*:**
A. Systolic is longer in high thorax and diastolic in low thorax
B. Diastolic murmur is longer than systolic murmur
C. Systolic murmur
D. Continuous murmur loudest near S_2
E. Murmur radiates throughout chest

ANSWERS

1	B	2	B	3	A	4	A	5	B	6		7	C
8	A	9	C	10	C	11	C	12	A,B	13	D	14	B
15	B,C	16		17	D	18	A,B,C	19	A,C	20	B	21	
22	A	23	D	24	B	25	A,B	26	A	27	B	28	
29		30	A,B	31		32	B	33	A	34	B,D	35	
36	A	37	B	38	A	39	C	40		41	C	42	D,E
43		44	B	45		46	B,C,D	47	B	48	C	49	A,B,C,D
50	A	51	A	52	D	53		54	A,B	55	A,B	56	A,C
57	A	58	C,D	59	A	60	A	61	B	62	B	63	D
64	C	65	A	66	A,B,C,D	67	A,B,C,D	68	A	69	C	70	D
71	A	72	A										

18

CMC VELLORE 2006

1. **In moderate HF, mortality is:**
   A. <5%
   B. 10%
   C. 20-30%
   D. 30-80%

2. **Post PTCA restenosis:**
   A. >70% luminal stenosis
   B. >40% diameter loss
   C. >0.72 mm diameter loss
   D. None of the above

3. **Primary prevention trial of statin**
   A. WOSCOPES B. 4S
   C. LIPID D. CARE

4. **WOSCOPE upon CHD mortality:**
   A. 31% B. 41%
   C. 25% D. 20%

5. **5-6 mm in ↓DBP results in ↓ in mortality:**
   A. U B. 25%
   C. 21% D. 35%

6. **In STEMI, true statement is:**
   A. Most cases occurred in prior occlusion <50%
   B. Most cases occurring with totally occluded coronary artery lead to transmural infarction
   C. High grade stenosis has high clearance of MI than low grade stenosis
   D. Infarct away from stenosis show dual occlusion simultaneously

7. **Arteriogenesis:**
   A. Opening of pre-formed vessels
   B. Formation of new vessels
   C. Maturation of preformed vessels

8. **Drug found to be useful in 2005 in STEMI:**
   A. Clopidogrel
   B. Valsartan
   C. Trimetazidine
   D. Aldosterone receptor blocker

9. **Drug used in severe AS:**
   A. Amlodipine B. Ramipril
   C. Digoxin D. Bisoprolol

10. **In IWMI with ↑JVP, Kussmaul sign+, PCWP 13 mm treatment:**
    A. IV frussemide
    B. Mod. Vol loading
    C. Rapid digitalization
    D. Dobutamine infusion

11. **Proximal RCA occlusion is least likely to be +ve with:**
    A. V3 V4 V5 showing q waves
    B. ST elevation more in lead III

12. **1 MET true is:**
    A. Resting oxygen consumption in 30 years old
    B. Resting oxygen consumption in 60 years old
    C. 3 to 5 mets show heavy labour
    D. O_2 consumption 3.5 ml/kg/min

13. **When should vasodilator be converted from iv to oral?**
    A. PCWP – 18-20 mmHg
    B. CI <1.5 ml/100 gm/min
    C. RAP 5-8 mmHg
    D. SVR 600-800 dyne

14. **PVR is:**
    A. 20-130 B. 100-300
    C. 120-160 D. 180-200

15. **PAEDP is:**
    A. 4-12 mmHg
    B. 20-25 mmHg

16. **RV enlargement is a feature of:**
    A. DORV
    B. TA
    C. PDA
    D. Pulmonary stenosis with intact IVS

17. Cardiomegaly without prominent aorta
A. PDA B. VSD
C. ASD D. AP window

18. Diastolic flow murmur in tricuspid area
A. TAPVC B. VSD
C. PDA D. AP window

19. ACE I related cough true is
A. Female 10% incidence
B. Male 20% incidence
C. Stops within 24 hours of stoppage
D. None

20. Wide split S2 in ASD is because of:
A. ↑ pulm flow than systemic flow
B. Markedly ↑ hang out
C. Due to reciprocal ↓ in systemic return from vein and ASD

21. In AF, true statement is:
A. Variable S1 heart sound
B. Pulse deficit
C. Variable height of a wave
D. S4 intermittent

22. Paradoxical split:
A. LBBB B. RBBB
C. LV paced beat D. RV paced beat

23. AF induced by:
A. Adenosine B. Amiodarone
C. Propafenone D. Quinidine

24. For Carvedilol, true statement is:
A. High dose block all three receptors
B. US carvedilol done in severe HF (NYHA IV)
C. ↑ survival 52%
D. All of the above

25. Class I indication of PPI:
A. Recurrent undiagnosed syncope with LBBB
B. RBBB with LAHB with ↑ PR asymptomatic
C. Asymptomatic cong CHB 18 years female resting HR 40/min QT 48 msec
D. IWMI with intermittent CHB
E. Old man with resting HR 56/min, TMT – 86/mt with poor exercise capacity

26. TMT C/I in all *except*:
A. Recent MI
B. USA with recent pain
C. Severe HOCM
D. Uncontrolled high BP
E. Severe AS

27. For TMT, true is:
A. Baseline used is PQ
B. J point depressed by >0.1 mV should be +ve
C. Relatively flat scope
D. ST↓ of 0.05 mV at 60-80 msec
E. Should be +ve in 3 consecutive leads

28. 58 years watching TV had syncope, gr 3/6 murmur in aortic area, radiating to carotid normal pulse, ECG, RBBB + LAHB, PR>.14 sec. diagnosis:
A. Vasovagal
B. AS
C. Mobitz type II
D. Post paralysis syncope

29. In HOCM pulse character is:
A. Pulsus alternans
B. Reverse pulsus paradoxus
C. Dicrotic
D. Bisferiens

30. Pulsus alternans:
A. Can be assessed only by BP instrument
B. Irregular
C. Occur after PVC
D. Shows mild CHF

31. Significant stenosis on angio:
A. >50% stenosis
B. >70% stenosis
C. >75% stenosis
D. >90% stenosis

32. MRI max range of normal pericardium:
A. 1 mm B. 2 mm
C. 3 mm D. 4 mm

33. ACE-I are must in MI in, all *except*:
A. Elderly
B. Reverted primary VT
C. AWMI
D. Global LV dysfunction

34. The infarcted area shows all except:
A. Dysynchrony B. Dyskinesis
C. Akinesis D. Hypokinesis
E. Hyperkinesis

35. Stroke volume is affected by all *except*:
A. HR B. Contractility
C. Preload D. Afterload

36. Least a agonist action:
A. Isoprenaline B. Adrenaline
C. Noradrenaline D. Dopamine

37. For dobutamine, all are true *except*:
A. +ve inotropic effect balanced by ↑ coronary flow
B. ↓ Peripheral vascular resistance
C. ↑ Survival in Cardiogenic shock
D. ↓ LVEDP
E. Less arrhythmia if titrtated with tachycardia

38. **For dopamine, all are true *except*:**
A. ↑ coronary blood flow
B. a action if dose >10mg/kg

39. **HOCM - drug of first choice:**
A. β blocker B. Digoxin
C. CCBs D. Diuretics

40. **True regarding valsalva maneuver strain phase are, all *except*:**
A. ↑ murmur of HOCM
B. ↓ murmur of AS
C. ↑ Duration of MVP
D. ↑ cervical venous hum

41. **Chronic subdural hematoma:**
A. ACA
B. MCA
C. PCA
D. Circle of Willis
E. Meningeal artery

42. **Lung volumes true all *except*:**
A. TLC = VC+RV
B. TLC = IRC+ERV+RV
C. VC=IRV+RV

43. **36 weeks pregnant female in labour pain on warfarin, treatment of choice is:**
A. Cesarean section
B. Cut-short of the second stage of labour
C. Normal vaginal delivery
D. Blood transfusion

44. **AR severity indicated by all *except*:**
A. PHT >500 msec
B. Mid systolic closure of MV
C. Late diastolic MR
D. Reversal in distal aorta

45. **For partial AV canal defect, all are true *except*:**
A. Cleft MV
B. Down's syndrome
C. Primum ASD
D. RAD

46. **All patients with acute STEMI to be given immediately:**
A. Aspirin
B. Thrombolytic
C. Heparin
D. β blocker
E. Thrombolytic+ heparin

47. **Aspirin true is all *except*:**
A. t ½ 15-20 min
B. Dose 30 mg leads to steady state in 3 weeks
C. Inhibits thromboxane A2
D. Blocks for 5 days
E. Mortality benefit equivalent to thrombolytics

48. **For Kussmaul sign true, statement is:**
A. Inspiratory ↓ in CVP
B. Pericarditis
C. Most often in RV failure

49. **Tamponade on ECHO true:**
A. RVOT <7 mm
B. Late diastolic RV collapse
C. Early diastolic RA collapse
D. All

50. **Carney complex diagnosis:**
A. One major + two minor
B. Two major
C. One clinical + 1 genetic
D. 8 criteria

ANSWERS

1	C	2		3	C	4	A	5		6	A	7	C
8	A	9	C	10	B	11	A	12	D	13	C	14	A
15	A	16	D	17	C	18	A	19	A	20	B	21	A,B
22	A,D	23	A	24	A	25	B	26	A	27	A	28	C
29	B	30		31	A	32	D	33	B	34	E	35	A
36	A	37	A	38	A	39	A	40	D	41	E	42	A
43	A	44	B	45	D	46	A	47	A,B	48	C	49	D
50	C												

19

GB PANT 2011

MEDICINE

1. **Hunt Hess Scale used for:**
   A. SAH
   B. CAD
   C. Dementia
   D. Psychological disorder

2. **SLE Activity Index, included all *except*:**
   A. Pyuria B. Seizure
   C. Myocarditis D. Fever

3. **Inherently resistant to colistin:**
   A. Pseudomonas B. E. coli
   C. Proteus D. Klebsiella

4. **Rapid sallow breathing index:**
   A. RR × Tidal Volume
   B. RR / Tidal Volume
   C. RR + Tidal Volume
   D. None

5. **CVP should be measured:**
   A. End expiration B. End inspiratory
   C. Mid expiratory D. Mid inspiratory

6. **Osmolality of enteral feed, not contributed by:**
   A. Mineral B. Carbohydrate
   C. Protein D. Fat

7. **Sulfur mustard toxicity all *except*:**
   A. Conjunctivitis
   B. Corneal damage
   C. Erythematous bullae
   D. Bradycardia

8. **Young male, microcytic hypochromic anemia, no iron deficiency, Hbs – 62%, HbA – 25%, HbA_{2-4}, HbF 8%:**
   A. Sickle cell disease
   B. Sickle cell trait
   C. Sickle βo that
   D. Sickle β plus thalassemia

9. **On PAC; prolonged APTT, corrected with 1:1 Plasma, past–history of surgery uneventful. Diagnosis is:**
   A. Vitamin K deficiency
   B. Factor VIII deficiency
   C. Factor XIII deficiency
   D. Factor XII deficiency

10. **Prenatal diagnosis of hemophilia A:**
    A. Point mutation of factor VIII gene
    B. Required fetal blood analysis through umbilical cord
    C. Not required in male fetus
    D. Family linkage analysis

11. **Poor prognostic factors for multiple myeloma:**
    A. Anemia
    B. ↑ creatinine
    C. Diffuse bone disease
    D. 139–

12. **Anemia of chronic disease:**
    A. ↓ Fe / ↓ TIBC / ↓ hepcidin
    B. ↑ Fe / ↑ TIBC / ↓ hepcidin
    C. ↑ Fe / ↑ TIBC / ↑ ferritin
    D. ↓ Fe / N TIBC / ↑ hepcidin

13. **↓ ed O_2 affinity:**
    A. ↓ pH / ↓ 2,3 DPG / ↑ temp
    B. ↑ pH / ↑ 23 DPG / ↑ temp
    C. ↓ pH / ↑ 23 DPG / ↑ temp

14. **According to ACR 2010 recommendation not a diagnostic criteria for RA:**
    A. Duration of joint pain
    B. Duration of morning stiffness
    C. No. of joints involved
    D. Increase ESR / (CRP)

15. **In OP poisoning, seen due to nicotinic cholinergic manifestation:**
    A. Lacrimation B. Sweating
    C. Salivation D. Bronchospasm

16. Type alfa error:
A. Null hypothesis true, rejected
B. Null hypothesis false, accepted

17. Drugs contraindicated in pregnancy for PEP for HIV:
A. Lamivudine **B.** Efavirenz
C. Zidovudine **D.** Nelfinavir

18. Dexamethasone in acute bacterial meningitis all *except*:
A. Used 20 min before first dose of antibiotics
B. Most effective in pneumococcal meningitis
C. After induced TNF, not effective
D. Does not ↑ penetration of vancomycin in CSF

19. ADPD all *except*:
A. USG— 100% sensitive after 3 hours
B. Type 2 early and poor prognosis
C. UTI and Pyelonephritis–Incidence ↑es
D. Screening for intracerebral aneurysm, its family history ICH is positive

20. Brugada syndrome — True:
A. β blocker DOC
B. ST ↑ in V_{4-6}
C. Quinolone—C/I
D. Fever induces ST changes

21. Not true:
A. Concentric constriction of visual field in long – standing papilledema
B. Tunnel vision—Always organic
C. Cortical blindness— Pupillary reflex normal
D. Visual acuity— Macular function

22. Vasopressors in sepsis all *except*:
A. NA and Dopamine— Initial vasopressor of choice
B. Low dose dopamine—Renal protection
C. MAP > 65
D. Arterial catheterization—as soon as possible

23. Pulse oximetry true:
A. Assesses O_2 content of blood
B. Does not—affected by nitroprusside
C. CO poisoning – useful
D. Emits two wavelength of monochromatic light

24. Not true of hypothyroidism:
A. CVT gain due to subcutaneous fat
B. CPS—common
C. ↑ PRL (Modest)
D. Skin thickness —↑ ed glycosaminoglycans

25. H. pylori all *except*:
A. Urea breath test not useful for early follow up
B. Bismuth triple therapy
C. Malt one
D. Always associated with chronic active gastritis

26. EMG finding in MND:
A. Normal NCV
B. Sensory studies normal
C. ↑ fasciculation

27. Short chain fatty acid, No. of C—atoms:
A. < 4 **B.** < 6
C. < 8 **D.** < 12

28. Positive AMPC test indicates:
A. Sensitive to both (penicillin + ceftriaxone)
B. Resistant to both
C. Sensitive to all antibiotics
D. Sensitive to penicillin, resistant to ceftriaxone

29. Leptospirosis all *except*:
A. Anicteric, more common in milder disease
B. Hemorrhagic pneumonia — Weil's disease (common)
C. Ceftriaxone does not cause herzeheimer reaction
D. Doxycycline—for prophylaxis

30. TB peritonitis true:
A. SAAG
B. Ascitic fluid ADA
C. SAFA
D. Ascitic fluid PCR for TB

31. Apnea duration in adult:
A. 10 sec **B.** 5 sec
C. 15 sec **D.** 20 sec

32. No. of criteria in CPIS:
A. 4 **B.** 5
C. 6 **D.** 7

33. CD < 100, on ATT, HAART to be started:
A. Immediately
B. After 2 weeks
C. After 2 months
D. Completion of ATT

34. Renin secretion ↑ed by:
A. ↑ NaCl in Asc. limb of LH
B. ↑ stretch afferent arteriole
C. Beta one receptor blocker
D. None

35. Influenza recommendation (2011) — True:
A. Given annually > 6 months with medical indication
B. Annually in > 6 months
C. Annually in > 65 years

36. P-Spikes used for:
A. Stem cell transplantation
B. Gene therapy
C. BM cell transplantation
D. None

37. True:
A. Cox 2 inhibitors—some antiplatelet activity
B. Aspirin loses analgesic effect, if given in enteric form
C. Diclofenac BM suppression
D. PCM equal analgesic effect than aspirin

38. Hepatitis B carries state (inactive)—all *except*:
A. Anti HBe Ag –ve
B. HBe Ag –ve
C. < 105 DNA (HBV)
D. Neuroinflammatory score < 4

39. End stage renal disease – Hb level to be kept at:
A. 10 – 11 B. 11 – 12
C. 12 – 13 D. 13 – 14

40. Framingham Heart Study, not a major criteria:
A. Hepatojugular reflux
B. CXR cardiomegaly and pulmonary edema
C. S_3
D. DOE

41. Turner's syndrome all *except*:
A. 45 XO
B. External genitalia (female) normal
C. Short stature
D. ↓ FSH

42. Anemia with Absent–Secondary renal character:
A. Kallmann syndrome
B. LH syndrome
C. Laurence-Moon Biedl syndrome
D. Klinefelter syndrome

43. Urine osmolality < 100, all *except*:
A. SIADH
B. Psychogenic polydipsia
C. Reset osmostat
D. Water intoxication

44. After 2–3 months of solid organ transplantation, most common cause of infection:
A. EBV B. Listeria
C. Toxoplasmosis D. MTB

45. Anorexia nervosa:
A. Depressive B. Bordering
C. Perfectionist D. Impulsive

46. Prasugrel is:
A. TXA_2 inhibitor
B. GP II b–III a inhibitor
C. PAR–1 antagonist
D. P_2Y_{12} inhibitor

47. Papilledema, caused due to toxicity of:
A. Vitamin A B. Vitamin D
C. Vitamin E D. Vitamin B_{12}

48. Acute arsenic poisoning causes:
A. Normal anemia
B. Neutropenia
C. Microcytic anemia
D. QT prolongation

49. Not involved in leprosy:
A. Pancreas
B. Testes
C. Eye
D. Larynx and pharynx

50. Nuclear radiation true—all *except*:
A. BM more sensitive than G1 mucosa
B. Marrow involvement—always required BMT
C. Cytopenia even on mild exposure
D. >100 Gy.—death within 48 hours

51. Radioactive iodine used in all *except*:
A. Follicular Ca B. Papillary Ca
C. Graves' disease D. Lymphoma

52. Mutations in deviation of diencephalon causes inferiors with which hormone?
A. ACTH B. PRL
C. Epinephrine D. Oxytocin

53. Idio crescentic GN type IV – True:
A. Granular deposits of Ig
B. No. of gene deposits with +ve ANCA
C. No. of gene deposits with –ve ANCA
D. Linear deposits of Ig with +ve ANCA

54. Daily recommended dose of Vitamin D in 75 years old:
A. 200 B. 400
C. 600 D. 800

55. Sympathetic NS stimulation causes all *except*:
A. Erection
B. Ejaculation
C. Increased red bladder tone
D. ↑ Gastric motility

56. Large duct pancreatitis – True all *except*:
A. Pain poorly responsive to pancreatic enzyme
B. ERCP – Markedly abnormal
C. Secretin test – Abnormal
D. Elastase level abnormal

57. Incidence of MS if sponge has MS:
A. 1 in 1000 B. 1 in 10000
C. None D. 1 in 50000

58. Major depression – duration:
A. 2 months B. 9 months
C. 6 months D. None

59. Essential tremor – True:
A. Improved by alcohol
B. Most prominent at rest

C. Head never involved
D. Non-progressive

60. **Heavy alcohol intake all *except*:**
A. ↑ GGT
B. ↑ CDT
C. ↑ Hyperurecemia
D. ↓ Thiamine

61. **Chronic daily headache, all *except*:**
A. Always > 9 hours daily
B. > 15 days/month
C. Chronic paroxysmal hemicrania can cause
D. Can be primary and secondary

62. **Ventricle pressure volume curve shifted to left by:**
A. AS B. MS
C. MR D. AR

63. **Poor prognostic factor in pulmonary hypertension:**
A. BNP < 100
B. 6 min walk test < 300 meter
C. Minimal right ventricular dysfunction
D. RAP < 6 mmHg

64. **Earliest change after R_x of Graves' disease:**
A. Normalisation of TSH
B. FT_3 / FT_4 ↓
C. Thyroid stimulating Ab. ↓
D. Peroxidase activity normal

65. **3rd generation TSH estimation—minimal level:**
A. 0.1 U/ml B. 0.01 U/ml
C. 0.001U/ml D. None

66. **Snake bite all *except*:**
A. Immobilisation better than tourniquet
B. Skin sensitivity omitted
C. Anticholinesterase inhibitor in neurotoxicity
D. ASVS given after signs of envenomation

67. **Fabry's disease:**
A. α galactosidase
B. Angiokeratoma and acroparesthesia from childhood
C. Early enzyme therapy—can prevent complication
D. All

68. **Familial HOCM gene:**
A. α myosin heavy chain
B. β myosin heavy chain
C. Myosin light chain
D. Myosin binding protein C

69. **G–6 PD all *except*:**
A. X linked
B. Diagnosed by peri. blood smear
C. Enzyme activity can be measured between episodes at hemolysis
D. Self-limiting even on continuation at offending drug

70. **Hyperparathyroidism — True:**
A. More common in female
B. Due to hyperplasia of 2 to 4 gland
C. May be associated with hypotension
D. Hypercalcemia/hypercalciuria — not always associated

71. **Coronary risk equivalent — all *except*:**
A. Documented aortic aneurysm
B. Renovascular hypertension
C. PAD
D. Carotid atherosclerosis

72. **C/I of continuous subcutaneous insulin infusion:**
A. Pregnancy
B. Painful neuropathy
C. Chronic infection
D. Progressive ischemia or proliferative retinopathy

73. **Not surrogate market of β cell function:**
A. Insulin
B. Proinsulin / Insulin ratio
C. HOMA—Beta
D. None

74. **Smoking all *except*:**
A. Passive smoking have effect on coronary atherosis
B. No effect on pregnancy
C. Causes breast cancer leukemia
D. Smoking cessation ↓ coronary risk

75. **Most common carcinoma in non-smoker:**
A. SECL
B. NSCLL
C. Adeno carcinoma

76. **Small fibre neuropathy:**
A. Proprioception
B. Temperature normal
C. Pain normal
D. DTR ↓ed

77. **Specificity true:**
A. True negative

78. **16 years female, headache, lethargy, short for age, bilateral temporal field visual defect, GH, ACTH, TSH (Low), PRL ↑ed, on radiography, retarded bone age, diagnosis:**
A. Optic chiasma glioma
B. Parasagittal meningioma
C. NPH
D. Craniopharyngioma

79. **True all *except*, TBM:**
   A. ATT for more than 9 months
   B. Ethambutol replaced by SM
   C. Corticosteroids should be given
   D. Continuation phase—H and R given

CARDIOLOGY

1. **True about valsalva maneuver audibility of heart sounds:**
   A. Heart sounds heard through 1 to 4
   B. 1 and 3
   C. 2 and 4
   D. 2 and 3

2. **RBBB camouflaged with LAHB is identified by:**
   A. Decreased duration of QRS

3. **Small fat r in V_1 significance:**
   A. DD of WQT
   B. Septal accessory pathway
   C. Complete LBBB

4. **Dronedarone true is:**
   A. Better than aminodine
   B. C/I in class I and II HF
   C. Given with meals
   D. Generally used in VTS

5. **Ebstein's anomaly cyanosis ↑ed by:**
   A. Sitting
   B. Prolonged standing
   C. Lying down
   D. None

6. **Pericardial rub:**
   A. Usually has an atrial component
   B. Dynamic
   C. Best heard in lower sternal border

7. **40 years treated for mediastinal tumor presented with SOB and ↑ JVP. Likely diagnosis:**
   A. Pulsus paradoxus

8. **Dicrotic notch coincides with which phrase of ECG:**
   A. Onset of T
   B. End of T
   C. P–Wave

9. **M_1:**
   A. S2 along with echo chase of MV
   B. Crossover of LV and RA pressure
   C. Occurs before actual closure of MV
   D. After closer of MV

10. **Young male with AR effect 65% equivocal symptoms, next step:**
   A. Stress test
   B. Follow up every 6 months
   C. AVR

11. **AS with MVR ideal R_x:**
   A. AVR with MVR
   B. AVR with MV valvulopathies
   C. AVR, mitral leak ↓es spontaneously
   D. MVR, follow AS for progress

12. **DCMP with Grade III MR with TR, on optimetal R_X but still on class–II CHF next few years progress:**
   A. MR_α ↓ on R_X
   B. Repair both MV and TV
   C. Mitral valve repair

13. **MVO_2 70%, AORTA 94%, PA 80%, QP/QS**
   A. 0.5 : 1
   B. 1 : 1
   C. 2 : 1
   D. 4 : 1

14. **Adenosine:**
   A. A_3 causes coronary vasodilation
   B. Usually diff. various types of SVT
   C. A_1, acts on sinus
   D. Aminophylline inhibits A_1 A_2 action

15. **Ranolazine:**
   A. Acts on atrial Na+ channel
   B. Metabolic agent used in chronic angina

16. **Eplerenone:**
   A. Incorrect match
   B. Liddle syndrome – amiloride
   C. Liddle syndrome – triamterene
   D. Gordon syndrome – thiazide
   E. Gordon syndrome – spironolactone

17. **Diastolic murmur starts after a gap from P_2. What is likely?**
   A. Eisenmenger still requires surgery
   B. PDA with PS
   C. PAH

18. **Ejection click (Aortic) does not signify as significant stenosis when:**
   A. Elderly
   B. Louder than S_1
   C. Soft A_2

19. **A patient on ACE–inhibitors develop dry cough not responding to anti-histaminics. Next step:**
   A. Change to Losartan

20. **HF on triple therapy metoprolol 60 mg BD, Remipril 5 mg/BD, lasix 40 mg, EF 40%:**
   A. Still have class 2 dyspnea and effort intolerance
   B. ↓ β–blocker
   C. Add. aldosterone antagonist
   D. ↑ diuretics

21. **A patient with TG = 250, HDL = 38, LDL 105, preferred food:**
   A. ↓ fatty fish consumption
   B. ↑ fruits

C. ↑ vegetables
D. ↑ refined grams

22. **Resistant HTN deposits:**
A. 3 drugs including a diuretic

23. **Resistant HTN is addressed in:**
A. Simplicity-2

24. **Coronary risk equivalents all *except*:**
A. Renovascular hypertension
B. Aortic aneurysm
C. DM
D. Carotid atherosclerosis

25. **A medical student undergone CXR normal examination CXR shows abnormal convexity in left upper border. ECG shows q in V_1 to V_2. What is expected in future?**
A. MR
B. Conduction disease
C. RCMP

26. **Female presents with acute SOB and signs of a acute LVF. BNP ↑, ECHO EF 50%:**
A. E^1/A^1
B. TDI
C. PFT

27. **Stage with HF. What according to 2 ACC/AHA is addressed:**
A. Taking weight and volume in every follow-up
B. Advice for device therapy
C. Renal BNP
D. Six-minute corridor walking

28. **A father brought ECG of a 10 years old boy who had history of easy fatigability, no record available:**
A. ECG shows V_1 to V_4 R, V_5 → R/S diagnosis
B. Severe PS
C. Undiagnosed TOF
D. Cannot be TOF
E. Closed VSD

29. **Patient presented with STEMI 30 minutes back. PCI center is 3 hours away, what will you do?**
A. Give TNK and send to PCI
B. Referred to PCI immediately
C. Air transfer to PCI
D. TNK and wait for 90 min

30. **IWMI RCA complete occlusion with thrombosis with ostial LAD 90%, 2d Echo–RWMA in inferior wall:**
A. RCA stent with or with out thrombectemy
B. Stenting in both RCA and LAD

31. **A patient with STEMI at 4 A.M. given 300 mg way of clopivas 350 mg, Aspirin and 0.6 ml of Enoxaprin PCI due at 10 A.M. Best adjunctive therapy:**
A. 0.3 ml of enoxaparin with GP IIb IIIa
B. 0.6 ml enoxa
C. Bivalirudin
D. UFH with GP IIb/IIIa

32. **2 years TOF given BT, had seizure at the end of transfusion peripheral pulses N, saturation 84% cause:**
A. Hypocalcemia B. Cyanotic spell

33. **Patient with long haul travel and headache, multiple peripheral pulmonary embolism with N hemodynamics. Best R_X:**
A. UFH B. Thrombolysis
C. PFO closing D. IVC filter

34. **Carotid sinus hyposensitivity is diagnosed by:**
A. > 3 sec. pass / > 50 mm BP fail
B. > 3 sec. / > 30 min BP
C. > 5 sec. / < 50 min BP
D. > 5 sec. / < 30

35. **LVH in LBBB is D_X by:**
A. QRS > 0.16 sec
B. $SV_2 + RV_6 > 45$ min
C. Left atrial enlargement
D. All of the above

36. **Hypertension in middle age obesity findings are:**
A. Isolated diastolic HTN
B. Mild systolic + Diastolic
C. Essential HTN

37. **Old age changes:**
A. ↓ in caliber of large arteries
B. ↑ HR
C. ↑ LV thickness
D. ↓ Myocyte size

38. **Pericarditis:**
A. Troponin normal without + CKMB
B. Inc. Trop I and CKMB
C. Normal enzymes
D. All

39. **Maximum risk with AF:**
A. Recent embolisation within 1 month
B. Recent MVR within 1 month
C. Recent onset AF
D. DVT within 1 month

40. **All are coronary risk equivalent *except*:**
A. Fatality risk > 5% in 10 years
B. MI and death > 20% in 10 years
C. DM with CAD
D. All

41. **60 years female DM_2 undergoing intestine surgery. What is true regarding perioperative risk?**
 A. 5% incidence of MI
 B. Most events are symptomatic
 C. More than 2/3rd cases are trop T positive

42. **LCX disease is diagnosed by what changes in OVR?**
 A. Isoelectric ST with upright T
 B. ST ↑ > 1 mm with T ↓
 C. ST ↑ > 1 mm with T ↑
 D. ST ↓ > 1 mm

43. **IWMI thrombolysed had pansystolic murmur, which disappear in evening rounds after thrombolysis. Next R_x?**
 A. ↓ vasodilation
 B. Surgery reference
 C. IABP
 D. All

44. **A patient of STEMI thrombolysed following which PSM developed color Doppler not works. Now what will you do for diagnosis with therapeutic implications?**
 A. Coronary and LV angiogram
 B. Clinical sense and get surgery reference
 C. Right heart catheterization

45. **Raised left jugular venous pressure is seen in:**
 A. Persistent LSVC
 B. Acute MR

46. **A HTN patient on ACE-inhibitors BP 110/70 developed SOB gross pedal edema with clear chest D_X:**
 A. CCP B. Hypertensive HF
 C. RCMP

47. **Patient with DM 2 BP 150/100 proteinuria present. E REST 2.1 on Aspirin, rosarvastat tab 20 mg/d and OHA. Next drug to be added:**
 A. Amlodipine B. Chlorthiazide
 C. Telmisartan

48. **Drug not used in ALLHAT:**
 A. Lisinopril B. α–blocks
 C. Chlorthiazide D. Amlodipine

49. **Prospective cohort all *except*:**
 A. Relatively inexpensive
 B. Framingham study 13 good example
 C. Large sample size
 D. None

50. **Which rules out concealed pathway?**
 A. RP < 70 msec

51. **Fascicular VT all *except*:**
 A. β-blocker is DoC
 B. Verapamil can be given
 C. Adenosine sensitive
 D. RBBB with sup. axis

52. **Brugada syndrome mechanism:**
 A. Phase O depolarization
 B. Phase 2 depolarization
 C. Repolarization
 D. Phase and depolarization

53. **Sinus node current not included:**
 A. I Na+ B. If
 C. ITO D. L–Ca^{2+}

54. **RFA is best in:**
 A. AF with FVR B. Parahisian
 C. AVNRT

55. **Left post accessory pathway aberrancy is diagnosed by:**
 A. LBBB B. RBBB/Rs in V_1
 C. RBBB/ Rs in V_1

56. **What finding in pulse oximetry clinically diagnosis of tricuspid atresia?**
 A. Dip of O_2 saturation in LA
 B. Saturation in LA, LV, RV, PA and risk is equal

57. **57 years old patient of with complete TGA develop syncope. Likely cause:**
 A. RV dysfunction
 B. CHF
 C. Complete heart block
 D. PS

58. **Ventricularization and dampening is seen in all *except*:**
 A. Small caliber of catheter
 B. Ostial disease
 C. Deep engagement of catheter
 D. Entry into conus branch of RCA

59. **Best view for left coronary bifurcation:**
 A. LAO caudal B. LAD caudal
 C. RAO caudal D. RAD caudal

60. **Which innocent murmur changes to organic?**
 A. Bicuspid aortic valve
 B. MVP syndrome

61. **Finding in CXR in right aortic atresia:**
 A. Uplifting of right bronchial
 B. Trachea to right side of bronchial
 C. Indentation to bronchus
 D. None

62. **Bilateral right sidedness is shown by:**
 A. Polysplenia
 B. Bilateral finger like atrial appendage
 C. Small wide bilateral bronchial
 D. Right bronchial supplying left bilobed lung

63. Late presentation of left of right ASD is due to:
A. Less pressure difference between LA and RA
B. ↑ Pulmonary vascular resistance
C. ↑ RV compliance

64. RV not dilated in VSD because:
A. Shunt is in systole (L→R)
B. LV compresses RV
C. Shut size decreases in diastole

65. Fetus to adult pulmonary vascular resistance is reached in:
A. 2–3 weeks B. 3–6 weeks
C. 6–10 weeks D. Any

66. True:
A. PVR reaches to adult level early in full term neonatal
B. Late in pre-term
C. Delayed in VSD
D. None

67. SPO_2 → SVC 70%, RV 80%, RA 76%, PA 90% LV 90%:
A. TGA
B. Blalock-Taussig shunt
C. TOF

68. SPO_2 =, RA 58%, RV 58%, SVC 70%, aorta 90%, PA 80%:
A. TGA B. PS
C. TOF D. Aortic stenosis

69. RV systolic pressure with intact ventricular septum:
A. Severe PS

70. Pulmonary ejection sound:
A. Attenuates with inspiration

71. Fetal circulation O_2 saturation. Ductus arteriosis 55%:
A. SVC 60%
B. IVC 70%
C. Ductus venosus 76%

72. In fetus correct is:
A. RV systolic pressure is ↑ true LV
B. RV and LV pressure is equal

73. RP > PR:
A. Differentiates various SVTS
B. Differentiates AVNT from AVRT
C. AVNT vs atrial tachycardia
D. Aortic patency vs AT

74. 35 years old with AOE, BMI–24, Non-DM_2, Non-HTN, TMT positive, MDCT normal, TG = slightly ↑ HDL 45. Next step:
A. CAG to R/V microvascular angina
B. Repeat TMT
C. Stress thallium
D. Reassure and treatment statin in fibrates

75. Female with postprandial and early morning angina had 3 episodes of transient ST ↑ in whole and had NTVT:
A. CCB B. β-blocker
C. ICD

76. Risk of SCD is seen in:
A. Early repolarization
B. Na channel abnormalities
C. All

77. Microvascular angina not medicated by:
A. Hs–CRP B. Endothelin
C. ICAM D. IL–18

78. Acute R_X of AF all *except*:
A. Flecainide B. Sotalol
C. Amiodarone D. Vernakalant

79. STEMI patient developed CHB acutely, undergone TPI in 5 days, reversed to sinus rhythm on ECA shows RBBB with left axis. Next R_X:
A. EPS to find HV interval
B. Loop event reader
C. Holter
D. PPI

80. IABP not cause:
A. ↑ of systolic pressure
B. ↑ of diastolic pressure
C. ↑ of mean pressure
D. ↑ CO

81. Best measure to assess gradient in AS:
A. Peak to peak
B. Mean
C. Instantaneous
D. None

82. A patient of AS with EP 25% (80 years old and what finding in dobutamine stress echo?
A. 3 m/s, what suggest feasibility of AVR
B. ↑ CO with no change in valve area
C. ↑ CO with ↑ of valve area
D. ↑ CO

83. Small equiphasic qrs in aVL significance:
A. Maximum vector is perpendicular
B. Reversal V_1 load

84. Which one is minor criteria of Framingham?
A. Vital capacity

85. Positive hepatojugular reflux can be seen in:
A. Obstructed SVC below azygous
B. Obstructed SVC above azygous
C. Hemiazygous vein

20

GB PANT 2009

1. **Calcium found in:**
   A. RBC B. WBC
   C. Plasma + RBC D. Plasma
2. **Hyposegmented neutrophil:**
   A. Puet-Flower
   B. Schwarzmann-Blackfan
   C. Sokel's index
3. **$T_H^o \rightarrow T_H^2$:**
   A. ILI B. IL-4
   C. TNF D. GM-CSF
4. **Intracorpuscular hemolysis all *except*:**
   A. PNH
   B. Spherocytosis
   C. Microangiopathic
   D. Haemoglobinopathy
5. **Shortest acting BZD:**
   A. Lorazepam B. Oxazepam
   C. Triazolam D. Trifluoperazine
6. **Drug does not inhibit conversion of $T_4 \rightarrow T_3$:**
   A. Methimazole B. PTU
   C. Amiodarone D. β blocker
7. **Drug does not given initially in young adult in recent d_x parkinsonism:**
   A. Levodopa B. Amantadine
   C. Selegiline D. Ropinirole
8. **Least nephrotoxic:**
   A. Amikacin B. Genta
   C. Streptomycin D. Netilmycin
9. **Proto oncogenes true:**
   A. Differentiation and growth of cells regulation
10. **Y chromosome:**
   A. Binomial variation in human Y chromosome 3 fails
   B. 1degree relative variable length seen
   C. Unexpressed gene 30%
   D. Long segment of Y length variability
11. **Sickle cell anemia glutamine at 6th:**
   A. Valine
12. **In depression PET scan ↓ signal is seen in:**
   A. Frontal B. Parietal
   C. Temporal D. Occipital
13. **Fibromyalgia all *except*:**
   A. More common in female
   B. Tender point 11 out of 18
   C. EEG shows disturbed REM pattern
   D. Musculoskeletal and neurological examination normal
14. **OA all *except*:**
   A. More common in female
   B. Initially involves cartilage
   C. Bone crepitation in characteristic
   D. Most common is idiopathic
15. **Gout all *except*:**
   A. More common than female
   B. 30% may have N uric acid and during acute attack
   C. 90% having overproduction mechanism than excretion
   D. Colchicine should not be informed in conjunction (mixed) with dextrose
16. **Marker of osteoblastic activity all *except*:**
   A. Alkaline phosphate
   B. Osteocalcinin
   C. Peptide-procollagen
   D. Hydroxyproline
17. **Thyrotoxicosis due to I_2:**
   A. Job-Basedow
18. **All are radiolucent renal stones *except*:**
   A. Urate
   B. Cystine
   C. Xanthine
   D. Allopurinol

19. **P. vera true all *except* (Polycythemia vera):**
   A. Arise from multi potent haematopoietic progenitor cells
   B. Hyperuricemia
   C. Splenomegaly
   D. Bone marrow aspiration is diagnostic

20. **Multiple myeloma all *except*:**
   A. ↑ ALP

21. **Anorexia nervosa all *except*:**
   A. Hyperuricemia
   B. Bradycardia
   C. MV prolapse
   D. Hypertension

22. **I_2 natural:**
   A. I^{123} B. I^{125}
   C. I^{131} D. I^{127}

23. **Insulin structure:**
   A. Senger
   B. Best and Benten

24. **Central hypothyroidism all *except*:**
   A. TSH is not a reliable diagnostic Mackay
   B. Adrenal insufficiency should be r/o before treatment
   C. TSH is used for treatment monitoring
   D. Craniopharyngioma C_A most common cause

25. **Max potassium:**
   A. Rectum fluid
   B. Distal small intestine (ileum)
   C. Pancreatic juice
   D. Bile

26. **Cholera stool all *except* (Rice water):**
   A. Mucous fleck B. Non-billous
   C. -ve blood D. Odour

27. **CFTR gene in C/F all *except*:**
   A. Most common mutation absent CFTR
   B. Autosomal recessive
   C. Characteristics feature in ↓ electrophysiological difference
   D. Pathway chloride not settled cre properly

28. **2° messenger:**
   A. ATP B. Urine
   C. Catt D. C–GMP

29. **Intrauterine growth all *except*:**
   A. IGF–1
   B. GH
   C. Insulin
   D. Epidermal growth factor, TGF, family

30. **Papillary necrosis all *except*:**
   A. DM B. SLE
   C. TB D. Cirrhosis liver

31. **Acute pyelonephritis differential by uncomplicated UTL by all *except*:**
   A. ↑ LDH–5
   B. Colony count >10 raise to power 8
   C. Antibodies to Tamm-Horsfall protein

32. **Membranous GN deposit:**
   A. Subepithelial
   B. Subendo
   C. Subepi + Subepido
   D. Mesangio

33. **Community acquired pneumonia most common:**
   A. Pneumococcus
   B. Mycoplasma
   C. S. aureus
   D. Mixed

34. **Shigella severe due to:**
   A. S. dysenteriae
   B. Flexneri

35. **Anthrax all true *except*:**
   A. Gram +ve spore
   B. Spore germinate at site of inoculation
   C. Pulmonary infiltrate atypical
   D. PEP > 2 months

36. **Anti-snake venom:**
   A. Recombinant
   B. Equine
   C. Duck

37. **Acute arsenic poisoning all *except*:**
   A. Toxic level > 9 umo I/L
   B. Rapidly by clears from blood
   C. X-ray abdomen C/I

38. **Alcohol legal intoxication:**
   A. 80–100 mg/dl B. 25
   C. 50–60 D. 100–120 mg/dl

39. **Mercury intoxication all *except* (Acute):**
   A. Tremor + polyneuropathy
   B. Hypotension
   C. Pink disease and acrodynia
   D. Erythrism

40. **Pseudohyponatremia all *except*:**
   A. Hypo-osmolality
   B. SIADH → NV hyponatremia
   C. NSAID potentiates vasopressin induced hyponatremia
   D. Nicotine stimulates vasopressin leads to ↓ Nat.

41. **Most common cause of nystagmus:**
   A. Cerebellar
   B. Vestibulo labrinthine
   C. Drug induced
   D. Brain stem

42. **TBM CSF not compatible:**
A. Acellular
B. Polymorphonuclear pleocytosis
C. ↓ Glucose
D. AFB–nt

43. **Smoking least A/W C_A:**
A. Larynx B. Pharynx
C. Stomach D. Oesophagus

44. **TB risk factor least in:**
A. HIV B. JI bypass
C. CRF on H/D D. DM

45. **Prinzmetal angina all *except*:**
A. Focal spasm at site of spasm in association atherosclerosis
B. Nitrates + CCB helpful
C. BB sometimes helpful
D. Mortality is < 5% at 5 years

46. **Cyanide poisoning:**
A. Amyl nitrate B. Thiosulfate
C. Na nitrate D. Fomapizil

47. **ASD all *except*:**
A. Sinus venosus type association anomalous pulmonary
B. Secundum association MVP in 25%
C. Small ASD often association DOE
D. Not association with atrial arrhythmia

48. **Athletic all *except*:**
A. Isotonic and isometric exercises both do not increase LV thickness
B. Both – ↑ses LV mass
C. Isotonic ↑ses and diastolic diameter
D. Hypertrophy reverts after stopping exercise

49. **Magenta tongue:**
A. B2

50. **Most common gas:**
A. N2

51. **50 years female severe chest pain, vomiting, intermittent dysphagia angio normal:**
A. 24 hours PH B. Manometry
C. Barium D. ↓ UG/E

52. **Case → finishing ↑ JVP ,↑ 5HIAA all *except*:**
A. Has involved liver
B. Tight tricuspid value
C. Often involves left side
D. Due to 5 HT brady

53. **D–dimer all *except*:**
A. High + predictive value

54. **K secretion in kidney not depends (from CD):**
A. Proximal Na absorption
B. Distal flow rate
C. Electrochemical gradient
D. Glucocorticoids

55. **In symptomatic distribution:**
Mean = Median

56. **All *except*:**
A. Mean for numerical data for symm curve
B. Median → ordinal data → skewed
C. Mode for bimodal
D. S_D shows variability from median

57. **DNA-enhancer:**
A. Long DNA segment (75–150 base-pain)
B. Orientation and place independent
C. Stimulates M transcription in adjacent cell

58. **During dialysis hemolysis by all *except*:**
A. Cu
B. Temp
C. Hypoosmolality
D. ↑ Formaldehyde

59. **Not a side effect of GH therapy:**
A. Gynaecomastia
B. Hypoglycemia
C. Epiphyseal slippage

60. **21 OH deficiency in prenatal diagnosis of CAH R_X in:**
A. Dexa
B. Beta
C. Hydro
D. Predinisolone

61. **Apo-A associated with:**
A. HDL
B. LDL
C. VLDL
D. Chylomicron

62. **For ketones dipstick test based in:**
A. Gerheardt's
B. Rothra with glucose oxidase
C. Glucose oxidase

ANSWERS

1	D	2	A	3	B	4	C	5	C	6	A	7	B
8	C	9	A	10		11		12	A	13	C	14	A
15	C	16	D	17		18		19	D	20	A	21	A
22	D	23	A	24	C	25	A	26		27	A	28	D
29	B	30	B	31	C	32	A	33	A	34	A	35	B
36	B	37	C	38	A	39	B	40	A	41	C	42	A
43	C	44	D	45	C	46	D	47	C	48	A	49	
50		51		52	C	53		54	D	55		56	
57	A	58	A	59		60	D	61	A	62	B		

21

GB PANT 2007

1. **Which of the following mutation results RCMP?**
   A. Trop I
   C. Trop C
   C. Tropomyocin
   D. Lamin A/C

2. **Regarding ARVD all of the following are true *except*:**
   A. Pulmonary HT is seen
   B. Fibrofatty deposits results from myocyte apoptosis
   C. Mutation in ryanodyne receptors in sarcoplasmic reticulum is responsible
   D. Cardiac MRI is useful in diagnosis

3. **Which of the following is not reversible direct thrombin inhibitor?**
   A. Lepirudin
   B. Bivaluridin
   C. Desirudin
   D. Argatroban

4. **All of the following are seen in Noonan's syndrome *except*:**
   A. Lymphoedema
   B. Pulmonary stenosis
   C. 45 XO

5. **Which of the following congenital anomaly is having maximum IE risk:**
   A. Bicuspid aortic valve
   B. Ebstein's anomaly
   C. VSD
   D. Pulmonic stenosis

6. **During stage II of Valsalva maneuver which physiological effect is seen:**
   A. Decreased BP and ↑ HR
   B. ↑ HR and ↑ BP
   C. ↓ HR and ↓ BP
   D. ↑ BP and ↓ HR

7. **Which of the following is a dangerous cardiac coronary anomaly:**
   A. LCA originating from right aortic sinus with inter arterial course
   B. ALCAPA
   C. Split RCA
   D. LCx originating from right aortic sinus

8. **In NYHA classification following is not a symptom:**
   A. Angina
   B. Cyansis
   C. Dyspnea
   D. Palpitation

9. **Phasic ejection click of aortic valve is seen in:**
   A. PS
   B. TOF
   C. Systemic hypertension
   D. AS

10. **Wide split second heart sound is seen in:**
    A. LV pacing
    B. PDA
    C. LVOT obstruction (severe)
    D. LSVC to LA with intact septum

11. **Wide pulse pressure is seen in:**
    A. PDA with PR
    B. Severe hypertensive TR
    C. Adult TOF
    D. As with MR

12. **Normotensive TR is seen in all *except*:**
    A. Carcinoid
    B. MS with functional TR
    C. IE
    D. Tricuspid valve prolapse

13. **BP in lower limbs is significantly more than in upper limb:**
    A. Takayasu arteritis

B. Coractation of aorta with AR
C. Femoral AV fistula
D. Bilateral RAS

14. **Cannon "a" wave is seen in:**
A. VVI B. DDD
C. Severe TS D. PSVT

15. **Syncope is not a characteristic manifestation of:**
A. HOCM B. Severe PS
C. CoA D. MS

16. **Hand grip causes:**
A. Increase S3 murmur
B. Increase AS murmur
C. Increase HOCM murmur
D. Decrease MS murmur

17. **All are true for PDA *except*:**
A. Pulmonary end is dilated
B. No infective endocardtitis in PDA without murmur
C. Device closure is done for PDA <8 mm
D. Maternal rubella is a cause in a neonate

18. **Nocturia is seen in all *except*:**
A. Diabetes mellitus
B. CHF
C. Hypertension
D. VSD

19. **R in V_1 is seen in all except**
A. VSD
B. Duchenne's muscular dystrophy
C. Posterior wall MI
D. Situs inversus with dextrocardia

20. **ACE inhibitors cause abrupt increase in serum creatinine in:**
A. Hypotension B. CHF
C. B/L RAS D. All of the above

21. **True about ACE inhibitors is all *except*:**
A. Increase renin
B. Increase angiotensin 1
C. Decrease renal blood flow
D. Increase bradykinin

22. **Digoxin level is increased in all *except*:**
A. Phenytoin B. Amiodarone
C. Erythromycin D. Verapamil

23. **Cardioselective beta blocker is:**
A. Sotalol B. Bisoprolol
C. Nadolol D. Pindolol

24. **Drug to be given in first 24 hours of MI:**
A. ACE inhibitors B. CCB
C. Statin D. Digoxin

25. **Drug beneficial in mortality in CHF:**
A. Digoxin
B. Spironolactone
C. Oral anticoagulants
D. All of the above

26. **Antioxidant effect is seen with all *except*:**
A. Carvedilol B. Vitamin D
C. Allupurinol D. Probucol

27. **Statin may cause all *except*:**
A. Decreased stent thrombosis
B. Stabilizes plaque
C. Decrease senile osteoporosis
D. Improves endothelial function

28. **Anterolateral papillary muscle is supplied by:**
A. LAD and LCx B. LAD
C. LCx D. RCA

29. **Vein draining into RA through coronary sinus are all *except*:**
A. Thebesian vein
B. Small cardiac vein
C. Anterior cardiac vein
D. Vein of Marshall

30. **Spontaneous contrast in LA is seen in:**
A. RCMP
B. Acute MI
C. Severe TS
D. RA myxoma

31. **Superior axis deviation is seen in all *except*:**
A. RSOV to RV
B. TOF with large inlet VSD
C. ECD
D. Tricuspid atresia

32. **Penetrating injury most commonly affects:**
A. RV B. LV
C. RA D. IVS

33. **Cyanosis with decreased blood flow is seen in:**
A. Ebsteins anomaly
B. Tricuspid Atresia with non restrictive VSD without PS
C. Taussig Bing anomaly
D. TGA

34. **Enlarged LA is seen in:**
A. Lutembacher's syndrome
B. ASD-OS
C. Corpulmonale
D. Ebsteins anomaly

35. **Oxygen step up in RV is seen in:**
A. PDA with PR
B. RSOV into LA

C. Sinus venosus ASD
D. Cortriatriatum

36. **Downs syndrome: most commonly associated with:**
A. ECD
B. TOF
C. PS
D. Pulmonary artery stenosis

37. **CHF in first week of life is seen in all *except*:**
A. Severe MR
B. Coarctation of aorta
C. VSD
D. Congenital MS

38. **WPW in congenital heart disease is associated with:**
A. RSOV
B. TGA
C. Ebstein's
D. Uhl's anomaly

39. **Markers of myocardial infarction are all *except*:**
A. Troponin C
B. Myosin light chain
C. LDH
D. CK-MB

40. **In diabetes mellitus: Goal of anti lipid therapy is (without CAd):**
A. LDL <100 and TG <150 mg%
B. LDL <100 and TG <200 mg%
C. LDL <130 and TG <200 mg%
D. LDL <160 and TG <150 mg%

41. **Pregnancy: following are suggestive of heart disease:**
A. Diastolic murmur at apex
B. LVS3
C. Systolic murmur grade 2/6 in pulmonary area
D. Edema

42. **Poor prognosis in pregnancy is seen in:**
A. PPH
B. CoA
C. OS-ASD
D. MR

43. **Most dangerous coronary anomaly:**
A. ALCAPA
B. Left coronary from right aortic sinus with interarterial course
C. LAD from right aortic sinus with retroaortic route
D. RCA from Lt aortic sinus

44. **Amyl nitrate inhalation increases murmur of:**
A. HOCM
B. TOF
C. PDA
D. MR

45. **Treatment of cyanotic spell is all *except*:**
A. Morphine
B. Esmolol
C. Phenylephrine
D. Frusemide

46. **Pacing: true is:**
A. Pacemaker mediated tachycardia is seen in VVI pacing
B. DDD pacing causes less of atrial arrhythmia than VVI
C. Biventricular pacing in HOCM is beneficial
D. VVI is useful in CHF

47. **Atrial fibrillation: true is:**
A. Risk of thromboembolism is smore in non valvular than valvular
B. Biatrial pacing is useful in prevention of intermittent AF
C. Rhythm control is definitely better than rate control
D. Aspirin and warfarin are equally efficacious in preventing stroke

48. **Infective endocarditis: highest risk is associated with:**
A. Bicuspid aortic valve
B. Ebstein's anomaly
C. PPH
D. OS-ASD

49. **IE: Indication for surgery are all *except*:**
A. Unstable prosthesis
B. Intractable CHF
C. NVE relapse after optimal antimicrobial treatment
D. Vegetation > 1mm with embolic phenomenon

50. **BMV balloon size:**
A. Height of person in cm/10+10 mm
B. Height of person in cm/10+5 mm
C. Height of person in mts +10 mm
D. Height of person in cm/8+10 mm

51. **Familial myxoma: true are all *except*:**
A. Endocrine disorder
B. Present in elderly
C. Multiple
D. Biatrial

52. **Continuous murmur is seen in all *except*:**
A. Truncus arterisus
B. Lutembacher syndrome
C. Severe RVOT obstruction
D. Arteriovenous fistula

ANSWERS

1	C	2		3	C	4	A	5		6	A	7	C
8	A	9	C	10	B	11	A	12	D	13	C	14	A
15	A	16	D	17	C	18	A	19	A	20	B	21	A.B
22	A	23	A	24	A	25	B	26	A	27	A	28	C
29	B	30		31	A	32	D	33	B	34	E	35	A
36	A	37	A	38	A	39	A	40	D	41	E	42	A
43	A	44	B	45	D	46	A	47	A,B	48	C	49	A
50	C												

22

GB PANT 2006

1. **All are branches of RCA *except*:**
   A. OM
   B. PDA
   C. PLV
2. **Normal ECG in MI:**
   A. 5% B. 10%
   C. 15% D. 20%
3. **Past MI with poor prognosis:**
   A. 1° VT
   B. 2° VT
   C. MR
   D. Aneurysm
4. **H wave in:**
   A. RCM B. RVMI
   C. CCP D. All
5. **Myocardial viability all *except*:**
   A. Contrast echo B. PET
   C. Stress echo D. TDI
6. **TMT to be done in:**
   A. MI (<5 days)
   B. Evaluation of CAD in valvular HD
   C. Routine evaluation of asymptomatic young
   D. Routine evaluation of post PCI
7. **Asymptomatic carotid artery stenosis stroke rate:**
   A. 2%/year B. 7%/year
   C. 5%/year D. 13%/year
8. **Carney complex clinical criteria all *except*:**
   A. Cardiac myxoma
   B. Cutaneous + myocardial
   C. Typical distribution of skin pigmentation
   D. 1st degree relative
9. **Hyperhomocysteinemia all *except*:**
   A. HRT
   B. CRF
   C. Statin (Fenofibrate)
10. **Decrease restenosis all *except*:**
    A. Gp IIb IIIa inhibitors
    B. Everlimus ES
    C. Brachy therapy (r)
    D. Methotrexate
11. **Systolic HTN *except*:**
    A. Alcohol withdrawal
    B. Beri beri
    C. Thyrotoxicosis
    D. AR
12. **Infectious causes of atherosclerosis are all *except*:**
    A. CMV B. H. pylori
    C. Chlamydia D. Mycoplasma
13. **LVEF 30%, poorest diagnosis:**
    A. AS B. AS + MS
    C. AR D. Chronic MR
14. **False negative ABI in all *except*:**
    A. PVD of upper limb
    B. Calcific and non-compressible AS
    C. Small cuff
    D. HTN LVF
15. **Hypertensive emergency like conditions are:**
    A. Encephalitis
    B. Hypercalcemia
    C. Anxiety with hyperventilation
    D. All
16. **Parenteral vasodilator drugs for hypertensive emergency are all *except*:**
    A. Phentolamine B. Enalapril
    C. Nicardipine D. Fenoldopam
17. **RCM cause all *except*:**
    A. Hemochromatosis
    B. Fabry's disease
    C. Glyogen storage disease
    D. Gaucher's disease

18. **Kawasaki disease all *except*:**
A. Coronary aneurysm in 20%
B. Steroid ineffective
C. Pericarditis
D. Rare in India

19. **Severity of MS in presence of AR:**
A. Overestimated
B. Underestimated
C. Depends on heart rate

20. **Not seen in IE:**
A. MCD B. MPGN
C. FSG D. RPGN

21. **IE absolute indication for surgery are all *except*:**
A. Unstable prosthesis
B. Perivalvular leak
C. CHF

22. **Absolute indication of surgery in IE are all *except*:**
A. Large hypermobile veg > 10 mm
B. Relapse of PVE
C. Fistula to pericardiac sac

23. **Rheumatic fever increase manifestation in elderly:**
A. Arthritis
B. Carditis
C. Chorea
D. Subcutaneous nodules

24. **Pulsus paradoxus all *except*:**
A. Pericardial effusion
B. CT
C. CCP
D. PE

25. **C/I of TMT all *except*:**
A. MI > 5 days
B. Advanced HB
C. Symptomatic AS
D. Uncontrolled HTN

26. **MV calcification all *except*:**
A. Males common
B. Stroke
C. LV inlet obstruction

27. **Type C lesion all *except*:**
A. Ostial
B. > 20 mm
C. Degenerated venous graft

28. **Takayasu related with all *except*:**
A. Rheumatoid arthritis
B. UC
C. PPH
D. Rheumatic fever

29. **Contrast nephropathy prevented by all *except*:**
A. NAC B. Saline
C. Ionic solution D. Theophylline

30. **All released from endothelium *except*:**
A. Fibrinogen B. VWF
C. Bradykinin D. Endothelin

31. **Surgery for dissection all *except*:**
A. Proximal B. AR
C. Isolated arch D. Marfan's

32. **Compensatory short term mechanism of LV dysfunction are all *except*:**
A. Increase preload
B. Increase HR and ejection
C. Blood flow redistribution to vital organs
D. Increase cardiac energy expenses

33. **Square wave sign on valsalva all *except*:**
A. ASD B. CHF
C. HOCM D. MS

34. **Severe AS asymptomatic N LV function treatment by:**
A. AVR B. Ross
C. Echo follow up D. Valvotomy

35. **TAPVC (obstructive) all *except*:**
A. N cardiac size
B. Ground glass appearance
C. Split S2
D. M > F

36. **Neonatal cyanosis seen in all *except*:**
A. TOF
B. TGA
C. HLHS
D. TAPVC with obstruction

37. **Cyanosis + increase Qp + LV volume overload all *except*:**
A. TAPVC B. TGA
C. ECD D. Truncus

38. **TGA at 2 weeks treatment:**
A. Arterial switch
B. Atrial switch
C. Rastelli

39. **Accessory pathway not seen in:**
A. TGA B. Ebstein
C. MVP D. TAPVC

40. **Increase step up of O_2 at RA level not seen in:**
A. VSD with TR B. Gerbode defect
C. PAPVC D. LSVC to RA

41. **HCM true *except*:**
A. Digoxin increase gradient and murmur
B. Isoproterenol and squatting have same effect

C. Valsalva decrease murmur
D. Post extrasytole increase gradient

42. **All are seen in RA/*except*:**
A. Eustachian
B. Thebasian
C. Ligament of marshall

43. **Most common coronary anomaly:**
A. Separate LAD/LCX
B. LCA from right
C. RCA from left sinus
D. LCX from RCs - 20%

44. **Least energy for cardioversion:**
A. VT
B. Sinus tachycardia
C. AF
D. Mahaim tachycardia

45. **VT (Monomorphic) with structurally N heart are all *except*:**
A. CPVT
B. Propranolol sensitive idiopathic VT
C. Idiopathic LV VT
D. RVOT VT

46. **Entrainment seen in:**
A. RV extrasystole VT
B. RVOT VT
C. Fascicular VT
D. Idiopathic LVOT VT

47. **Late manifestation of RF:**
A. EM
B. Arthritis
C. Carditis
D. Subcutaneous nodule

48. **Short RP tachycardia are all *except*:**
A. AVNRT
B. AVRT
C. AT
D. AT with increase PR

49. **Blocks accessory pathway all *except*:**
A. IA B. IC
C. Amiodarone D. IV

50. **Anti-arrhythmic of choice in pregnancy:**
A. IA
B. IC
C. BB
D. DC cardioversion

51. **Selective beta-blocker without ISA are all *except*:**
A. Acebutalol
B. Betaxolol
C. Esmolol
D. Bisoprolol

52. **Vasodilator BB are all *except*:**
A. Carvedilol
B. Labetalol
C. Bucindolol
D. Bisoprolol

53. **Statin trial in ACS all *except*:**
A. Prove it
B. Miracle
C. A to Z
D. Prosper

54. **Secondary prevention trial in ICD all *except*:**
A. CAT
B. Maveric
C. AVID
D. CIDS

55. **Geneva risk score are all *except*:**
A. Hypertension
B. Prior DVT
C. Cancer
D. HF

56. **Tangier's disease all *except*:**
A. Autosomal recessive
B. Increase HDL
C. Peripheral lipid deposition
D. Risk of CAD low

57. **Reverse redistribution on thallium:**
A. CAD
B. Amyloidosis
C. Sarcoidosis
D. Fabry's

58. **Least common in AIDS:**
A. Kaposi
B. IE
C. Myocarditis
D. Atherosclerosis

59. **Cilostazol all *except*:**
A. PDE III inhibitor
B. Vasodilator
C. Anti-platelet
D. Not well tolerated

ANSWERS

1	A	2	A	3	B	4	D	5	D	6	B	7	A
8	D	9	A	10	A	11	B	12	C	13	D	14	D
15	D	16	B	17	D	18	C	19	A	20	A	21	B
22	A	23	A	24	A	25	A	26	A	27	A	28	D
29	C	30	A	31	C	32	D	33	C	34	C	35	C
36	C	37	A	38	A	39	D	40	D	41	C	42	C
43	C	44	D	45	A	46	C	47	D	48	C	49	D
50	D	51	A	52	D	53	D	54	B	55	A	56	A
57	D	58	A	59	D								

23

GB PANT 2005

1. **U wave is seen in all *except*:**
   A. AR   B. CAD
   C. Hypothermia   D. Hypokalemia

2. **Intracoronary thrombus can be caused by all *except*:**
   A. Aspirin   B. Ticlopidine
   C. Clopidogrel   D. Abciximab

3. **All are gene polymorphism in metabolic syndrome *except*:**
   A. BAR2   B. LDL
   C. INS VNRT   D. K121 q

4. **Azygos vein drain into:**
   A. SVC   B. IVC
   C. Right atrium   D. Right ventricle

5. **Smallest valve is:**
   A. Aortic valve   B. Mitral valve
   C. Tricuspid valve   D. Pulmonary valve

6. **Catheter, which is used to hook coronary artery?**
   A. Amplatz   B. NIH
   C. Pig tail catheter   D. Judkins

Which drug is withdrawn from the market because of its side effects causing rhabdomyolysis?
   A. Rosvastatin   B. Simvastatin
   C. Pravastatin   D. Cerivastatin

8. **All of the following are used for postoperative AF prophylaxis *except*:**
   A. Over drive pacing
   B. Beta blockers
   C. Amiodarone
   D. Sotalol

9. **Following is the TOF palliative procedure:**
   A. Kono procedure
   B. Rastelli's procedure
   C. Nick's procedure
   D. Brock's procedure

10. **Chauusat's criteria are used in:**
    A. Glenn's operation
    B. Fontan's operation
    C. BT shunt
    D. Ross procedure

11. **All are types of long RP/short PR tachycardia *except*:**
    A. SNRT
    B. Atrial tachycardia
    C. ANRT
    D. Atypical AVNRT

12. **Probe patent foramen ovale is seen in:**
    A. 0-5%   B. 0-10%
    C. 10-20%   D. 20-35%

13. **All are class side effects of ACE inhibitors *except*:**
    A. Renal failure
    B. Angioneurotic edema
    C. Dysguisea
    D. Proteinuria

14. **In all of the following conditions dicrotic pulse is seen *except*:**
    A. Accelerated hypertension
    B. Hypertensive individual with low peripheral vascular resistance
    C. Hypovolemic shock
    D. Septic shock

15. **Following is true about ezetimibe:**
    A. 10mg atorvastatin + 10 mg ezetimibe = 80 mg simvastatin
    B. Inhibit cholesterol absorption
    C. Inhibit biliary cholesterol formation
    D. Inhibit triglyceride absorption

16. **All are true about nitrate *except*:**
    A. Causes rebound angina on discontinuation
    B. Dilate epicardial coronary arteries
    C. Should not be given with sildenafil
    D. Reduces afterload more than preload

17. **Giant coronary artery aneurysm is seen in:**
A. SLE B. Syphilis
C. PAN D. Sarcoidosis

18. **All are true about coronary arteries *except*:**
A. RCA arising from anterior coronary sinus
B. Left dominance is less than right side dominance
C. Sinus artery arises from left coronary artery
D. Septal artery is the branch of anterior descending artery

19. **All are true about TMT *except*:**
A. SVT is relative indication to stop
B. 2/4 angina is absolute indication to stop
C. Sinosis and pallor is absolute indication to stop
D. Inability to measure BP is an absolute indication to stop

20. **All are absolute indication to stop the TMT *except*:**
A. Hypertensive response
B. Patient desire to stop
C. Ataxia and palor
D. Sustained VT

21. **All are non-coronary causes of ST depression during TMT *except*:**
A. WPW syndrome
B. Glucose overload
C. Excessive exercise
D. Long QT syndrome

22. **Total pulmonary resistance is:**
A. 20 to 130 B. 100 to 300
C. 700 to 1400 D. 10 to 20

23. **All are secondary trials *except*:**
A. MADIT B. AVID
C. CASH D. CIDS

24. **All are indicators of inappropriate hypertension *except*:**
A. Age between 30 to 40 years
B. BP > 180/110
C. Presence of LVH in ECG
D. Abdominal bruit

25. **Following is seen in DORV:**
A. Sub pulmonic conus reabsorption
B. Subaortic conus reabsorption
C. None of the above
D. Both of the conus reabsorption

26. **Beck triad is:**
A. Muffled heart sound + Hypertension + distended neck veins
B. Muffled heart sound + Hypotension + distended neck veins
C. Muffled heart sound + Decreased JVP + hypotension
D. Loud S1+ distended neck veins with hypertension

27. **Echo finding in patients of MS is:**
A. Anterior motion of the posterior leaflet
B. Posterior motion of the posterior leaflet
C. Immobile posterior leaflet
D. Anterior motion of the anterior leaflet

28. **Which of the following is branch of left circumflex artery?**
A. Obtuse marginal
B. Acute marginal
C. Anterior septal
D. Cornus artery

29. **All are seen in metabolic syndrome *except*:**
A. Increased fibrinogen
B. Increased fibrin
C. Impaired glucose tolerance
D. Obesity

30. **Which of the following is WHO criteria added to definition of metabolic syndrome?**
A. Hyperalbuminemia
B. Impaired glucose tolerance
C. Decreased HDL
D. Obesity

31. **Best preventive treatment for contrast-induced nephropathy is:**
A. N-acetyl cysteine
B. Theophylline
C. Saline hydration
D. Mannitol

32. **All are true about treatment of HOCM *except*:**
A. Beta blockers are the drugs of choice
B. Alcohol septal ablation decreases the gradient
C. MVR suffice in patient having septal hypertrophy >16 mm
D. Septal myomectomy done if alcohol septal ablation fails

33. **Metabolic syndrome is associated with:**
A. Hypothyroidism
B. Acromegaly
C. PCOD
D. Cushing's disease

34. **Which is the wrong combination?**
A. Merit HF trial - metaprolol
B. CIBIS - bisoprolol
C. ESSENCE - enalapril
D. EPHESUS – epelerenone

35. **All are true about ARVD *except*:**
A. Epsilone waves are seen in ECG
B. Autosomal recessive
C. Male predominant
D. Most common cause of death ventricular arrhythmia

36. **All are true about hypereosinophilic syndrome *except*:**
A. Increased eosinophils in peripheral blood
B. Lymphadenopathy is seen
C. Heart involvement is uncommon
D. Can cause restrictive lung disease

37. **In patients of chronic stable angina all of the following treatments are useful *except*:**
A. Aspirin B. Beta blocker
C. ACE-inhibitors D. Statins

38. **All are true about cardiac tamponade *except*:**
A. Pulsus paradoxus seen
B. Kussmaul's sign is seen
C. Muffled heart sounds
D. RA collapse on echo

39. **Assymmetrical septal hypertrophy seen in the following conditions *except*:**
A. Inferior wall MI
B. Antroseptal MI
C. HOCM
D. Posterior wall MI

40. **Pulmonary stenosis is associated with all *except*:**
A. Turner's syndrome
B. Noonan's syndrome
C. Crest syndrome
D. Watson syndrome

41. **Which gas is used in IABP?**
A. Oxygen B. Room air
C. Nitrogen D. Helium

42. **Decreases afterload provides the compensatory mechanism in:**
A. Mitral stenosis
B. Mitral regurgitation
C. Aortic stenosis
D. Aortic regurgitation

43 **H wave in JVP corresponds to:**
A. Isovolumic contraction
B. Isovolumic relaxation
C. Ejection phase
D. Diastasis

44. **Renovascular hypertension is seen in all of the following condition *except*:**
A. Fibromuscular hyperplasia
B. Takayasu artertitis
C. Renal artery embolization
D. Atherosclerosis

45. **Most common heart disease is:**
A. Coronary artery disease
B. Sudden cardiac death
C. Rheumatic heart disease
D. Hypertension

46. **Absolute contraindication for IABP:**
A. Acute MR B. VSD
C. Severe AR D. Severe AS

47. **Intracranial bleed is least common in:**
A. Putamen B. Pons
C. Thalamus D. Cerebellum

48. **Control of hypertension decreases the incidence of all of the following *except*:**
A. Sudden cardiac death
B. Stroke
C. CAD
D. Heart failure

49. **All of the following infections are associated with coronary artery disease *except*:**
A. CMV
B. H pylori
C. Coxsackie B virus
D. Chlamydia

50. **All of the following are criteria for diagnosis of metabolic syndrome *except*:**
A. Obesity
B. BP > 130/85
C. LDL > 200
D. Impaired glucose tolerance

51. **Type B coronary lesion is:**
A. Irregular contour
B. Concentric
C. > 3 months total occlusion
D. Friable SVG graft

52. **All of the following leads to square root response on valsalva maneuver *except*:**
A. ASD B. MS
C. CHF D. PVA

53. **In MVP infective endocarditis prophylaxis is indicated in all *except*:**
A. Severe MR on auscultation
B. Valve thickness >5 mm
C. Only click no MR
D. Severe MR on echocardiography

54. **All of the following are phosphodiesterase inhibitor *except*:**
A. Milrinone B. Amrinone
C. Epinephrine D. Cilostazole

55. Presence of PND indicates:
A. Alveolar edema
B. Interstitial edema
C. Pedal edema
D. All of the above

56. All of the following are causes of pulmonary edema due to starling force *except*:
A. CHF
B. Overperfusion pulmonary edema
C. Mitral stenosis
D. Radiation pulmonary edema

57. Branheim sign is seen in:
A. Coronary AV fistula
B. Systemic AV fistula
C. Pulmonary AV fistula
D. All of the above

58. All of the following are causes of pulmonary hypertension *except*:
A. HIV
B. Portal hypertension
C. Hypothyroidism
D. Anorectic drugs

59. Which of the following drug is contraindicated in pregnancy?
A. Hydralazine B. Enalapril
C. Beta blockers D. Methyl dopa

60. In HIV patient incidence of all of the following are increased *except*:
A. Lymphoma
B. Kaposi's sarcoma
C. Infective endocarditis
D. Dilated cardiomyopathy

61. Longest contractile protein is:
A. Actin B. Titin
C. Myosin D. Collagen

62. Which of the following is phosphodiesterase inhibitor with carcinoma sensitization property?
A. Levosimenden B. Milrinone
C. Amrinone D. Cilostazole

63. TNF alpha antagonist is:
A. Etarnacept B. Interferon alpha
C. Cyclosporin D. SN 560

64. Following causes QT prolongation *except*:
A. Amiodarone B. Sotalol
C. Flecanide D. Digoxin

65. Following statements are true regarding free wall rupture *except*:
A. Incidence more in anterior wall MI
B. Common in patients with previous MI
C. Common in old age
D. Common in hypertensive individual

66. Severity of MS is proportional to:
A. Intensity of the murmur
B. Loud S2
C. Length of the murmur
D. Presence of opening snap

67. Drug of choice for HACEK organism infective endocarditis is:
A. Vancomycin B. Ceftraxone
C. Ampicillin D. Rifampicin

68. Pericarditis is caused by all of the following *except*:
A. Doxorubicin
B. Emetine
C. Methysergide
D. None of the above

69. All are true about non-ionic contrast *except*:
A. Less tendency to form clots
B. Less nephrotoxic
C. Preferred in patients with deranged kidney function test
D. Less chances of arrhythmia

70. Which of the following investigation is most sensitive and specific for myocardial viability test?
A. Treadmill test
B. Doppler echocardiography
C. SPECT scan
D. PET scan

71. False regarding ANP is:
A. A and B are clearance receptor
B. C is clereance receptor
C. ANP is vasodilator
D. Increased concentration is seen in patients of heart failure

72. Potassium sparing diuretic is:
A. Furosemide
B. Indapamide
C. Triamterene
D. Hydrochlorothiazide

73. All are secondary prevention trial *except*:
A. Care B. Lipid
C. 4S D. AFCAPS

74. All are cyanotic congenital heart disease *except*:
A. Truncus arteriosus
B. TGA
C. RSOV
D. TOF

75. **Diastolic murmur is seen in all of the following *except*:**
A. Large VSD B. Large PDA
C. Small PDA D. Severe MR

76. **Most specific for MI within 48 hours is:**
A. Indium antibodies
B. SPECT scan
C. TMT
D. MRI

77. **Catheter used to selectively hook the coronary artery is:**
A. Amplantz
B. NIH
C. PIG tail
D. Multipurpose catheter

78. **For the prevention of contrast nephropathy best is:**
A. Mannitol
B. IV saline
C. Furosemide
D. Soda bicarbonate

79. **Thermodilution technique uses:**
A. Simpson's formula
B. Steward Hamilton formula
C. Laplace principle
D. Bernoulli's principle

80. **Bisferien's pulses seen in all *except*:**
A. Dilated cardiomyopathy
B. AR
C. AS + AR
D. HOCM

81. **Skin manifestation of infective endocarditis is:**
A. Erythema marginatum
B. Erythema nodosum
C. Janeway lesions
D. Tendon xanthomas

82. **All of the following are true about renovascular hypertension *except*:**
A. Renal bruit is heard
B. Flash pulmonary edema is seen
C. Retinopathy is uncommon
D. Aorto arthritis is one of the causes

83. **Myocardial infarction with cardiogenic shock treatment of choice is:**
A. Thrombolytic therapy
B. CABG
C. PTCA with IABP
D. Heparin with aspirin

84. **False regarding true cardiac aneurysm is:**
A. VT is seen
B. Thromboembolism can occur
C. Increased incidence of rupture
D. Cardiomegaly on chest X-ray

85. **Absolute contraindication for PTCA is:**
A. LAD disease
B. Left main unprotected disease
C. Ejection fraction <40%
D. Double vessel disease

86. **Infective endocarditis prophylaxis is indicated in:**
A. Flexible bronchoscopy
B. Sclerotherapy of esophageal varices
C. Cesarean section
D. Upper GI endoscopy

87. **Dichrotic pulse is seen in all *except*:**
A. Septic shock
B. Hypovolemic shock
C. CHF
D. Elderly hypertensive

88. **Pulmonary vascular resistance is:**
A. 5-150
B. 20-130
C. 10-300
D. 750-2000

89. **All of the following catheters are used in coronary angiography *except*:**
A. Judkins
B. Sones
C. Corand's
D. Amplantz

90. **Least common in SLEs:**
A. Pericardial effusion
B. Pericarditis
C. Myocardial infarction
D. Pulmonary artery hypertension

91. **All are causes of early systolic murmur:**
A. Small muscle VSD
B. Chordal rupture
C. TR with MS
D. VSD with pulmonary arterial HT

92. **In pulmonary artery hypertension all are decreased *except*:**
A. Prostacyclin
B. Endothelin
C. NO
D. cAmp

93. **Gangrene with palpable pulse is seen in:**
A. DM
B. Lerich's syndrome
C. Thromboembolic obstruction
D. All of the above

94. Restenosis rate in drug eluting stent is:
A. 0-2%
B. 4-8%
C. 10%
D. 12%

95. Thrombolytic with shortest half-life is:
A. Streptokinase
B. rTPA
C. Reteplase
D. Tenecteplase

96. All are causes of acute infective endocarditis *except*:
A. S aureus
B. Beta hemolytic streptococcus
C. HACEK
D. Pneumococcus

97. Torsade de pointes is seen with all *except*:
A. Procainamide
B. Sotalol
C. Mexilitene
D. Disopyramide

98. Continuous murmur is seen in:
A. Cerebral AV malformation
B. VSD with MS
C. Pulmonary artery stenosis
D. ALCAPA

99. All are beta-blockers with vasodilatory properties *except*:
A. Carvidilol
B. Labetalol
C. Bucindolol
D. Bisoprolol

100. Acute AR not useful is:
A. NTG
B. Nitroprusside
C. Surgery
D. Labetalol

ANSWERS

1	B	2		3	B	4	A	5	D	6	D	7	D
8		9	B	10	B	11	C	12	D	13	C	14	A
15	B	16	D	17	A	18	C	19	B	20	A	21	D
22	B	23	A	24	A	25	C	26	B	27	A	28	A
29	B	30	A	31	C	32	C	33	C	34	C	35	B
36	C	37	D	38	B	39	A	40	C	41	D	42	B
43	D	44	C	45	D	46	C	47	D	48	C	49	C
50	C	51	A	52	D	53	C	54	C	55	B	56	B,D
57	B	58		59	B	60	C	61	B	62	A	63	A
64	D	65	B	66	C	67	B	68	A	69	A	70	
71	A	72	C	73	D	74	C	75	C	76	A	77	A
78	B	79	B	80	A	81	C	82	C	83	C	84	C
85	B	86	B	87	D	88	B	89	C	90	C	91	C
92	B	93	C	94	B	95	B	96	C	97	C	98	C
99	D	100	A										

24

JAIPUR 2009

1. **In high TG's all are given *except*:**
   A. Protocol B. Cholestyraquine
   C. Fibrate D. Statin
2. **Hyperhomocysteinemia seen in all *except*:**
   A. Lipid lowering B. Hypothyroidi
   C. CRF D. HRT
3. **Oral GP IIb IIIa inhibitor:**
   A. Ximelifiban B. Lamifiban
   C. Tirofiban D. Eptifibatide
4. **Not a GP IIb IIIa inhibitor:**
   A. Tirofiban B. Eptifibaride
   C. Abciximab D. Fondaparinaux
5. **Balloon size:**
   A. (Ht/10) +10 B. (Ht+10) /10
6. **PTE all are true *except*:**
   A. Pulmonary infarction
   B. Paradox embolism
   C. Syncope
   D. Pneumothorax
7. **Atherosclerosis RAS predominantly involve:**
   A. Ostial B. Midsegmental
   C. Distal D. Lobar
8. **RCA branches are all *except*:**
   A. OM B. AM
   C. PDA D. PLV
9. **Type C lesion, all true *except*:**
   A. Ostial
   B. Regenerated graft with friable lesion
   C. Length > 20
   D. Total occlusion > 3 months old
10. **Reverse thallium redistribution seen in:**
    A. CAD
    B. Fabry's disease
    C. Amyloidosis
    D. Sarcoidosis
11. **Mason-Likar modification all true *except*:**
    A. Absent q in inferior leads
    B. LAD (Left axis deviation)
    C. New q in aVL
    D. Increased voltage in limb leads
12. **Oasis 6 –inc all *except*:**
    A. Allergic
    B. Catheter thrombosis
    C. Hemorrhagic shock
    D. Bleeding
13. **Invasive vs conservative strategy in all trials all *except*:**
    A. Ictus B. FRISCH II
    C. Vanqish D. Freedom
14. **Myocardial viability assessment by all *except*:**
    A. CME
    B. TDI (Tissue Doppler)
    C. PET
    D. Stress echo
15. **Normal coronary blood flow seen in:**
    A. Stunned
    B. Hibernating
    C. Myocardial bridge
    D. MI
16. **Non-cardiac surgery, acute MI occurs most commonly in:**
    A. < 5 hours B. 6-24 hours
    C. 3-5 days D. > 1 week
17. **TMT is not routinely done in all *except*:**
    A. Post MI <5 days
    B. Routine testing in asymptomatic individuals
    C. Routine testing in post PTCA patients
    D. CAD testing valvular heart disease
18. **Not produced by endothelium:**
    A. Fibrinogen B. VWF
    C. Bradykinin D. Endothelin

19. Asymptomatic carotid stenosis, annual risk of stroke:
A. 2% B. 5%
C. 7% D. 13%

20. Normal ECG in AMI is seen in:
A. 5% B. 10%
C. 20% D. 30%

21. Ventricular septal rupture in MI:
A. A/w HTN
B. Present in killip IV
C. More common with IWMI
D. Females and elderly males

22. Thrombolytic with maximum risk of non-cerebral bleed:
A. STK B. tPA
C. TNK D. rTPA

23. Post CABG MI diagnosed by raised troponin levels more than:
A. >5 times B. >7 times
C. >3 times D. >10 times

24. Universal definition of MI includes MI due to stent thrombosis as:
A. I B. IIb
C. IVa D. IVb

25. Early marker of evolving hypertension:
A. Decreased nocturnal dipping
B. Increased pulse pressure
C. Salt sensitivity
D. Hypertensive response to exercise

26. Post MI – worst prognosis:
A. 1° VT B. 2° VT
C. MR D. LV aneurysm

27. In stent restenosis prevented by all *except*:
A. Gp IIb/IIIa inhibitors
B. Methotrexate
C. Gamma radiation
D. Everolimus releasing stent

28. Infection associated in atherosclerosis are all *except*:
A. CMV B. Chlamydia
C. H. pylori D. Mycoplasma

29. Aortic dissection surgery done in all *except*:
A. Marfan with disease
B. Isolated aortic arch
C. AR
D. Proximal aorta

30. AR with MS, severity is:
A. Under estimated B. Overestimated
C. Normal D. No relation

31. IE absolute indicator of surgery are all *except*:
A. Unstable prosthesis
B. Prosthetic relapse
C. Perivalvular ext.
D. CHF due to valve dysfunction

32. Loud S1 causes are all *except*:
A. MR B. Tachycardia
C. High output D. MS

33. In cardiac tamponade all are seen *except*:
A. Prominent Y
B. Pulsus paradoxus
C. Raised JVP

34. Pulmonary oedema with normal PCWP:
A. HAPE B. LV dysfunction
C. CRF D. MS

35. Asymptomatic AS with normal LV:
A. Follow up echo B. AVR
C. BAV D. Nothing

36. Pulsus paradoxus seen in all *except*:
A. Pericardial effusion
B. Pulmonary embolism
C. CCP
D. Tamponade

37. Lunule with nodule seen in:
A. AV value B. Semilunar value
C. RA D. LA

38. Which of the following not seen in right atrium?
A. Ligament of Marshall
B. Eustachian
C. Thebasian
D. Crista terminalis

39. Severity of MR all are true *except*:
A. Loudness B. MDM
C. S_3 D. Split S_2

40. Cardiomyopathy + loss of pubic hair + CHB seen in:
A. Hemochromatosis
B. Addison's
C. Kearns Sayre syndrome
D. Klinefelter's

41. See saw murmur seen in:
A. TOF with absent pulmonary valve
B. TOF with PDA
C. TOF with P. atresia
D. TOF with P. stenosis

42. Best balloon vulvotomy in:
A. AS B. MS
C. PS D. TS

43. Coronary aneurysm seen in all *except*:
A. FMD B. Syphilis
C. SLE D. Atherosclerosis

44. Which is a late manifestation of RF?
A. Arthritis
B. Carditis
C. Erythema marginatum
D. Subcutaneous nodules

45. Which is common in RF in adult?
A. Arthritis
B. Carditis
C. Subcutaneous nodules
D. Chorea

46. Murmur of HOCM:
A. Valsalva decreases the murmur
B. Squatting and isoproterenol have same action
C. Digitalis inc gradient and murmur
D. Post VPC gradient decreases

47. Mitral annular calcification all true *except*:
A. MR
B. LV in flow obstruction
C. Males more
D. Associated with stroke

48. EF 30%, worst prognosis, seen with:
A. AS with MR B. MR
C. AS D. AR

49. Most common coronary anomaly is:
A. Separate LCX and LAD
B. LAD from right sinus
C. Right coronary from left sinus
D. LCX from right sinus

50. TGA at 2 weeks treatment is:
A. Arterial switch
B. Atrial switch
C. Rastelli's
D. Balloon atrial septostomy

51. Step up in RA seen in all *except*:
A. PAPVC
B. LSVC to RA
C. VDD with TR
D. Gerbode's defect

52. Infradiaphragmatic TAPVC all are true *except*:
A. M > F
B. Normal sized heart
C. Split S_2
D. Ground glass on CXR

53. Wellen's syndrome:
A. T-wave inversion or biphasic in V_1–V_3
B. ST depression
C. Notch at J point with ST elevation
D. Tall symmetrical T wave

54. Fetal death seen in all *except*:
A. Ebstein's B. TGA
C. PSVT D. CHB

55. Bypass tracts are more commonly seen in all *except*:
A. Ebstein's B. TGA
C. TAPVC D. MVP

56. Vasodilatary β blocker all *except*:
A. Bisoprolol B. Bucindolol
C. Carvedilol D. Labetalol

57. Investigation preferred in patient developing syncope while swimming:
A. ECG B. HUTT
C. ECHO D. EPS

58. Dual chamber pacing not done in:
A. Sick sinus syndrome
B. DCM
C. HCM

59. ECG – V_4 placed in:
A. Left 5th IC space at MCL
B. Between V_3 and V_5
C. Anterior axillary line - V_5
D. Apex

60. Least voltage cardioversion is required in:
A. VT
B. AF
C. Atrial flutter
D. Sinus tachycardia

61. Sustained VT is defined as hemodynamically unstable or occurring for more than:
A. 15 sec B. 20 sec
C. 25 sec D. 30 sec

62. β-blockers in associated with:
A. Catecholamine toxicity
B. Down regulation of β-receptors

63. R/S more than one in V_1 not routinely seen in:
A. Duchenne
B. Post-wall MI
C. Ebstein's anomaly

64. Atrial myxoma not seen:
A. Hypoalbuminemia B. Clubbing
C. Polycythemia D. ↑ ESR

65. A and V wave:
A. In RA, A is taller V
B. In RA, A < V
C. In LA, A is > V
D. In LA, V > A

66. **Eplerenone is:**
A. Selective aldosterone antagonist
B. TNF-α receptor agonist
C. GH agonist
D. Testosterone antagonist

67. **Oximetry : RA = 69, LA = 70, PA = 68, Aorta = 70:**
A. TAPVC B. TOF
C. Large VSD D. DORV

68. **Square root response not seen in:**
A. ASD B. MS
C. CHF D. PPH

69. **Kawasaki's, all true all *except*:**
A. Aneurysm in 20%
B. Pericarditis can occur
C. Steroids not useful
D. Rare in India

70. **Takayasu a/w all *except*:**
A. Rheumatic fever
B. Rheumatoid arthritis
C. PPH
D. Ulcerative colitis

71. **Tangier disease true are all *except*:**
A. Autosomal recessive
B. Inc. HDL
C. CAD risk not much increased
D. Cholesterol deposits in tissues

72. **BE = – 30, HCO_3^- = 5, pH = 7.09, wt = 50 kg. How much [HCO_3^-] to be given in 1st hour:**
A. 250 B. 350
C. 600 D. 900

73. **CIN like presentation can occur by all *except*:**
A. Saline B. Ionic contrast
C. Theophylline D. NAC

74. **Least common in HIV:**
A. Kaposi's sarcoma
B. IE
C. Pericardial effusion
D. Myocarditis

75. **Cirrhosis liver presents with all *except*:**
A. PPH B. Haemoptysis
C. Hypoxemia D. AV fistula

76. **About magnesium all true *except*:**
A. In MI not useful
B. Useful in TDP
C. In eclampsia act through dopamine receptors

77. **Rheumatoid arthritis a/w all *except*:**
A. PPH
B. Lymphoma
C. Microcytic anemia
D. Scleritis

78. **Not seen in CHF:**
A. Inc. ESR
B. Inc.TNF
C. Inc. Na
D. Inc. adrenomedullin

79. **TG lowering drug all *except*:**
A. Probucol
B. Cholestyramine
C. Fibrate
D. Statin

ANSWERS

1		2	A	3	A	4	D	5	A	6	D	7	A
8	A	9	A	10	A	11	B	12	B	13	D	14	B
15	A	16	B	17	A	18	A	19	A	20	A	21	A
22	A	23	A	24	D	25	A	26	B	27	B	28	D
29	B	30	A	31	C	32	A	33	A	34	A	35	A
36	A	37	B	38	A	39	A	40	C	41	A	42	C
43	B	44	D	45	A	46	C	47	C	48	B	49	C
50	A	51	B	52	C	53	A	54	B	55	C	56	A
57	A	58	A	59	A	60	A	61	D	62	B	63	C
64	A	65	A	66	A	67	A	68	D	69	D	70	C
71	B	72	A	73	B	74	A	75	A	76	A	77	A
78	C	79	B										

25

JAIPUR 2006

1. **Statin not metabolised by Cyp 450:**
   A. Pravastatin **B.** Atorvastatin
   C. Simvastatin **D.** Cerivastatin

2. **Maximum not patient thiemopyridial derivative is ascand AMI:**
   A. CURF
   B. COMIT
   C. AMTER

3. **Anticoagulant not required in:**
   A. Abiocor **B.** Heart mate
   C. Novacor **D.** Abiomed

4. **RAS – atherosclerotic are all *except*:**
   A. ACEI should not be given
   B. Creatine increase – consistent with bilateral RAS
   C. 30% seen with CA

5. **Renovascular HTN all *except*:**
   A. CT angio and spiral CT is IOC
   B. More common in black
   C. Acute elevation of creatine should be considered as diagnostic
   D. Elevated renin in 50%-80% cases

6. **25/M, chest pain, cocain 2 hours before IWMI and JVP elevated, management ECG shows:**
   A. TPA **B.** Angio
   C. Phentolamine **D.** NTG

7. **IABP - major hemodynamic change:**
   A. Increase Co
   B. Decrease afterload
   C. Increased contractility
   D. Increase HR

8. **Septal aneurysm seen:**
   A. a/w PFO **B.** PAPVC
   C. Sinus V **D.** ASD

9. **Decrease vascularity in Cx-R:**
   A. ASD + VSD **B.** ASD + PDA
   C. TA + ASD **D.** RCS + VSD

10. **Correct in female all *except*:**
    A. Aspirin prevent more MI then stroke
    B. CAD - attributed to obesity

11. **4 MI - female, more common than male *except*:**
    A. ST elevation **B.** DM
    C. HTN **D.** CHF

12. **EF - <30% after AMI, AF present DOC is:**
    A. Amiodarone
    B. Sotalol
    C. Flecainide

13. **Exercise test not useful *except*:**
    A. Digoxin
    B. Paced rhythm
    C. VPC with ST change
    D. Severe anaemia with MVP

14. **Increase cholesterol:**
    A. Coconut oil **B.** MUFA
    C. PUFA **D.** Stearic acid

15. **TG least effectively decreased by:**
    A. Statin **B.** Niacin
    C. Fish oil **D.** Fat < 10%

16. **HIT-II Mit (Non STMJ, after UFH for 2 days, PLC, 2,28000 ↓ decrease 16000, Hemogen):**
    A. Continue heparin **B.** Replace LMWH
    C. DTI **D.** GPIIb/IIIa

17. **USA – Least common risk:**
    A. LV dysfunction
    B. TropT
    C. Prolonged chest pain
    D. New onset

18. **Homocystinuria:**
    A. Trials show improvement in CAD risk following folic acid
    B. Risk marker rather than risk factor
    C. Only high HC level are risk factor

19. Silent ischemia:
A. < 2.5% patient
B. Cercadian rhythm
C. Some patients need revascularisation
D. Most of the cases are related to vasospasm

20. AT2 receptor causes:
A. Myocardial growth
B. Increase NE
C. Apoptosis
D. Increase aldosterone

21. Trial associated with nebolol:
A. Senior
B. Aspire
C. No trial

22. Patient with AMI and hypertension – DOC:
A. ARB
B. CCB
C. Diuretics

23. HOCM - true all *except*:
A. Q-JVP
B. MR-20-30% in non-obstructive HOCM
C. 20-40% - Exercise produces hypotension
D. MRI does not have adv. over echo

24. C/I cardiac transplant are all *except*:
A. VO_2 11-15
B. Recurrence USA
C. Recurrent VT
D. Recurrent fluid imbalance

25. Recent trial least effective ant HTN:
A. ACEI B. BB
C. CCB D. Diuretics

26. BNP true all *except*:
A. Increase CO
B. Sympathetic inhibition
C. Less arrhythmogenic than dobutamine
D. Concentration > 4.1 mg/ml

27. 35/m, systolic murmur in 2 ICS, valsalva-murmur decrease, premature beat increase:
A. PS B. Bicuspid AV
C. HOCM D. MVP

28. All true *except* in tamponade:
A. Pulsus paradoxus
B. Rapid y descent
C. Electrical alternans

29. MVA when PHT = 110 is:
A. 2
B. 1.5
C. 9.5

30. Severe AR - most significant criteria:
A. Increase pulse pressure
B. S4
C. Austin flint murmur
D. Apical shift

31. Suggestive of austin flint murmur rather than MS is:
A. S1 loud B. OS
C. S3 D. BP 150/60

32. CIN - best treatment:
A. Hemofilteration
B. Isotonic saline
C. Saline + NAC

33. Bicuspid AV a/w all *except*:
A. A. dissection
B. Aneurysm
C. Myxometous degeneration MV
D. IE

34. Not found in supravalvular ASA:
A. Hemozygous hypexchol
B. Ejection click, commonly found

35. Asymptomatic non obs. HOCM - DOC:
A. Beta-blocker B. Disopyramide
C. CCB D. Septal ablation

36. True about Ebstein are all *except*:
A. Quardapte
B. ASD/PFO seen
C. Tacklers
D. Danvidon's and carpenter operation most commonly done

37. Infant with cyanosis, LVH and normal axis:
A. TA B. PA
C. TAPVC D. PDA

38. PDA:
A. Most patient die of CHF
B. Repair > 8 mm by surgery

39. In neonate not a cardial cause of cyanosis:
A. Truncus B. Meth Hb
C. LSVC to LA D. T APVC

40. L-TGA – seen:
A. Atria inverted
B. Ventricle inverted
C. Abnormal connection of SVC to LA from pulm end

41. AF + 1 convert to sinus rhythm:
A. Ibutilide
B. Amiodarone
C. Sotalol

42. **Adenosine not used in:**
A. AFL
B. At tachycardia
C. AVNRT
D. AVRT

43. **Catecholamine induced tachycardia all true *except*:**
A. Both AR/AD
B. Bidirectional
C. Amiodarone useful
D. Structurally normal heart

44. **Rate drop pacemaker used:**
A. Sleep induced bradycardia
B. AF with block
C. Athlete heart
D. Vasovagal syncope

45. **AF cardioverted, unreasonable:**
A. Wait and watch for recurrence
B. Sotalol
C. Flecainide
D. RFA

46. **ACEI not excreted fecally:**
A. Fosinopril
B. Perindopril
C. Trandipril

47. **HIV true all *except*:**
A. CCP
B. Lymphoma
C. DCMP
D. PAH

48. **FDG - true *except*:**
A. Better in fasting
B. Glucose monitoring useful
C. Diabetic require insulin
D. Oral glucose loading

49. **14-week pregnancy, wide split fixed S2, systolic murmur at base and diastolic murmur at TA prominent C + V wave T/T:**
A. Termination
B. Follow up and treatment
C. 2nd trimester surgery is
D. Surgery in 3rd trimester

50. **Worst prognosis:**
A. Nonsmoker, BP 150/90, HDL 30, TG 280
B. Smoker, 120/80, 50, 210
C. NS, 130/80, 50, 195
D. NS, 170/90

51. **Least risk in pregnancy:**
A. PPH
B. Marfan's with aortic dilatation
C. MVP, MR
D. Eisenmenger

52. **History of syncope 8 years, twice/year diagnostic test:**
A. Loop recorder
B. EPS
C. TMT
D. Echo

26

JAIPUR 2005

1. **U wave increased in amplitude in all *except*:**
   A. Digoxin B. Quinidine
   C. Flecanide D. Isopropranolol

2. **In middle aged asymptomatic man, TMT is positive in:**
   A. 1-8% B. 5-10%
   C. 10-20% D. 40%

3. **Bachman bundle between SA node and AV node is:**
   A. Anterior internodal bundle
   B. Middle internodal bundle
   C. Posterior internodal bundle
   D. Interatrial bundle

4. **AV node development in fetus starts at:**
   A. 3rd week B. 4th week
   C. 5th week D. 6th week

5. **Digoxin is contraindicated in all of the following *except*:**
   A. AR
   B. WPW
   C. Diastolic dysfunction
   D. HOCM

6. **LV end diastolic volume is:**
   A. 50-90 ml/m^2 B. 90-120 ml/m^2
   C. <30 ml/m^2l D. 30-50 ml/m^2

7. **Coronary blood flow in basal condition is:**
   A. 50-70 ml B. 20-30 ml
   C. 10-30 ml D. 30-50 ml

8. **Patient of mitral stenosis in NYHA class-I, 5 years survival rate is:**
   A. 85% B. 70%
   C. 62% D. 15%

9. **Post mitral valve replacement in MS patient 10 year survival rate is:**
   A. 80% B. 70%
   C. 50% D. 100%

10. **Premenopausal women with atypical chest pain having = 3mm ST depression during TMT test, predictive value of CAD is:**
    A. 50% B. 70%
    C. 90% D. 100%

11. **Mean Lerman scratch is heard in:**
    A. Pericarditis
    B. Diabetes
    C. Hyperthyroidism
    D. hypothyroidism

12. **Sensitivity of TEE for infective endocarditis vegetation detection is:**
    A. 90% B. 99%
    C. 80% D. 100%

13. **Umbilical vein SpO_2:**
    A. 80% B. 40%
    C. 30% D. 10%

14. **Halitosis occurs with:**
    A. ACE Inhibitors
    B. Nitrate
    C. Beta blockers
    D. Statins

15. **Post perfusion syndrome occur due to:**
    A. Coxsackie- B virus
    B. CMV
    C. Staph aureus
    D. Influenza

16. **Nocturnal angina occurs with:**
    A. MR B. MS
    C. AR D. AS

17. **Syncope is least common in:**
    A. MS B. MR
    C. AS D. AR

18. **Postoperative ASD, second heart sound should be:**
    A. Wide and fixed split
    B. Normally split

C. Narrow split
D. Single S2

19. **Difference between VT from SVT in favor of VT is:**
A. Variable S1
B. Heart rate > 160 beats/min
C. Respond to carotid sinus massage
D. CHF in VT

20. **True about syncope is:**
A. Vasovagal occurs without warning
B. Fall in elderly most commonly due to syncope
C. Is a characteristic presentation in pericardial effusion
D. Exercise increase syncope in MR

21. **All are correct about massive pulmonary embolism *except*:**
A. RV systolic pressure > 65 mm Hg
B. Hemoptysis rare with infarction
C. Normal SpO_2 precludes pulmonary embolism
D. Chest X-ray and ECG may be normal

22. **Two-week post aortic valve replacement patient present with severe acute flank pain, fever - 100º F, Heart Rate - 100 beats/min, TLC - 14500/dl; DLC -P80 L15, 5% band forms, urine analysis - 15 RBC/HPF, protein - 3+, most probable diagnosis is:**
A. Renal infarction
B. Focal glomerulonephritis
C. Diffuse glomerulonephritis
D. Renal abscess

23. **About alcoholic cardiomyopathy true is:**
A. Global systolic dysfunction occurs early
B. Rarely associated chest pain, presence of which suggests CAD
C. More common in mixed drinkers than beer and wine
D. Uncommon in patient with alcohol cirrhosis and portal hypertension

24. **Regarding tricuspid valve disease true is:**
A. Associated endocarditis suggest IV drug abuser
B. TR causes more ascitis than TS
C. TS occur without mitral disease in RHD
D. TR is most commonly due to RHD

25. **Which is the systemic vasodilator and pulmonary vasoconstrictor?**
A. Serotonin B. Histamine
C. Tolazoline D. PGE2

26. **TORIC study involves:**
A. Torsemide B. Ramipril
C. Nerestide D. Ezetimibe

27. **True about beta blockers in heart failure is:**
A. Carvidelol better than metoprolol
B. Carvidelol = Metoprolol
C. Carvidelol less useful than metoprolol
D. None of the above

28. **Aortic dissection during pregnancy occurs most commonly in:**
A. 1st trimester
B. 2nd trimester
C. 3rd trimester
D. Rare during pregnancy

29. **All are true about anorexia nervosa *except*:**
A. Bradycardia
B. Hypertension
C. Hypercholesteremia
D. Syncope

30. **Pacing in myocardial infarction indicated in all *except*:**
A. IWMI with CHB with stable BP
B. Symptomatic infranodal block
C. RBBB with LAD in AWMI
D. CHB persisting 48 hours after AWMI

31. **In all reentry in mechanism of arrhythmia, *except*:**
A. Torsade de pointes
B. PSVT in WPW
C. VT
D. Atrial flutter

32. **Normal HV interval in:**
A. 35-55 sec B. 10-20 sec
C. 70-90 sec D. 30-200 sec

33. **Child with HOCM and family history of sudden cardiac death what should be done?**
A. No competitive sport
B. Non contact competitive sports allowed
C. Isometric sports allowed
D. Isotonic sports allowed

34. **Old hypertensive patient with LBBB with AWMI, BP - 140/80 mm Hg, HR – 80/min all should be done *except*:**
A. IV metoprolol followed by oral metoprolol
B. ACE inhibitor should be started
C. Pacing should be done
D. Admitted in ICU

35. **All are correct regarding CHF *except*:**
A. HTN is most common cause
B. Prognosis better in diastolic than systolic heart failure
C. Frank starling curve shift to down and right
D. LVF in independent of preload and dependent on afterload

36. All decrease BP *except*:
A. Isometric exercise
B. Sodium intake < 2gm/day
C. Calcium supplements
D. Calorie < 1000 Kcal/day

37. Bicuspid valve development to AS in:
A. 25% B. 33%
C. 65% D. 70%

38. Myocardial loss producing diastolic dysfunction is:
A. 20% B. 10%
C. 8% D. 12%

39. Which is correct regarding abnormal pulse?
A. Hyperkinetic pulse occurs in patient with increased stroke volume
B. Dicrotic pulse has two systolic peaks
C. Collapsing pulse seen in AS
D. Parvus et tardus seen in AR with AS

40. All are true about aortic dissection, *except*:
A. =25% mortality in 1st 24 hours
B. Conservative treatment preferred for uncomplicated proximal and distal dissection
C. Associated significant AR need AVR in all cases
D. Surgery better in proximal dissection

41. Statement true about atrial tachycardia with AV block is:
A. Digoxin with hypokalemia can cause
B. P wave simulates normal p wave (NSR) morphology
C. Respond to carotid sinus massage
D. Irregularly irregular pulse

42. All are true about ECG changes in myocarditis, *except*:
A. Increased QRS voltage
B. CHB
C. ST-T change
D. Tachycardia

43. Regarding myocardial contusion all are true *except*:
A. Increased technetium pyrophosphate uptake
B. CHF
C. Pericarditis ECG changes are present
D. Increased CPK MB levels

44. Regarding fibrinolytics true is:
A. APSAC more fibrin specific than STK
B. Patency rates approximately same for STK and t-PA in earlier angiography studies
C. GISSI-2 mortality same for t-PA and STK
D. t-PA and APSAC can be given repeatedly

45. Penetrating injury involving free wall most commonly in:
A. RV B. LV
C. RA D. LA

46. All are true regarding development of heart, *except*:
A. Aortic valve and ventricle develop from bulboventricular loop
B. Loop inversion gives rise to c-TGA
C. Sinus venosus, atria, aortic root develop from bulbo-ventricular loop and are intrapericardial
D. Ductus arteriosus develop from sixth aortic arch

47. Cardiac fluoroscopy voltage used is:
A. 51-70 B. 30-50
C. 90-120 D. None of the above

48. Regarding JVP true is:
A. Decrease in inspiration
B. Measured at suprasternal notch
C. Increase with anxiety like BP
D. 2 positive waves and 3 negative waves

49. PND does not occur with:
A. CCP
B. Left atrial myxoma
C. Supra mitral ring
D. Left ball valve thrombus

50. All are true about cardiac asthma, *except*:
A. All bronchial veins are tributaries of pulmonary vein, so pressure increases simultaneously in both
B. PND denotes interstitial and pulmonary edema denotes alveolar edema
C. Cardiac asthma occurs in subclinical heart disease with less severe cyanosis than bronchial asthma
D. Dyspnea occurs before cough

51. Square wave sign is seen in all *except*:
A. ASD B. MS
C. AS D. CHF

52. All are true regarding platelets, *except*:
A. Adhesion in first event in primary hemostasis
B. Activation produces release of granular contents
C. Specific receptors are involved in adhesion and aggregation
D. Platelet binds to fibrillar collagen in endothelial damage

53. CABG coagulation defect not found is:
A. Anti thrombin III deficiency
B. Fibrinolysis activation
C. Protamine reaction
D. Platelet dysfunction

54. True about angina is:
A. CABG improves survival in left main disease
B. Angioplasty improves symptom and subsequent survival

C. Due to total occlusion of LAD
D. No role of statins

55. **All are true about post MI perfusion imaging, *except*:**
A. Perfusion defects decreases with time
B. Thallium is impractical for looking for effect of thrombolytic therapy
C. PET scan can be used
D. MRI is useful

56. **All are true regarding beta myosin heavy chain, *except*:**
A. Myosis has 2 heavy chains and 4 light chains
B. Beta MCH mutation seen in HCM
C. Beta MHC is less than alpha MHC in adult and had less ATPase activity
D. ATPase activity is in head region of beta MHC

57. **Autosomal recessive is:**
A. Familial ASD
B. Holt Oram
C. Supravalvular AS
D. Ellis van Crevalled

58. **Regarding BP measurement true is:**
A. 1st Kortkoff sound indicates SBP
B. Inter observation variation in less in IV phase than V phase
C. Small cuff show falsely low BP
D. All are true

59. **First CABG done by:**
A. Kolosov and Favalloro
B. Garrett, Denis, DeBakey
C. Kerns and Little
D. None of the above

60. **String galvanometer discovered by:**
A. Protamie B. Ethovein
C. Marshard D. Pastuer

61. **Augmented limb lead increases voltage by:**
A. 25% B. 50%
C. 75% D. 100%

62. **False about ASD is:**
A. Ostium primum in usually associated with rsR, RVH and normal axis
B. All ASD have prolong PR interval
C. In children with large L → R shunt, cardiac catheterization show normal right sided pressure
D. ESM and MDM at lower sternal border

63. **Tumor associated with sudden cardiac death is:**
A. Fibroma B. Mesothelioma
C. Lymphoma D. Myxoma

64. **All are peripheral signs of wide pulse pressure *except*:**
A. De Musset sign
B. Hill sign
C. Square root sign
D. Pistol shot sounds

65. **Regarding cardiac metastasis all are true *except*:**
A. Endocardium and valves are less affected
B. Single cardiac mass is usually benign
C. Chylous pericardial effusion usually seen with breast carcinoma
D. Most common primary is bronchial carcinoma

66. **False positive TMT seen with all *except*:**
A. WPW syndrome B. Digoxin
C. Phenothiazine D. Hypokalemia

67. **Cardiac transplant is done when annual predicted survival is:**
A. <50% B. <25%
C. <10% D. <90%

68. **Type C RVH is seen with:**
A. COPD B. PS
C. IWMI D. PPH

69. **Endomyocardial fibrosis common in:**
A. Northern India
B. Southern India
C. East India
D. West India

70. **Regarding S1 true is:**
A. Paradoxical split seen in RBBB
B. Loud in LGL syndrome
C. Decreased intensity in MVP
D. Severe calcification and MS increases the S1 intensity

71. **Lipoprotein A associated with which apolipoprotein:**
A. B-100 B. B-48
C. A D. E

72. **Branham sign seen with:**
A. Systemic AV fistula
B. SLE
C. Bronchial collaterals
D. Rheumatic fever

73. **Regarding palpitation true is:**
A. Is due to pre-extra systolic beat
B. Is due to post-extra systolic beat
C. Common in MS
D. All

74. **Best view for LMCA calcification is:**
A. PA view B. LAO 60°
C. RAO 45° D. Left lateral

75. **Development of sudden acute symptomatic MR is seen in all *except*:**
   A. Marfan's syndrome
   B. IE
   C. Rheumatic fever
   D. MI

76. **Norepinephrine levels in heart failure is:**
   A. >500 pg/ml B. >1000 pg/ml
   C. > 2000 pg/ml D. > 10000 pg/ml

77. **Bainbridge reflex is:**
   A. Increased heart rate with increased vascular resistance
   B. Decreased heart rate with increased vascular resistance
   C. Increased heart rate with decreased vascular resistance
   D. Decreased heart rate with decreased vascular resistance

78. **Regarding MI true is:**
   A. Early Ventricular Fibrillation worse than late VF
   B. Early VF decreases the mortality
   C. Mortality with early and late VF is same
   D. None

79. **Conduction system development in fetus begins at:**
   A. 4th week
   B. 8th week
   C. 3rd week
   D. 20th week

80. **All are seen in heart failure *except*:**
   A. Increased norepinephrine levels
   B. Increased sodium
   C. Increased ANP
   D. Increased endothelin levels

81. **Eruptive xanthoma seen with:**
   A. Type I hyperlipidemia
   B. Type II hyperlipidemia
   C. Type IIIa hyperlipidemia
   D. Type III hyperlipidemia

82. **Most common tumor in children's:**
   A. Myxoma B. Rhabdomyoma
   C. Angiosarcoma D. Lymphoma

ANSWERS

1	C	2	B	3	A	4	D	5	A	6	A	7	A
8	A	9	B	10	A	11	C	12	B	13	A	14	B
15	B	16	C	17	B	18	A	19	A	20	C	21	C
22	A	23	D	24	A	25	B	26	A	27	A	28	C
29	B	30	A	31	A	32	A	33	A	34	C	35	A
36	A	37	B	38	C	39	A	40		41	A	42	A
43	C	44	C	45	A	46		47	C	48	A	49	A
50		51		52		53		54		55	C	56	D
57	D	58	A	59	A	60	B	61	B	62	C	63	
64	C	65	C	66	C	67	B	68		69	B	70	B
71	A	72	A	73	B	74	B	75	C	76	C	77	
78	B	79		80	B	81		82					

27

JAYADEVA 2011

1. **Which country men and women currently have the highest life expectancies in the world?**
   A. China B. America
   C. India D. Japan

2. **What is the murmur of rheumatic mitral regurgitation?**
   A. A low-pitched diastolic rumble with an opening snap, best heard at the apex
   B. A decrescendo, high-pitched diastolic murmur heard best at the lower left sternal border, starting almost with the second heart sound
   C. A holosytolic, high-pitched murmur that starts with the first heart sound and continues through the second heart sound, best heard at the apex and radiates either to the axilla or lower left sternal border
   D. A mid-systolic high-pitched murmur best heard at the apex and left sternal border, accompanied by one or more systolic clicks in half the cases

3. **Genomics is the study of gene function through the parallel measurements of genomes, most commonly using the techniques of:**
   A. cDNA microarrays
   B. Oligonucleotide arrays
   C. Serial analysis of gene expression (SAGE)
   D. All of the above

4. **Cardiovascular diagnostic criteria phenotypic manifestations include MVP, endocarditis, dysrhythmia, dilated annulus, MR, TVP, AR, aortic dissection and dilatation of the aortic root. The syndrome is:**
   A. Marfan's syndrome
   B. Ehlers-Danlos syndrome
   C. Down's syndrome
   D. Turner's syndrome

5. **Recognized abnormal response to the Valsalva's maneuver in heart failure includes:**
   A. Absence of phase IV overshoot
   B. The square response
   C. Both
   D. None

6. **Common diagnostic criteria for complete left bundle branch block include all *except*:**
   A. Broad, notched R waves in lateral precordial leads (V_5 and V_6) and usually leads I and aVL
   B. Absent septal Q waves in left-sided leads
   C. Small or absent initial R waves in right precordial leads (V_1 and V_2) followed by deep S waves
   D. Wide and deep S waves in left precordial leads (V_5 and V_6)

7. **According to ACC/AHA guidelines: Absolute contraindication to exercise testing include all *except*:**
   A. Acute myocardial infarction (within 2 days)
   B. Left main coronary stenosis
   C. High risk unstable angina
   D. Symptomatic severe aortic stenosis

8. **Incidence of coronary heart disease and sudden cardiac death is lowered by omega 3 fatty acids due to:**
   A. Anti-platelet and anti-inflammatory effects
   B. Enrichment of membrane phospholipids
   C. Reduction in risk for abnormal cardiac electrical conductivity
   D. All of the above

9. **Stunned myocardium include all *except*:**
   A. Responsible for postoperative pump dysfunction following cardiopulmonary bypass
   B. Also occurs after demand induced ischaemia
   C. Can be induced pharmacologically using adenosine
   D. Areas of stunned myocardium can coexist in the irreversibly injured myocardium

10. **Atrial infarction is:**
A. Common on left side then on right side
B. Frequently in atrial appendage than in lateral wall of atrium
C. Frequently in posterior wall of atrium
D. Linked to increased secretion of natriuretic peptide

11. **Relative contraindications to diagnostic cardiac catheterization include all *except*:**
A. Valvular heart disease
B. Acute gastrointestinal bleeding
C. Acute stroke
D. Acute renal failure

12. **Bezold-Jarisch reflex is associated with:**
A. Cerebral arteries
B. Hepatic artery
C. Coronary arteries
D. Pulmonary arterioles

13. **All are true thromboangiitis obliterans (TAO) *except*:**
A. TAO is a non-segmental vasculitis that affects the proximal arteries, veins and nerves
B. The precise cause of TAO is not known
C. No specific laboratory tests other than biopsy can diagnose TAO
D. The cornerstone of treatment is cessation of tobacco use

14. **Aspirin:**
A. Selective inhibitor of both Co_x- and Co_x-2
B. Antiplatelet effect lasts for the life time of platelets approximately 7–10 days
C. Plasma half-life is 1 hour
D. Does not prolong the bleeding time

15. **Difference between pre-eclampsia and chronic hypertension:**
A. After 20 weeks of pregnancy
B. Before 20 weeks of pregnancy
C. Elevated blood pressure after delivery
D. Left ventricular hypertrophy more common

16. **The most common side effect of β-blockers:**
A. Bronchospasm
B. Fatigue
C. Depression
D. Decreased sexual dysfunction

17. **β-adrenoceptor blocking drug with alpha blocking activity is:**
A. Propranolol B. Bisoprolol
C. Bucindolol D. Atenolol

18. **Least lipid soluble β-blocker is:**
A. Metoprolol B. Atenolol
C. Propranolol D. Timolol

19. **The key sensitive feature on physical examination in a patient with severe aortic stenosis is:**
A. Palpation of carotid upstroke (parvus and tardus)
B. Systolic pressure may be normal or increased
C. Pulse pressure may be normal or increased
D. A systolic thrill

20. **What is Gorlin formula for the calculation if stenotic mitral valve area?**
A. Valve area (cm^2) = (cardiac output/heart rate) × diastolic filling period/37.7 × square root of mean gradient across valve
B. Valve area (cm^2) = cardiac output/square root of mean valve gradient
C. Valve area (cm^2) = (cardiac output/heart rate) × systolic period/44.3 × square root of mean valve gradient
D. None of the above

21. **A seventy-year-old man is admitted to the hospital with chest pain of 3 hours duration. ECG demonstrates anterior ST elevation for which he is given aspirin, r–TPA, heparin and intravenous nitroglycerin. His symptoms resolve. Serum chemistries reveal a peak CPK of 1800 and a CK–MB fraction of 15%. He is eventually transferred out of the CCU and his hospitalization is uneventful until day 5, when he develops sudden, severe shortness of breath. BP is 110/75 and his pulse is 125 and regular. Examination reveals a new systolic murmur. What would the most appropriate therapeutic intervention be?**
A. Intravenous nitroglycerine
B. Intravenous sodium nitroprusside
C. Surgical repair of VSD
D. Intra-aortic balloon counterpulsation

22. **A 65-year-old female presents to the hospital with sudden crushing chest discomfort and moderate shortness of breath. Her initial ECG reveals 2 mm ST depression in leads V_1–V_4 with inverted T waves. She has bibasilar rales in the lower half of both lungs on auscultation. CXR reveals moderate pulmonary edema. Serial ECG's and CPK's confirm a non-Q wave myocardial infarction. With diuretics, her pulmonary edema resolves within 24 hours. What is the most appropriate management strategy at this point?**
A. Observation
B. CT angiography
C. Cardiac catheterization with coronary angiography
D. Medical treatment

23. **Effort syncope is seen in:**
A. Severe LMCA stenosis
B. Straight back syndrome
C. Pulmonary AV fistula
D. Persistent LSVC to LA

24. **Oxygen step up in RV is seen in:**
A. PDA with PR
B. RSOV into LA
C. Sinus venosus ASD
D. Cortriatriatum

25. **Absence of ischemia is noticed in the following coronary anomalies *except*:**
A. Split RCA
B. Ectopic RCA from right cusp
C. Anomalous left coronary artery from the pulmonary artery
D. Ectopic RCA from left cusp

26. **Pacing: true is:**
A. Pacemaker mediated tachycardia is seen in VVI pacing
B. DDD pacing causes less of atrial arrhythmia than VVI
C. Biventricular pacing in HOCM is beneficial
D. VVI is useful in CHF

27. **Counterclockwise QRS is seen in all *except*:**
A. DORV
B. Tricuspid atresia
C. Pulmonary atresia
D. ECD

28. **In Mason-Likar modification, all are true *except*:**
A. Q waves appears in aVL
B. Voltage increases in inferior leads
C. Absent Q waves in inferior leads
D. There is left axis deviation

29. **Worst prognosis arrhythmia that may be due to acquired/congenital LQTS:**
A. Torsade de pointes
B. Ventricular tachycardia
C. Ventricular fibrillation
D. Monomorphic ventricular tachycardia

30. **Decrease amplitude in fast flushing method for measurement of invasive intra-arterial pressure indicates:**
A. High damping coefficient with low systolic BP
B. High damping coefficient with high systolic BP
C. Low damping coefficient with low systolic BP
D. Low damping coefficient with high systolic BP + Diastolic BP

31. **Hamilton Stewart equation used for calculation of:**
A.. Cardiac output B. Blood volume
C. Chamber pressure D. Valve area

32. **A 45-year-old male presenting with acute ASML treatment of choice would be:**
A. Aspirin + Reopro + PTCA/Stent
B. Aspirin + Reopro + LMWH
C. Aspirin + Reopro + Tenecteplase
D. Aspirin + PTCA/Stent + Clopidogrel

33. **Inhalation of 100% oxygen in normal person causes:**
A. Proportional increase in SaO_2 + PaO_2 + Venous oxygen saturation
B. Proportional increase in SaO_2 + PaO_2 + but not Venous oxygen saturation
C. Proportional increase in SaO_2 but not PaO_2 and Venous oxygen saturation
D. Proportional increase in PaO_2 but not SaO_2

34. **PGE infusion is used to keep PDA patent in all *except*:**
A. Pulmonary atresia with intact septum
B. Severe CoA
C. Corrected TGA
D. Hypertrophic obstructive cardiomyopathy

35. **Restenosis with drug-eluting stent:**
A. 0–2% B. 4–8%
C. 10% D. 12%

36. **Abio Cor is:**
A. Total artificial heart
B. Micromed debakey ventricular assist device
C. Anti-apoptotic heart
D. Paracorporeal pulsatile device

37. **Large anterior wall MI apical thrombus; drug to be given lifelong are *except*:**
A. Aspirin B. β-blockers
C. ACE inhibitors D. Warfarin

38. **Reverse pulsus paradoxus is seen in all the following *except*:**
A. Hypertrophic cardiomyopathy
B. Positive pressure ventilation
C. Isorhythmic dissociation
D. Diaphragmatic palsy

39. **TMT is used in all *except*:**
A. Diagnosis of unstable angina
B. Post CABG
C. Males with atypical symptoms
D. Post MI with stent implantation

40. **VY descent in Wiggers cycle corresponds to:**
A. End of early diastolic filling
B. End of ejection

C. End of isovolumetric relaxation
D. Onset of isovolumetric relaxation

41. **Drug of choice for aspirin allergy is:**
A. Dipyridamole B. Ticlopidine
C. Sulfinpyrazone D. Clopidogrel

42. **Brockenborough phenomenon is:**
A. Decrease systolic pressure in post ectopic beat
B. Decrease pulse pressure in post ectopic beat
C. Decrease diastolic pressure in post ectopic beat
D. Decrease aortic systolic pressure in post ectopic beat

43. **Treatment for NSTEMI includes all *except*:**
A. Thrombolysis B. Antiplatelets
C. β-blockers D. Anticoagulants

44. **ACE inhibitor is contraindicated in:**
A. Unilateral renal artery stenosis
B. Bilateral renal artery stenosis
C. Renal failure with 2–3 mg%
D. Diabetic nephropathy

45. **TPI in AWMI is done in all *except*:**
A. RBBB with LAHB
B. Transient 2: 1 block
C. Transient CHB
D. AMI with LBBB

46. **Most common cause of low output heart failure in the world is:**
A. Anaemia B. Beriberi
C. Thyrotoxicosis D. Chagas' disease

47. **On average, how long does a patient with severe aortic stenosis have to live after developing symptoms of heart failure?**
A. One year B. Two years
C. Three years D. Five years

48. **MI in presence of LBBB is diagnosed by all *except*:**
A. > 3 mm ST in increased V_1 V_2
B. Q in I aVL, V_5 V_6
C. Slurring upstroke in V_3 V_4
D. Primary SI–T changes in V_5 V_6

49. **Poor prognostic factors for SCD in HOCM are:**
A. Age < 30 years
B. VT on Holter
C. Family history positive
D. Severity of gradient across LVOT

50. **Restenosis will be least with:**
A. Concentric lesion < 10 mm
B. > 10 mm
C. Prox graft stent (SVG)
D. Total occlusion

51. **Renal osteodystrophy can be differentiated from nutritional and genetic forms of Vitamin D deficiency effect by having:**
A. Hypophosphatemia
B. Hyperphosphatemia
C. Hypocalcemia
D. Hypercalcemia

52. **All of the following are known to worsen hyperkalemia in a patient renal failure *except*:**
A. Spironolactone B. ACE inhibitors
C. Furosemide D. Amiloride

53. **All are true statements about "Behcet's syndrome", *except*:**
A. Recurrent aphthous ulcerations are a sine qua non for the diagnosis
B. In endemic areas the syndrome is associated with HL A–B5
C. Neurological involvement are seen in 80%
D. Superficial or deep peripheral vein thrombosis

54. **All of the following are Jones Major Criteria for rheumatic fever, *except*:**
A. Erythema nodosum
B. Migratory polyarthritis
C. Sydenham's chorea
D. Subcutaneous nodules

55. **Which one of the following drugs is the most common cause of progressive multifocal leukoencephalopathy?**
A. Natalizumab B. Cituximab
C. Rituximab D. Bevacizumab

56. **Tumor lysis syndrome is associated with all of the following laboratory features, *except*:**
A. Hyperkalemia
B. Hypercalcemia
C. Hyperuricemia
D. Hyperphosphatemia

57. **A high amylase level in pleural fluid suggests a diagnosis of:**
A. Tuberculosis
B. Malignancy
C. Rheumatoid arthritis
D. Pulmonary infarction

58. **All of the following are true about retinoic acid syndrome *except*:**
A. Vitamin A toxicity
B. Pulmonary features of dyspnea
C. Due to mature neoplasm cell adhering to alveoli/pulmonary capillary infiltrates
D. Cause 10% of mortality rate

59. **Antidote of paracetamol is:**
A. N-acetylcysteine
B. Methylene blue
C. EDTA
D. No effective antidote known

60. **Pseudoporphyria can be induced by all *except*:**
A. Methotrexate B. Infliximab
C. Naproxen D. 5-Fluorouracil

61. **Which one of the following is the correct statement regarding findings in JVP?**
A. Cannon wave: Complete heart block
B. Slow '*y*' descent: Tricuspid stenosis
C. Giant '*c*' wave: Tricuspid stenosis
D. Increased JVP with prominent pulsations: SVC obstruction

62. **A woman presents with amenorrhoea, infertility and galactorrhea. On CT scan, there is enlarged sella turcica. The diagnosis of the disease can be established by investigation of the following:**
A. Prolactin levels B. ADH levels
C. TSH levels D. LH levels

63. **All of the following are true about Warfarin therapeutic usage *except*:**
A. The INR is maintained between 2 and 3
B. It is very useful in the prophylaxis of thromboembolism
C. Its effect is monitored by observing the clotting time
D. Used in DVT

64. **Management of febrile neutropenic patients on anti-cancer therapy include all *except*:**
A. Colony stimulating factors
B. Transfusion of granulocytes
C. Antibiotic prophylaxis
D. Repeated hand washing

65. **Adverse effects of amiodarone include all *except*:**
A. Corneal deposits
B. Thyroid dysfunction
C. Pulmonary fibrosis
D. Hypertension

66. **All of the following are associated with kerosene poisoning *except*:**
A. Signs minimal
B. Gastric lavage is done
C. Antibiotics not routinely indicated
D. Present with pneumonitis

67. **Least extrapyramidal side effects are seen with the following drug:**
A. Clozapine B. Haloperidol
C. Thioridazine D. Trifluoperazine

68. **All of the following causes Guillain-Barré syndrome, *except*:**
A. Mycoplasma B. Legionella
C. EBV D. Campylobacter

69. **Chorea is commonly seen in all the following systemic diseases *except*:**
A. SLE
B. Hyperthyroidism
C. Infections including HIV
D. Addison's disease

70. **All are seen in dengue hemorrhagic fever *except*:**
A. Leucopenia
B. Relative lymphocytosis
C. Decreased hematocrit level
D. Thrombocytopenia

71. **Hemolytic uremic syndrome causing most commonly anti-cancer drug is:**
A. Mitomycin C
B. Ifosfamide
C. Vincristine
D. Cyclophosphamide

72. **Hemorrhagic cystitis is caused by:**
A. Polyoma virus B. Adenovirus
C. Coxsackie virus D. Parvovirus

73. **All are true regarding non-typhoidal salmonella fever *except*:**
A. Most commonly due to consumption of poultry related foods
B. Typically presents as enterocolitis
C. Very small infective dose required to produce salmonellosis
D. Non-response to routine treatment

74. **Not seen in association with hepatitis C virus:**
A. Lichen planus
B. Essential cryoglobulinemia
C. Porphyria cutanea tarda
D. PAN

75. **An elderly patient with hypertension with diabetes, proteinuria without renal failure, the anti-hypertensive of choice is:**
A. Furosemide B. Methyldopa
C. Enalapril D. Propranolol

76. **A 10-year-old boy gets drowned and stays under water for 20 minutes, what should you do?**
A. Barbiturate infusion
B. Steroid administration
C. Cardiac massage
D. Wait and watch

77. A boy can climb up and down stairs one step at a time jump, build a tower of 10 cubes, open a door, use 3 words in a sentence. What is his minimum age?
A. 20 months
B. 24 months
C. 30 months
D. 36 months

78. The Baby-Friendly Hospital Initiative (BFHI) is not an initiative:
A. Every 4 hourly breast-feeding
B. Give breast-feeding to infants within 4 hours of caesarean
C. Initiate breast-feeding within a half-hour of birth
D. Encourage breast-feeding on demand

79. A 6-month-old infant presents with an early feature of vomiting, more severe diarrhea, mild to moderate fever and dehydration. The possible infection is due to:
A. Norwalk virus
B. Rota virus
C. Shigella
D. E. coli

80. Which is not an indication for bone marrow transplantation?
A. Severe combined immunodeficiency disease
B. Wiskott-Aldrich's syndrome
C. Ataxia telangiectasia
D. Chronic granulomatous disease

81. All of the following are true regarding HbH disease *except*:
A. Deletion of 3 of the 4 alpha-globin genes
B. Hypochromia and microcytosis
C. More common in Africa
D. Does not precipitate in circulating RBCs

82. Congenital rubella syndrome is associated with all *except*:
A. Blindness
B. Neural deafness
C. Hutchinson's teeth
D. Hepatosplenomegaly

83. Growth disturbance is seen in all of the following *except*:
A. Osteopetrosis B. Diaphysial aclasia
C. Achondroplasia D. Osteomalacia

84. What is the cutoff point for mid-arm circumference in estimation of the body's muscle mass?
A. 10.5 cms B. 11.5 cms
C. 12.5 cms D. 13.5 cms

85. Umbilical discharge in a child is commonly due to:
A. Patent vitellointestinal duct
B. Patent urachus
C. Umbilical hernia
D. Umbilical adenoma

86. In Dubin Johnson syndrome what is not seen?
A. Alkaline phosphatase
B. Reversal of coproporphyrin ratio
C. OCP exacerbate
D. Conjugated hyperbilirubinemia

87. Young child with febrile seizures develops status epilepticus. What should be ideally done?
A. Start anti-convulsants after taking detailed history from attendant
B. Clonazepam I.V.
C. Diazepam per rectal
D. No treatment required, just maintain the airway

88. "Constrictive pericarditis" is a feature of all *except*:
A. Pyogenic pericarditis
B. Tuberculous pericarditis
C. Rheumatic pericarditis
D. Neoplastic pericarditis

89. Percentage of HbF in a 6-month-old infant is:
A. 10% B. 30%
C. 50% D. 60%

90. Antibiotic prophylaxis to a child with rheumatic heart disease should be given minimum till:
A. At least 5 years after onset
B. Lifelong
C. Till 17 years
D. Till 21 years

ANSWERS

1	D	2	C	3	D	4	A	5	C	6	D	7	B
8	D	9	C	10	B	11	A	12	C	13	B	14	B
15	A	16	B	17	C	18	B	19	A	20	D	21	C
22	C	23	A	24	A	25	C	26	B	27	C	28	D
29	C	30	A	31	A	32	A	33	C	34		35	B
36	A	37	D	38	D	39	A	40	A	41	D	42	B
43	A	44	B	45	D	46	D	47	B	48	A	49	
50	A	51	B	52	C	53	C	54	A	55	A	56	B
57	B	58	A	59	A	60		61	A	62	A	63	C
64	B	65	D	66	B	67	A	68	B	69	D	70	C
71	A	72	B	73	C	74	D	75	C	76	C	77	D
78	A	79	B	80	C	81		82	C	83	D	84	
85	A	86	A	87	C	88	C	89	A	90	B		

28

JAYADEVA 2010

1. **The drug to be avoided in patients with known coronary artery disease when treat muscular skeletal symptoms:**
   A. Acetaminophen
   B. Non-acetylated salicylates
   C. Non-Cox-2 selective non-steroidal anti-inflammatory drugs
   D. Cox-2 selective non-steroidal anti-inflammatory drug

2. **In CHF, angiotensin receptor blockers are a reasonable alternative to ACE inhibitors in ACEI intolerant patients due to the following reasons *except*:**
   A. Angioedema
   B. Irritant cough
   C. Renal insufficiency
   D. Skin rash

3. **Rapid 'Y' descend in JVP excludes the diagnosis of:**
   A. Cardiac tamponade
   B. RV myocardial infarction
   C. Restrictive cardiomyopathy
   D. Constrictive pericarditis

4. **The following are normally branches from the left anterior descending artery *except*:**
   A. Recurrent lateral artery
   B. Posterior ascending artery
   C. Left atrial circumflex artery
   D. Septal artery

5. **In setting of acute MI, severe systemic hypoxemia due to intracardiac shunting can occur with:**
   A. RV myocardial infarction
   B. Ventricular septal rupture
   C. LV papillary muscle rupture
   D. LV free wall rupture

6. **Current role of GP IIb/IIIa inhibitors in acute STEMI:**
   A. Immediately on arrival to all patients proceeding for primary angioplasty
   B. Half dose fibrinolytic agent with full dose GP IIb/IIIa inhibitor as reperfusion strategy
   C. GP IIb/IIIa inhibitor in the cath lab, just prior to primary angioplasty
   D. GP IIb/IIIa agents as an alternative to fibrinolytic agents in all low risk STEMI patients

7. **Regarding Dressler's syndrome – Not true:**
   A. Usually occurs 1-8 weeks after MI
   B. Leukocytosis is a feature
   C. Aspirin is the drug of choice
   D. NSAIDs and steroids are helpful in refractory cases

8. **The boundaries of 'Triangle of Koch' does not include:**
   A. Tendon of Todaro
   B. Coronary sinus
   C. Tricuspid annulus
   D. Crista terminalis

9. **Which statement is false?**
   A. Anterior mitral leaflet has a significantly larger surface area compared to posterior mitral leaflet
   B. Anterior mitral leaflet has close to double the width from annulus to its free margin, compared to posterior mitral leaflet
   C. Anterior leaflet occupies only half the annular circumference as compared to posterior mitral leaflet
   D. Closure line of both mitral leaflets is not at the margins of the leaflets but a few mm within

10. **Which of the following is not associated with coronary sinus?**
   A. Vein of Marshall/Ligament of Marshall
   B. Thebesian valve

C. Rahib's ASD
D. Pectinate muscle

11. **Initial drugs of choice, for a young black American with essential hypertension when compared to whites:**
A. Beta blocker and diuretics
B. ACEI and diuretics
C. Calcium channel blockers and beta blockers
D. Diuretics and calcium channel blocker

12. **Regular pulse with changing pulse volume:**
A. Complete heart block
B. Atrial based pacemaker (AAI) for severe sinus bradycardia
C. CHB with atrial fibrillation
D. 2 : 1 AV block

13. **Not a risk factor for aortic dissection:**
A. Diabetes mellitus
B. Pregnancy
C. Coarctation of aorta
D. Bicuspid aortic valve

14. **Most common splanchnic artery aneurysm:**
A. Hepatic artery
B. Splenic artery
C. Superior mesenteric artery
D. Inferior mesenteric artery

15. **Most common site of peripheral arterial aneurysm from the following:**
A. Iliac arteries
B. Femoral arteries
C. Popliteal arteries
D. Posterior tibial arteries

16. **Risk factors for aortic aneurysm rupture include the following *except*:**
A. Male gender
B. Hypertension
C. Aneurysm diameter
D. Rate of increase in aneurysm diameter

17. **In mitral regurgitation jet spectral envelop, if the time taken for the MR jet velocity to attain velocity 3 m/s from velocity 1 m/s is 30 mili-seconds, then dp/dt is:**
A. 1200 mmHg/sec
B. 1066 mmHg/sec
C. 920 mmIIg/sec
D. 1080 mmHg/sec

18. **Identify the condition with the highest cardiac output and the widest difference in arteriovenous oxygen content:**
A. Systemic arterior venous fistula
B. High altitude dwellers
C. Severe anaemia
D. Maximal exercise

19. **When SVC O_2 saturation is 40% with arterial saturation 98% one must suspect:**
A. Hypoventilation
B. Low cardiac output state
C. High altitude physiology
D. Variation in normal basal resting hemodynamics

20. **Flow murmur of across the mitral valve is not a feature of:**
A. Anemia
B. Pulmonary arteriovenous fistula (pulmonary)
C. Thyrotoxicosis
D. Systemic arteriovenous fistula

21. **Described as a crescendo-decrescendo murmur:**
A. Graham Steel murmur
B. Murmur of acute AR
C. Murmur of AR due to everted aortic cusps
D. Pulmonary regurgitation due to absent pulmonary valve

22. **Which of these statements is not true for arterio sclerosis of hypertension?**
A. It has diffuse distribution along the course of the vessel
B. It affects the arterial media
C. It is primarily due to collagen fragmentation and loss of collagen
D. It is one cause of age related rise in arterial systolic pressure

23. **Most common mechanical complication resulting in cardiogenic shock:**
A. LV free wall rupture
B. LV septal rupture
C. RV infarction
D. LV pump failure

24. **Least common organism isolated in early prosthetic valve endocarditis, from the following:**
A. Staph aureus
B. Gram negative bacilli
C. Streptococci
D. Fungi

25. **LV wall stress peaks in:**
A. Early systole B. Mid systole
C. End systole D. End diastole

26. **Which of the following events occurs farthest from aortic component of second heart sound?**
A. Physiological third heart sound
B. Third heart sound of LV systolic dysfunction
C. Tumor plop of LA myxoma
D. Pericardial knock of constrictive pericarditis

27. If systolic time interval is defined as the ratio of LV ejection time to pre ejection time, then systolic time interval is likely to be the least in:
A. Severe systemic hypertension
B. Aortic stenosis with preserved LV function
C. Dilated cardiomyopathy
D. Low gradient AS with LV dysfunction

28. Which of the following is a cyanotic condition?
A. Hemi anomalous pulmonary venous connection
B. Post Hemi Fontan surgery
C. Hemitruncus
D. AV canal defect

29. A typical well defined left anterior descending artery is not a feature of:
A. Double outlet RV
B. Transposition of great vessels
C. Single ventricle
D. Corrected transposition of great vessels

30. In the fetus, amongst the following, blood snowing across .... has are highest oxygen saturation.
A. Aortic isthmus
B. The tricuspid valve
C. The pulmonary veins into LA
D. Right hepatic vein

31. Kearns Sayre syndrome is characterized by the triad which includes the following *except*:
A. Cardiomyopathy
B. External ophthalmoplegia
C. Pigmentary degeneration of the retina
D. Cardiac conduction blocks

32. In the infant, aorta to pulmonary artery shunt through PDA will result in stepdown in oxygen saturation in pulmonary artery in:
A. Truncus arteriosus
B. Tricuspid atresia
C. Transposition of great vessels
D. Obstructed TAPVC

33. The most important difference between a mild form of tetralogy and severe form of Tetralogy of Fallot is:
A. Marked difference in RVOF gradient
B. Marked difference in RVOF impedance
C. Marked difference in RV systolic pressure
D. Marked difference in RV filling pressure

34. A widely patent aortic valve may remain completely closed during the entire cardiac cycle after:
A. Arterial switch surgery for TGA
B. Double switch surgery for corrected TGA
C. Damus Kaye Stansel procedure
D. Post Fontan surgery

35. Cyanosis completely disappear with administration of 100% oxygen in:
A. Central hypoventilation
B. Simple TGA
C. Methemoglobinemia
D. Sulfhemoglobinemia

36. Highly specific for RV hypertrophy in a neonate:
A. Tall 'R' with inverted 'T' waves in V1 beyond first week of life
B. Deep 'S' with upright 'T' waves in V1 within 7 days of life
C. Tall 'R' waves with upright 'T' waves in V1 beyond first week of life
D. Tall 'R' waves with upright 'T' waves in the V1 at birth

37. Prostaglandin (PGE1) infusion to maintain ductal patency may not be useful in:
A. Hypoplastic left heart syndrome
B. Hypoplastic right heart syndrome
C. Interrupted aortic arch
D. Obstructed TAPVC

38. Which statement is false for sinus of valsalva aneurysm from right sinus, as compared to those from the non-coronary sinus?
A. More commonly associated with VSD
B. More likely to rupture into RA than RVOF
C. More commonly associated with aortic incompetence
D. Far more common than aneurysm from non-coronary sinus

39. Highest fatality to mother with pregnancy is associated with:
A. Surgically corrected TOF
B. Fontan repair
C. Surgically corrected TGA
D. Eisenmenger syndrome

40. Beta-blocker with beta 1 selectivity and intrinsic partial agonist activity:
A. Pindolol B. Nadolol
C. Acebutalol D. Esmolol

41. First heart sound (S1) can be constant in intensity in complete heart block, when associated with the following, *except*:
A. On DDD pacing B. On VDD pacing
C. VVIR pacing D. Atrial fibrillation

42. Sinus node artery, AV nodal artery and acute marginal artery, all three can arise from:
A. Dominant right coronary artery
B. Dominant left circumflex artery

C. From either
D. From neither

43. Is not included as a feature of LAHB:
A. QRS axis between –45 and –90
B. RS pattern in II, III and aVF
C. QRS duration 120 ms
D. Persistent 'S' waves in V_6

44. Anti-arrhythmic drug which causes QRS widening, without significant QT lengthening:
A. Sotalol B. Amiodarone
C. Quinidine D. Flecainide

45. The most useful information with regard to autonomic nervous system function is obtained during .... and .... phases of valsalva maneuver.
A. Phase I and III B. Phase II and III
C. Phase I and IV D. Phase II and IV

46. When blood pressure elevation during pregnancy is noted at 12-16 weeks of gestation, one must suspect:
A. Gestational hypertension
B. Chronic/essential hypertension
C. Pre eclampsia
D. Eclampsia

47. Thiazide diuretic cause the following changes in serum/blood:
A. Increase HCO_3 B. Increase Cl–
C. Increase Na+ D. Increase Mg++

48. The following drugs have been found to be therapeutically useful in treatment of active Takayasu's arteritis, *except*:
A. Cyclophosphamide
B. Methotrexate
C. Colchicine
D. Prednisolone

49. Drug of choice for cyclosporine induced hypertension:
A. Beta-blocker
B. Calcium channel blocker
C. ACE inhibitors
D. Diuretics

50. Popliteal artery entrapment syndrome is often linked to:
A. Soleus muscle
B. Gastrocnemius muscle
C. Quadriceps muscle
D. Sartorius muscle

51. Turbulence of flow of fluid in duct/pipe is inversely related to:
A. Velocity of flow
B. Diameter of the pipe
C. Viscosity of the fluid
D. Density of the fluid

52. Hemodynamic changes in pregnancy include:
A. Increase in systematic vascular resistance
B. Increase in cardiac output
C. Maximal increase in left atrial pressure in mitral stenosis in first trimester
D. Non-tolerance of regurgitatnt lesion

53. Evaluation of pregnant lady with hypertension and aortic coarctation should include:
A. Chest X-ray, electrocardiogram and echo Doppler studies
B. Electrocardiogram, echo Doppler studies and CT angiogram
C. Electrocardiogram, echo Doppler studies and MR angiogram
D. Cardiac catheterization and assessment of hemodynamics

54. The disorder where you would consider pregnancy to be contraindicated is:
A. Mitral regurgitation
B. Aortic regurgitation
C. Atrial septal defect
D. Pulmonary arterial hypertension

55. Which of the following is not a predictor of sudden death in an otherwise healthy individual with no structural heart disease or metabolic dearrangement?
A. Markedly prolonged PR interval of 0.36 ms
B. QTc 0.245 ms
C. QTc 580 ms
D. Epsilon wave in right precordial leads

56. The body organ with the most adverse ratio of oxygen consumption to blood supply:
A. Kidney B. Heart
C. Liver D. Brain

57. Acute exposure to high altitude results in:
A. Increase arterial $PaCO_2$
B. Increase arterial in PaO_2
C. Increase systemic vascular resistance
D. Increase in cardiac output

58. The organisms predominating in hospital acquired pneumonia are:
A. P. aeruginosa
B. Acinetobacter spp.
C. MDR enterobacteriaceae
D. All of the above

59. **The most effective management of catheter related urinary tract infection is:**
A. Removal of the catheter
B. Systemic antibiotic treatment
C. Topical metal antimicrobial
D. Drainage bag disinfectants

60. **Preparation for surgery for patients with pheochromocytoma include:**
A. Alpha-blockade
B. Volume expansion
C. High-salt diet
D. All of the above

61. **The most important treatment of non-alcoholic fatty liver disease is:**
A. Weight loss
B. UDCA (Ursodeoxycholic acid)
C. Glitazones
D. Statins

62. **H. pylori is a cofactor in the development of all *except*:**
A. Duodenal or gastric ulcers
B. Gastric cancer
C. Gastric mucosa-associated lymphoid-tissue (MALT) lymphoma
D. Barrett's esophagus

63. **In COPD corticosteroid treatment that is likely to benefit severely symptomatic patients is:**
A. 40 mg of prednisone taken once daily for 10 to 14 days
B. 40 mg of prednisone taken once daily for upto 8 weeks
C. 10 mg of prednisone taken once daily for 10 to 14 days
D. Not beneficial at all

64. **Effective drugs used in treatment of hepatic encephalopathy include all *except*:**
A. Lactulose
B. Rifaximin
C. Neomycin
D. Vitamin supplementation

65. **The standard background therapy for patients with heart failure is:**
A. Angiotensin-converting-enzyme (ACE) inhibitors + Beta blockers
B. ACE inhibitors + Calcium channel blockers
C. Beta blockers + Digoxin
D. Beta blockers + Spironolactone

66. **The most common cause of Cushing's syndrome is:**
A. Secretion of corticotrophin from the pituitary gland
B. Adrenal tumours
C. Iatrogenic administration of exogenous glucocorticoids
D. Ectopic production of corticotrophin

67. **Asthmatic attacks may be triggered by all of the following *except*:**
A. Viral respiratory infections
B. Airborne allergens
C. Cold air
D. Food

68. **In patients with COPD, prognosis can be improved by all *except*:**
A. Cessation of smoking
B. Oxygen therapy
C. Lung volume reduction
D. Use of mucolytic agents

69. **Lung abscess is a common complication of infection caused by:**
A. Anaerobic bacteria
B. Influenza virus
C. Mycoplasma pneumoniae
D. Legionella pneumophilia

70. **The classic form of HCV-related glomerular disease is:**
A. Membranoproliferative glomerulonephritis
B. Membranous glomerulonephritis
C. Fibrillary glomerulonephritis
D. Focal segmental glomerulosclerosis

71. **Most common is HIV-associated nephropathy is:**
A. Mesangio capillary glomerulonephritis
B. Collapsing glomerular lesions in the kidney biopsy
C. Chronic renal failure
D. Hypertensive nephrosclerosis

72. **In patients who have HIV and HCV co-infection the most appropriate treatment option is:**
A. Combination of pegylated interferon (pegiinterferon) alfa and weight-based ribavirin for 24 weeks
B. Combination of pegylated interferon (peginterferon) alfa and weight-based ribavirin for 48 weeks
C. Use of HAART alone
D. None of the above

73. **The emergency treatment options for acute stroke within 3-4 hours include:**
A. Intravenous recombinant tissue plasminogen activator (rt-PA)
B. Endovascular interventions
C. Mechanical embolectomy

D. Intra-arterial thrombolysis

74. Definite indications for initiation of anti-retroviral therapy include all *except*:
A. Acute infection syndrome
B. Chronic infection with symptoms
C. Asymptomatic diseases CD4+ T-cell count <350/μL
D. All of the above

75. Which one of the following tests measure biosynthetic liver function?
A. Blood ammonia
B. AST and ALT
C. Serum prothrombin time
D. Serum bilirubin

76. The duration of treatment with oral anti-coagulants in patients with first episode of idiopathic of DVT and pulmonary embolism is:
A. 3-6 months B. 6-12 months
C. 12-24 months D. Lifelong

77. In nosocomial urinary tract infections, the following are true *except*:
A. Treatment of candiduria is indicated in obstruction
B. Recovery of S. aureus in urine culture should be treated with systemic antibiotics
C. Irrigation of catheters with antimicrobial agents is recommended
D. In chronic indwelling bladder catheterization, it is necessary to replace the catheter and obtains fresh sample for culture

78. The most common presentation of primary hyperparathyroidism is:
A. Peptic ulcer
B. Proximal limb weakness
C. Renal stones
D. Asymptomatic

79. Oral anticoagulant induced skin necrosis is associated with:
A. Antithrombin III deficiency
B. Plasminogen deficiency
C. Protein C deficiency
D. Protein S deficiency

80. Which one of the following is not a high anion gap acidosis?
A. Ketoacidosis
B. Lactic acidosis
C. Chronic renal failure
D. Diarrhoea

81. The severity of beta thalassemia can be ameliorated by:
A. Co inheritance of alpha thalassemia
B. Co inheritance of Hb E
C. Presence of iron deficiency
D. Presence of iron overload

82. Polycythemia vera rubra is characterised by:
A. Splenomegaly
B. Hyperviscosity symptoms
C. Presence of JAK 2 mutation
D. Elevated levels of plasma erythropoietin

83. Which of the following organisms would be most likely to cause infection in a splenectomised patient?
A. Streptococcus pneumoniae
B. Hemophilus influenza
C. E. coli
D. Plasmodium vivax

84. Protein conjugate pneumococcal vaccine rather than capsular polysaccharide vaccine is recommended in:
A. Adults more than 65 years
B. Patients with CSF leak
C. Children less than 2 years
D. Patients with HIV

85. In Wernicke's aphasia, which of the following is preserved?
A. Comprehension
B. Repetition of spoken language
C. Naming
D. Fluency

86. WHO defines anaemia in women as a hemoglobin level of:
A. Less than 14 gm/dl
B. Less than 13 gm/dl
C. Less than 12 gm/dl
D. Less than 11 gm/dl

87. The following is true of tuberculous arthritis *except*:
A. It involves large weight bearing joints
B. Normal chest X-ray
C. Absence of fever
D. Coexisting osteomyelitis

88. Clinical identification of metabolic syndrome does not include:
A. Waist circumference as indicator of abdominal obesity
B. LDL cholesterol
C. Triglyceride level
D. Fasting blood glucose

89. **Significant action on dopaminergic receptors:**
A. Dobutamine B. Dopexamine
C. Vasopressin D. Epinephrine

90. **Beta blockers are recommended as first line anti-arrhythmic therapy in the following *except*:**
A. Long QT syndrome
B. RVOF VT
C. Brugada syndrome
D. Arrhythmogenic RV dysplasia

91. **Gooseneck deformity in angiography is a feature of (a) Common atrium (b) Partial AV canal defect (c) Complete AV canal defect:**
A. a, b, c B. a, b
C. b, c D. c, a

92. **Bivaluridin's indicators include the following, *except*:**
A. In patients with heparin induced thrombocytopenia
B. For medical management of STEMI in place of heparin
C. For primary PCI in STEMI
D. For PCI in NSTEMI

93. **Proarrhythmic effect is typically occurrence of monomorphic VT rather than torsade de pointes:**
A. Flecainide B. Sotalol
C. Quinidine D. Dofetilide

94. **Which statement/s is/are true for Streptokinase compared to tissue plasminogen activator?**
A. Direct plasminogen activator
B. Longer half life
C. Fibrin selective
D. None true

95. **Drug with K+ channel blocking and Na+ channel enhancing action:**
A. Flecainide B. Ibutilide
C. Dofetilide D. Azimilide

96. **Association with 22q11 deletion is not a feature of:**
A. TOF
B. TGA
C. Truncus arteriosus
D. Type B aortic interruption

ANSWERS

1	D	2	C	3	A	4		5	A	6	C	7	D
8	D	9	A	10	D	11	D	12	D	13	A	14	B
15	C	16	A	17	B	18		19	B	20	B	21	D
22	C	23	D	24	A	25	A	26	A	27	A	28	B
29	D	30	D	31	A	32	D	33	A	34		35	A
36	C	37	D	38	B	39	D	40	C	41	C	42	A
43	D	44	D	45	D	46	B	47	A	48	C	49	A
50	B	51	B	52	B	53	C	54	D	55	D	56	B
57	D	58	D	59	A	60	D	61	A	62	D	63	A
64	D	65	A	66	C	67	D	68	D	69	A	70	B
71	B	72	B	73	A	74	D	75	C	76	D	77	C
78	D	79	C	80	D	81	A	82	D	83	A	84	C
85	D	86	C	87	C	88	B	89	B	90	C	91	A
92	B	93	A	94	B	95	B	96	B				

29

JAYADEVA 2009

1. **Which of the following foodstuff is a rich source of molybdenum?**
   A. Yeast
   B. Margarine
   C. Legumes
   D. Garlic

2. **Migratory necrolytic erythema is seen in:**
   A. Peutz-Jegher's syndrome
   B. Sarcoidosis
   C. Glucoganomas
   D. Acute pancreatitis

3. **Microvesicular fatty liver is seen in all *except*:**
   A. Obesity
   B. Reye's syndrome
   C. Tetracyclines
   D. Acute fatty liver of pregnancy

4. **Hypervolemic hyponatremia is observed in:**
   A. Burns
   B. Capillary leak due to sepsis
   C. Diabetes mellitus
   D. Hyperaldosteronism

5. **Linezolid is:**
   A. Macrolide antibiotic
   B. MAO inhibitor
   C. Effective parenterally only
   D. Anti-pseudomonal drug

6. **Which of the following is a T-cell lymphoma?**
   A. Burkitt's lymphoma
   B. Follicular lymphoma
   C. Mycosis fungoides
   D. Hairy cell leukemia

7. **Yeast is rich in:**
   A. Thiamine
   B. Riboflavin
   C. Pantothenic acid
   D. Vitamin B_{12}

8. **The following are calcium channelopathies *except*:**
   A. Episodic ataxia
   B. Spinocerebellar ataxia 6
   C. Familial hemiplegic migraine
   D. Hypokalemic periodic paralysis

9. **The following can cause hypercalcemia *except*:**
   A. Prolonged immobilization
   B. Tumour lysis syndrome
   C. Sarcoidosis
   D. Multiple myeloma

10. **Bouchard nodes are seen in:**
    A. Distal interphalangeal joints in osteoarthrosis
    B. Proximal interphalangeal joints in osteoarthrosis
    C. Proximal interphalangeal joints in rheumatoid arthritis
    D. Gout

11. **Thalidomide is used in the treatment of:**
    A. Erythema nodosum leprosum
    B. Behcet's syndrome
    C. Refractory aphthous ulcers
    D. All of the above

12. **HAM test is done for:**
    A. Spectrin defect
    B. Complement defect
    C. GPI anchor protein
    D. Mannose binding protein

13. **In beta thalassemia the most common gene mutation is:**
    A. Intron 1 inversion
    B. Intron 22
    C. 619 bp deletion
    D. 3.7 bp deletion

14. **All are predominantly motor neuropathy *except*:**
    A. Guillain-Barré syndrome
    B. Porphyria
    C. Lead intoxication
    D. Arsenic intoxication

15. Acanthosis nigricans in an obese child suggests:
A. Polycystic ovary syndrome
B. Insulin resistance
C. Hypertension
D. Fatty liver

16. Following liver transplant, recurrence of primary disease in the liver most likely occurs in:
A. Primary biliary cirrhosis
B. Wilson's disease
C. α-1 antitrypsin deficiency
D. Auto immune hepatitis

17. Which of the following is true regarding Eaton-Lambert syndrome?
A. Commonly affects the occular muscles
B. Neostigmine is the drug of choice
C. Commonly associated with adenocarcinoma
D. Repeated electrical stimulation enhances muscle power

18. A young lady presents with recurrent abdominal pain and anaemia. Peripheral smear shows basophilic stippling of RBCs. Most likely diagnosis is:
A. Sickle cell anaemia
B. Coelic disease
C. Lead poisoning
D. Ankylostomiasis

19. All of the following statements about Creutzfeldt Jakob disease are true *except*:
A. A neuro degenerative disease
B. Caused by prions
C. Brain biopsy is specific for diagnosis
D. Myoclonus is rarely seen

20. Obesity associated with neonatal hypotonia, developmental dealy, hypogonalism is seen in:
A. Carpenter syndrome
B. Cohen syndrome
C. Prader-Willi syndrome
D. Cushing's syndrome

21. Prolonged HV interval (> 55 msec) is associated with greater likelihood of developing:
A. RBBB
B. LBBB
C. Bifascicular block
D. Trifascicular block

22. Brugada syndrome is:
A. X-linked recessive
B. Autosomal dominant
C. Autosomal recessive
D. X-linked dominant

23. Primary acrodermatitis enteropathica is:
A. Autosomal dominant inheritance
B. Due to defective intestinal zinc absorption
C. Defective selenium absorption
D. Commonly follows diarrhea

24. Vitamin E deficiency in premature infants is associated with:
A. Thrombocytopenia
B. Malabsorption
C. Haemolytic anaemia
D. Ataxia

25. Following statements with intestine P450 is true *except*:
A. Major P450 in small bowel enterocyte is CYP 3A4
B. Concentration of total P450 is highest in the jejunum
C. A number of drugs have decreased absorption when consumed with grape fruit juice
D. Active ingradient in grape juice is furano-coumarins

26. All are seen in cystinosis *except:*
A. Renal calculi
B. Photophobia and blonde hair
C. Fanconi syndrome
D. Presence of cystine within leukocytes

27. Bile salt stimulated lipase in breast milk protects the newborn against:
A. E. coli
B. Giardia lamblia
C. Tuberculosis
D. Chickenpox

28. All are causes of hypertension with hypokalemia *except*:
A. End stage renal disease
B. Conn's syndrome
C. Cushing's syndrome
D. Bilateral renal artery stenosis

29. The hormone that stimulates appetite is:
A. Cholecystokinin
B. Glucagon like peptide-1
C. Peptide YY
D. Ghrelin

30. Which of the following drugs can be safely prescribed in pregnancy?
A. Warfarin
B. Tetracyclines
C. Heparin
D. ACE inhibitors

31. **"Bucket handle" fracture of metaphysis is seen in association with:**
A. Scurvy
B. Syphilis
C. Sexual abuse
D. Osteogenesis imperfecta

32. **Most appropriate drug for treatment of bulimia nervosa is:**
A. Amitryptyline B. Fluoxetine
C. Lithium D. Sertaline

33. **'Adult concept of death' develops in a child between the ages:**
A. 2–6 years B. 6–12 years
C. 12–14 years D. 14–16 years

34. **Treatment of choice for Kawasaki's disease is:**
A. Methotrexate
B. Dapsone
C. Cyclosporine
D. IV immunoglobulins

35. **Acrodermatitis enteropathica is secondary to malabsorption of:**
A. Zinc B. Selenium
C. Copper D. Chromium

36. **"Sleep apnea" is defined as a temporary pause in breathing during sleep lasting atleast:**
A. 40 secs B. 30 secs
C. 20 secs D. 10 secs

37. **Which test is performed to detect reversible myocardial ischemia?**
A. Coronary angiography
B. MUGA scan
C. Thalium scan
D. Resting echocardiogram

38. **Tardive dyskinesia is a worrisome side effect following the use of:**
A. Serotonin reuptake inhibitors (SSRIs)
B. Stimulant medications
C. Atypical antipsychotics
D. Neuroleptics

39. **Leflunamide is most effective for the treatment of:**
A. Wegener's granulomatosis
B. SLE
C. Ankylosing spondylitis
D. Rheumatoid arthritis

40. **Serum alkaline phosphatase is classically increased in which of the following diseases?**
A. Osteoporosis
B. Multiple myeloma
C. Paget's disease
D. Hypoparathyroidism

41. **Serotonin reuptake inhibitor used in childhood depression is:**
A. Methylphenidate
B. Sertraline
C. Trihexyphenidyl HCl
D. Benztropine

42. **Plasmapheresis is the treatment of choice for:**
A. Henoch-Schölein purpura
B. Wegener's granulomatosis
C. Goodpasture's syndrome
D. Acute renal transplant rejection

43. **Biotin deficiency is associated with:**
A. Polyneuritis
B. Seborrhoea, dermatitits
C. Anaemia
D. Poor wound healing

44. **Renal damage due to amphotericin B are all *except*:**
A. Azotemia
B. Glomerulonephritis
C. Renal tubular acidosis
D. Hypokalemia

45. **Hyperkalemia is commonly seen in:**
A. Proximal renal tubular acidosis
B. Distal renal tubular acidosis
C. Use of Angiotensin II blocker
D. Bartter syndrome

46. **The drugs which do not provide mortality benefit in CCF:**
A. Spironolactone B. Beta blocker
C. Furosemide D. ACE inhibitors

47. **Prevalence of acute rheumatic fever during epidemics:**
A. 15% B. 25%
C. 3% D. 0.3%

48. **All are causes of pulsus paradoxus *except*:**
A. Acute severe asthma
B. Pericardial tamponade
C. Severe aortic stenosis
D. Massive pulmonary embolism

49. **IVP elevation is not a feature of:**
A. Right heart failure
B. Hypovolemia
C. ASD with mitral valve disease
D. Constrictive pericarditis

50. **Having apical impulse is not seen in:**
A. Aortic stenosis
B. Hypertension
C. Severe LV dysfunction
D. Thyrotoxicosis

51. Soft S1 is a feature of:
A. Decreased LV contractility
B. Short PR interval
C. Mitral stenosis
D. Atrial septal defect

52. All are causes of cyanosis with wide split S2 *except*:
A. TAPVC
B. Single atrium
C. Ebstein's anomaly of TV
D. Truncus arteriosus

53. S3 is not a feature of:
A. Severe MR
B. Pregnancy
C. Mitral stenosis
D. Large VSD with L-R shunt

54. All are causes of S4 *except*:
A. Acute MI
B. Atrial fibrillation
C. Aortic stenosis
D. Acute MR

55. All are causes of pansystolic murmur *except*:
A. Mild to moderate AS
B. MR
C. VSD
D. TR

56. All are causes of reduced intensity of MDM in MS *except*:
A. ASD
B. Severe PH
C. Mitral regurgitation
D. Obesity

57. All are causes of cyanosis with continuous murmur *except*:
A. Pulmonary AV fistula
B. Eisenmenger's PDA
C. TOF with functioning BT shunt
D. Pulmonary atresia with collaterals

58. All are citeria for RVH *except*:
A. R in V1 > 0.7 mv
B. R/S in V1 > 1 with R > 0.5 mv
C. R/S in V5 or V6 <1
D. Left axis deviation of QRS > - 30

59. Giant T wave inversion is not a feature of:
A. Acute pericarditis
B. Ischaemic heart disease
C. Apical cardiomyopathy
D. Cerebrovascular accident

60. Identify the correct statement:
A. Digitalis prolongs QT interval
B. Hypocalcaemia causes QT shortening
C. Systemic hypothermia causes osborn waves
D. Hyperkalemia causes prominent 'U' waves

61. All are features of severe MS *except*:
A. Resting mean pressure gradient > 10 mm HG
B. MVOA < 1.0 cm
C. Pressure 1/2 time < 220 msec
D. A2-OS interval < 80 msec

62. Following is not a feature of severe AR:
A. Vena contracta < 6 mm
B. Regurgitant volume > 60 ml
C. Regurgitant fraction > 50%
D. Austin-flint murmur

63. Most specific symptom of heart failure is:
A. Exertional dyspnea
B. Leg swelling
C. Nocturnal cough
D. PND

64. All are determinants of systemic BP *except*:
A. Cardiac output
B. Compliance of the pulmonary vasculature
C. Myocardial contractility
D. Systemic vascular resistance

65. All are true in heart failure *except*:
A. High pulse pressure is a marker of low cardiac output
B. Proportional pulse pressure correlates well with cardiac index
C. Low diastolic pressure is a feature of sepsis
D. Orthostatic hypotension signals volume deletion

66. Most common type of anaemia in heart failure is:
A. Anaemia of chronic disease normocytic normochronic anaemia
B. Iron deficiency anaemia
C. Dilutional anaemia
D. Megaloblastic anaemia

67. All are features of "Vulnerable plaque" *except*:
A. Thin fibrous cap
B. Large lipid core
C. Abundant smooth munch cubs
D. Numerous inflammatory cells

68. All are true regarding cardiac valves *except*:
A. Septal leaflet of TV has multiple direct chordal attachment to the IVS
B. Both mitral leaflets are normally similar in area
C. "Nodule of Arantius" is a normal finding on AV
D. Pulmonary valve is in fibrous continuity with TV

69. Identify the wrong statement:
A. Sinus node artery arises from RCA in 55% of people

B. His bundle has dual blood supply
C. Right and left bundle branches have single blood supply
D. AV node is situated in the triangle of Koch

70. **All are features of morphological RV *except*:**
A. Moderator band
B. Finely trabeculated apical zone
C. More apical attachment of AV valve
D. Crista supraventricularis

71. **Following is not a feature of pulmonary venous hypertension of chest X-ray:**
A. Multiple 'end-on' views of the pulmonary arteries
B. Kerly 'B' lines
C. Batwing appearance
D. "Cephalisation"

72. **HDL is increased by all *except*:**
A. Alcohol B. Niacin
C. β-blocker D. Exercise

73. **All are causes of dilatation of ascending aorta *except*:**
A. Bicuspid aortic valve
B. Marfan's syndrome
C. Syphytis
D. Parachute mitral valve

74. **Cardiomyopathy with a best prognosis:**
A. Peripartum cardiomyopathy
B. Dilated cardiomyopathy
C. Takotsubo cardiomyopathy
D. Cardiomyopathy due to HIV infection

75. **All are features of constrictive pericarditis *except*:**
A. Elevation and equilibration of pressure in all chambers
B. "Swinging" of heart on ECHO
C. Kussmaul's sign
D. Rapid 'Y' descent on JVP

76. **The drug which does not reduce PH:**
A. Aminorex B. Epoprostenol
C. Bosentan D. Sildenafil

77. **Identify the wrong statement regarding obstructive sleep apnea:**
A. It is strongly associated with obesity
B. It is highly prevalent in patients with metabolic syndrome
C. It has a strong association with cardiovascular disorders like hypertension, AF, CAD and heart failure
D. There is no effective treatment

78. **Following is not a high risk for pregnancy:**
A. Mitral regurgitation
B. Severe AS
C. Cyanotic heart disease
D. Marfan's syndrome with aortic root > 40 mm

79. **Identify the "Major" predictor of increased perioperative cardiovascular risk:**
A. Uncontrolled systemic hypertension
B. LBBB
C. Decompensated heart failure
D. History of stroke

80. **Cardiac involvement in SLE can cause all *except*:**
A. Libman Sach's endocarditis
B. Sclerosing inflammation of aortic root causing AR
C. Pericardial effusion
D. Congenital complete heart block

81. **Anti-proliferative drug which does not cause heart failure:**
A. Sirolimus
B. Doxorubicin
C. Cyclophosphamide
D. Mitomycin

82. **Hyperthyroidism can be associated with all *except*:**
A. Reversible pulmonary hypertension
B. Large pericardial effusion
C. Atrial fibrillation
D. Congestive heart failure

83. **All are causes of wide QRS tachycardia *except*:**
A. Preexited tachycardia
B. VT
C. Pacemaker tachycardia
D. AV nodal re-entrant tachycardia

84. **Following is a minor criteria in Jone's criteria for diagnosis of rheumatic fever:**
A. Raised ASLO tites
B. Polyarthritis
C. Raised ESR
D. Erythema marginatum

85. **Most common organism which causes native valve endocarditis in the community:**
A. HACEK group
B. Streptococcus viridans
C. Enterococci
D. Candida albicans

86. **"Vascular Rings" can be caused by all *except*:**
A. Anomalous origin of left subclavian artery
B. Anomalous origin of right subclavian artery
C. Right aortic arch
D. Double aortic arch

87. **Dual antiplatelet therapy is indicated in all *except* (Aspirin + Clopidogrel):**
A. After coronary stenting
B. Acute coronary syndrome
C. Patients with stable angina
D. Post MI patients

88. **The drug which does not decrease mortality in post MI patients:**
A. Enalapril B. Aspirin
C. Metoprolol D. Nifidepine

89. **Hyperkalemia is not a feature of:**
A. Metolazone
B. Ramipril
C. Amiloride
D. Eplerenone

90. **Most common cause of sudden cardiac death:**
A. Hypertrophic cardiomyopathy
B. Coronary artery anomalies
C. Coronary heart disease
D. ARVD

ANSWERS

1	C	2	C	3	A	4	C	5	B	6	C	7	A
8	A	9	B	10	B	11	C	12	C	13	B	14	D
15	B	16	B	17	D	18	C	19	D	20	C	21	D
22		23	B	24	C	25	D	26	A	27	B	28	A
29	D	30	C	31	C	32	B	33	B	34	D	35	A
36	D	37	C	38	D	39	D	40	C	41	B	42	C
43	B	44	B	45	C	46	C	47	C	48	C	49	B
50	D	51	A	52	D	53	C	54	B	55	A	56	C
57	B	58	D	59	A	60	C	61	C	62	A	63	D
64	B	65	A	66	C	67	C	68	D	69	C	70	B
71	A	72	C	73	D	74	C	75	B	76	A	77	D
78	A	79	C	80	B	81	A	82	B	83	D	84	C
85	B	86	C	87	C	88	D	89	A	90	C		

30

JAYADEVA 2008

1. **Burkitt's lymphoma commonly presents with:**
   A. Abdominal mass
   B. Anemia
   C. Recurrent infection
   D. Hyperviscosity symptoms

2. **First line therapy of idiopathic thrombocytopenic purpura in adults:**
   A. Danazol   B. Corticosteroids
   C. Azathioprine   D. Cyclosporine

3. **Heerfordt's syndrome includes all of the following *except*:**
   A. Lacrimal gland   B. Parotids
   C. Uveitis   D. Fever

4. **In haemophilia, which one is true:**
   A. Level of factor VIII: C and level of factor VWF–both reduced
   B. Level of factor VIII: C is normal but level of factor VWF is reduced
   C. Level of factor VIII: C is reduced but level of factor VVVF is normal
   D. None of the above

5. **In Plummer-Vinson syndrome following is true *except*:**
   A. Iron deficiency anemia
   B. Web is at upper esophageal sphincter
   C. Radiologically web is seen
   D. On esophagoscopy web is easily seen

6. **Following are H pylori associated diseases *except*:**
   A. Gastric adenocarcinoma
   B. Gastropathy
   C. Gastritis
   D. Gastric B cell lymphoma

7. **Which one of the following has better diagnostic value in heart failure?**
   A. ANP   B. C peptide
   C. BNP   D. Endothelia

8. **Treatment of choice in Chlamydia pneumoniae is:**
   A. Streptomycin   B. Erythromycin
   C. Cephalosporin   D. Cotrimoxazole

9. **VSD may occur in patients of STEMI in:**
   A. 1-2%   B. 5-10%
   C. 10-15%   D. 15-20%

10. **Which one of the following doesn't increase thyroxine binding globulin levels?**
   A. Pregnancy
   B. Oestrogen therapy
   C. Excess costeroids
   D. Phenothiazines

11 **The most potent glucocorticoid effect found in:**
   A. Hydrocortisone   B. Dexamethasone
   C. Prednisolone   D. Fludrocortisone

12. **The most common cause of hypocalcemia:**
   A. Renal failure
   B. Phosphate therapy
   C. Osteomalacia
   D. Rickets

13. **Which one is not related to T2DM?**
   A. Often overweight
   B. No HLA links
   C. Often immune disturbance
   D. C-peptide persists

14. **In celiac spree there is deficiency of all *except*:**
   A. Vitamin B_{12}
   B. Vitamin A
   C. Iron
   D. Folic acid

15. **Which of the following have hypergastrinemia with decreased acid output?**
   A. Zollinger-Ellison syndrome
   B. Peptic ulcer disease
   C. Pernicious anemia
   D. G-cell hyperplasia

16. **Which drug is not used in SIADH?**
A. Fludrocortisone B. Desmopressin
C. Hypertonic saline D. Demclocycline

17. **Headache with scalp tenderness seen in:**
A. Migrainous neuralgia
B. Giant cell arteroids
C. Cluster headache
D. Trigeminal neuralgia

18. **Tuberous sclerosis is commonly associated with all of the following *except*:**
A. Retinal phakomas
B. Renal tumours
C. Gliomas
D. Cardiac tumours

19. **Cyanosis may be seen in:**
A. Mercury B. Nitrates
C. Atropine D. Aspirin

20. **Amotivation syndrome seen with:**
A. LSD B. Cocaine
C. Cannabis D. Amphetamine

21. **On oesophageal manometry shows high amplitude waves, occasional peristaltic progression seen in:**
A. Systemic sclerosis
B. Achalasia
C. Gastro-oesophageal reflux spasm
D. Diffuse oesophageal spasm

22. **All can cause RPGN *except*:**
A. SLE
B. Post-streptococcal glomerulonephritis
C. Wegener's granulomatosis
D. Minimal change glomerulonephritis

23. **"Pseudo hyponatremia" occurs in:**
A. Hyperproteinemia
B. Mannitol use
C. Hypothyroidsm
D. Osmotic diuresis

24. **Pyrantel pamoate is effective in both:**
A. Amoebiasis and trichiriasis
B. Enterobiasis and ascariasis
C. Amoebiasis and strongyloides
D. Taenia solium and strongyloides

25. **Primary idiopathic polymyositis does not involve:**
A. Pelvic girdle muscles
B. Ocular muscles
C. Neck muscles
D. Pharyngeal muscles

26. **Which one of the following is not a feature of leptospirosis?**
A. Elevated CPK
B. Hepatorenal syndrome
C. Thrombocytopenia
D. More than 10 fold rise of transaminases

27. **Vitamin B_6 deficiency is associated with all of the following *except*:**
A. Cyclosporine B. Penicillamine
C. INH D. Cycloserine

28. **Which one statement is false?**
A. Eptifibatide – GP IIb / IIIa inhibitor
B. Ticlopidine – COX inhibitor
C. Warfarin – Vitamin K inhibitor
D. Ximelogatran - Direct thrombin inhibitor

29. **Post-exposure immunization with immunoglobulin recommended in the following *except*:**
A. Measles B. Rubella
C. Rabies D. Hepatitis A

30. **Pseudomembranous colitis is significantly high risk with:**
A. Clindamycin
B. Ceftriaxone
C. Piperacillin/Tazobactum
D. Ampicillin

31. **Which one skin manifestation is commonly linked to mycoplasma pneumonia?**
A. Erythema multiform
B. Erythema nodosum
C. Vesicular exanthems
D. Urticaria

32. **Which one drug is not used in treatment of chronic hepatitis B?**
A. IFN – L2 B B. Tenofovir
C. Adefovir D. Cidofovir

33. **Which one of the following is fusion inhibitor?**
A. Efavirenz B. Enfuviritide
C. Emtricitabine D. Fosamprenavir

34. **Least nephrotoxic amphotericin-B:**
A. Amphotericin B lipid complex
B. Liposomal amphotericin B
C. Amphotericin B colloidal dispersion
D. None of the above

35. **Which one of the following is least common mode of presentation in sarcoidosis?**
A. Abnormal routine chest X-ray
B. Pulmonary symptoms
C. Erythema nodosum
D. Cranial nerve palsies

36. **Erythema nodosum seen in all of the following *except*:**
A. Mycoplasma B. NSAIDs
C. Chlamydia D. Sulphonamides

37. Which one is chloride channelopathy?
A. Paramyotonia congenital
B. Hypokalemic periodic paralysis
C. Myotonia congenita
D. Hyperkalemic periodic paralysis

38. All are true about pulmonary embolism *except*:
A. Chest pain is the most common symptom
B. Most commonly presents within 2 weeks
C. More is the survival time, more is the chance of recovery
D. Arises from leg veins

39. All are true response of the murmur of Mitral valve prolapse to interventions *except*:
A. Standing upright increases
B. Recumbent decreases
C. Amyl nitrite decreases
D. Hand grip variable effect

40. All of the following are true about analgesic nephropathy *except*:
A. Hematuria
B. Pyuria
C. Proteinuria >l g/d
D. IVP shows "ring sign"

41. The following statements about corectopia are true, *except*:
A. It is abnormal shape of the pupil
B. It is abnormal pupillary position
C. It is abnormal fusion of the eyelids
D. It is usually accompanied by dislocation of thelens

42. Among the following infections which is the most common cause of external otitis (swimmer's ear):
A. Klebsiella pneumonia
B. S aureus
C. P aeruginosa
D. Fungi

43. The following statements about Cowden syndrome are correct, *except*:
A. It is an autosomal dominant condition
B. Usually presents in the first decade of life
C. May be associated with Thyroid goiter/Gastro-intestinal polyps
D. The lesiens found in this condition , are smooth, pink or whitish papules on the palatal, gingival, buccal and labial mucosae

44. Which of the following drug is used in severe intractable migraine attacks (status migrainosus)?
A. Flumarizine B. Prochlorperazine
C. Sodium valproate D. Gabapentin

45. The following statements about insulin dependent diabetes mellitus (IDDM) are true, *except*:
A. Autoimmune destruction of pancreatic P cells
B. Both genetic susceptibililty and environmental factors contribute to pathogenesis
C. Median age of onset of the disease is between 7 to 15 years
D. Children with IDDM are usually obese

46. In utero the heart starts beating as early as:
A. 18-20 days B. 20-22 days
C. 22-24 days D. 24-26 days

47. In fetal circulation the PO_2 of the blood entering the umbilical vein from the placenta is:
A. 20-25 mm Hg B. 25-30 mm Hg
C. 30-35 mm Hg D. 35-45 mm Hg

48. The most frequent congenital heart disease seen in fetal alcohol syndrome is:
A. Tetralogy of Fallot
B. Pulmonary stenosis
C. Atrial septal defect
D. Patent ductus arteriosus

49. 22q11 deletion is most commonly seen in:
A. Ventricular septal defect
B. Atrial septal defect
C. Pulmonary stenosis
D. Interrupted aortic arch

50. Upright T waves in the right sided chest leads may be normal:
A. On day 1 of life
B. In the first 48 hours of birth
C. In the first 7 days of life
D. In the first month of life

51. Identify the wrong statement:
A. Damage to left anterior fascicle is very common because of its delicate nature
B. Left posterior fascicle is thicker and is protected near the LV
C. ECG features of left septal fascicular block is absence of septal Q waves
D. QRS duration is prolonged in fascicular block

52. During stress testing all are true *except*:
A. In about 10% of patients ischemic response may appear only in the recovery phase
B. SY tin leads with abnormal Q waves is a marker of more extensive CAD
C. 'U' wave inversion is relatively specific for CAD
D. 'P' seudonormalisation of T waves are a non-diagnostic finding

53. Identify the wrong statement in normal diastolic filling pattern of LV:
A. E/A > 1.5
B. Deceleration time = 160-240 secs (septa)

C. EA (Mural annular velocity) < 10 cm/s
D. E/Ea < 8

54. **All are features of athlete's heart *except*:**
A. Symmetric hypertrophy
B. LV cavity dimension is decreased
C. Diastolic function is normal
D. Hypertrophy is rarely > 17 mm
E. None of the above

55. **Which is the wrong statement in cardiac myocyte?**
A. Myofibrils account for > ½ of the hearts weight
B. Atrial myocytes are larger than ventricular myocytes
C. About 1/4 to 1/3 is occupied by mitochondria
D. Purkinje cells are the modified myocytes

56. **Identify the wrong statement regarding aldosterone antagonist therapy:**
A. Useful in NY HA class If I – IV HF with EF < 35%
B. Painful gynaecomastia may develop in 5—10% of patients on eplerenone
C. Life threatening hyperkalemia is the major problem
D. Contraindicated if serum potassium is > 5.5 m/mol/L

57. **After heart transplantation all are true *except*:**
A. 1 year survival is 90-95%
B. Allograft CAD is seen in 50% by 5 years
C. Recipient heart is denervated
D. Allograft does not require immunosuppression

58. **Following is not a mechanism of arrhythmogenesis:**
A. Abnormal automaticity
B. Early after depolarization
C. Entrance and exit block
D. Re-entry

59. **Identify the wrong statement regarding exercise:**
A. 30 minutes of walking daily results in 30% reduction in vascular events
B. Decreases systolic BP
C. Improves insulin sensitivity
D. Decreases HDL cholesterol

60. **Features suggestive of phaeochromocytoma:**
A. Persistent hypertension
B. Sudden paroxysms
C. Abdominal bruit
D. Elevated serum creatinine level

61. **Identify the wrong statement:**
A. RV MI occurs in 50% of inferior MI
B. Isolated RV MI is seen in 3-5%
C. Atrial infarction is more common on left side than right
D. 5% of patients with acute MI have normal coronaries

62. **Biomarker which is most useful to detect myocardial injury?**
A. Myoglobi B. CPK
C. Troponin T D. CKMB

63. **Incidence of cardiogenic shock in S I LMI in recent trials:**
A. 7% B. 20%
C. 30% D. 40%

64. **Following is not a predictor of late VF in acute MI:**
A. Inferior MI
B. Persistent sinus tachycardia
C. Atrial fibrillation
D. Anterior MI with IVCD

65. **Contraindication for PTMC:**
A. MRI–II
B. Severe PH
C. LA appendage clot
D. Bicommisural calcification

66. **In HCM annual mortality is:**
A. 5% B. 1-2%
C. 10% D. 20%

67. **First human cardiac catheterization was done by:**
A. Andre Cournand
B. Mason Sone
C. Judkins
D. Warner's Forssman

68. **Following is not a feature of left isomerism:**
A. Bilateral morphologic left bronchi
D. Howell-Jolly bodies
C. Transverse liver
D. Levocardia

69. **Incidence of PFO in 4th decade is:**
A. 25% B. 45%
C. 50% D. 70%

70. **Wide split second heart sound is not a feature of:**
A. RV failure
B. Severe MR
C. Massive pulmonary embolism
D. LBBB

71. **The drug which has no survival benefit in patients with LV dysfunction:**
A. Dobutamine
B. Eplerenone
C. Enalapril
D. Carvedilol

72. Which is not true in the blood supply of different structures of the heart?

A. AV node is supplied by RCA in the majority
B. Conus branch supplies the RVOT
C. IVS is supplied by both LAD and RCA
D. Posteromedial papillary muscle has dual blood supply

73. Continuous murmur is not a feature of:

A. PDA with severe PH
B. Pulmonary AV fistula
C. Small ASD with severe MS
D. RSOV to RVOT

74. IABP is absolutely contraindicated in:

A. Post MI VSD
B. Intractable angina
C. Aortic dissection
D. High risk PTICA

75. Ductus arteriosus is embryologically derived from:

A. Dorsal aorta **B.** 6th aortic arch
C. 5th aortic arch **D.** 4th aortic arch

76. Incidence of stent thrombosis is reduced by:

A. Dual antiplatelet therapy
B. Statins
C. Drug eluting stents
D. Anticoagulation

77. Identify the wrong statement in EMF (End myocardial fibrosis):

A. Hallmark is fibrotic obliteration of the apex of the ventricle
B. Typically seen in tropical and subtropical countries
C. Most common in middle aged and elderly
D. Systolic function is preserved

78. Following is not a major criteria for diagnosis of infective endocarditis:

A. Positive blood culture
B. New valvular regurgitation
C. Predisposing Matt condition
D. Vegetation

79. Cannon 'a' waves are seen in all *except*:

A. Junctional rhythm **B.** VT
C. CHB **D.** Tricuspid stenosis

80. Paradoxic splitting of S2 is seen in all *except*:

A. LBBB
B. LV pacing
C. Serves AS
D. Systolic hypertension

81. All are true regarding atrial flutter *except*:

A. Occurs most often in patients with organic heart disease
B. Atrial rate between 250-350/min
C. Systemic embolisation is less common than in atrial fibrillation
D. Requires high energy (100-200 joules) DC shock

82. In acute AR:

A. S1 is soft or absent
B. Pulse pressure is always wide
C. S3 is uncommon
D. Diastolic murmur is long and loud

83. "Water bottle" configuration of cardiac silhouette is seen in:

A. AR
B. MS
C. Pericardial effusion
D. Hypertrophic cardiomyopathy

84. Feature of "Unstable plaque" all are true *except*:

A. Thin fibrous cap
B. Large lipid care
C. High content of macrophages
D. Abundant smooth muscle cells

85. Device closure of the shunts can be done for all *except*:

A. Mid muscular VSD
B. Ostium primum ASD
C. PDA
D. Ostium secundum ASD

86. Factor not predisposing to aortic dissection:

A. Cystic medial necrosis
B. Marfan's syndrome
C. Hypertension
D. Aorto arteritis

87. Regarding "Acrocyanosis" all are true *except*:

A. Persistent cyanosis of the hands and feet
B. Patients are asymptomatic
C. Tropic skin changes and ulcerations are common
D. Pharmacologic intervention is not indicated

88. Lymphedema is not a feature of:

A. Leopard syndrome
B. Turner's syndrome
C. Noonan's syndrome
D. Yellow Nail syndrome

89. HIV infection can cause all *except*:

A. Long QT interval
B. Pericardial effusion
C. Marantic endocarditis
D. Restrictive cardiomyopathy

90. Identify the correct statement in constriction pericarditis:

A. Prominent X descent in JVP is a common finding
B. Paradoxic pulse is seen in majority
C. 'Square root' sign is a feature
D. Septal bounce is absent

31

KOLKATA 2011

CARDIOLOGY

1. **Best non-invasive test for P.E. in case of clinical suspicion:**
   A. d-dimer
   B. MDCT with angiography
   C. MRI
   D. Doppler

2. **Diagnostic test of device:**
   A. Pulmonary angiography
   B. MDCT
   C. V/P scan
   D. MR angiography

3. **Ch. CCP not caused by:**
   A. Myxoedema B. CA breast
   C. Post CABG D. CRF on dialysis

4. **Obstructive sleep apnea defined as stoppage of air flow:**
   A. 10 sec. B. 20 sec.
   C. 30 sec. D. 40 sec.

5. **Syncope is not a symptom of:**
   A. AS B. MS
   C. PPH D. CHB

6. **Hyperkalemia features all *except*:**
   A. Sine wave B. Narrow T
   C. Narrow QRS D. Diminish P wave

7. **ATP recommendation, test not used in:**
   A. VLDL B. LDL
   C. Chylomicron D. TG

8. **Special for cholesterol profile about blacks:**
   A. ↓ Total ch., LDC ↓ Lp (a) ↑
   B. ↓ Total ch., HDL ↓ Lp (a) ↑
   C. ↓ Total ch., TG ↓ Lp (a) ↓
   D. ↓ Total ch., TG ↑, HDL ↓

9. **Newer risk factors for CAD in black:**
   A. Low renin hypertension
   B. LVH
   C. Hypovitaminosis D
   D. Na+/H ratio

10. **Drug least effective as monotherapy is HTN in blacks:**
    A. CCB B. Diuretics
    C. β blockers D. α blockers

11. **Hispanic paradox:**
    A. ↑ DM, HTN, obesity
    B. ↑ DM, obesity and ↓ HTN
    C. ↑ HTN, ↓ DM, obesity
    D. ↓ DM, HTN, obesity

12. **Prevalence of HTN is urban India/South India:**
    A. 10–15% B. 10–20%
    C. 20–40% D. 40–50%

13. **Severity of MS all *except*:**
    A. Loudness of S1
    B. PND
    C. A_2 – Os gap
    D. Duration of murmur

14. **Omega-3 fatty acids given in:**
    A. Severe hypertension
    B. TG > 500
    C. ↓ HDL
    D. LDL > 200

15. **↓ HDL-C disease not associated with:**
    A. Prolonged statin use
    B. Sedentary life style
    C. Anabolic steroids
    D. Diabetes

16. **TOF_1 systolic BP–110/40 velocity + 5 m^2, PAP:**
    A. 10 B. 20
    C. 30 D. 40

17. **AF with variable S_1 disappear in:**
    A. AF with FVR B. AF with SVR
    C. AF with CHB D. None

18. To terminate atrial flutter drug not used:
A. Amiodarone B. Lidocaine
C. Ibutilide D. Procainamide

19. Typical atrial flutter all *except*:
A. Positive wave is II, III, aVF
B. Counter clockwise is RA
C. Ventricular rate 2 : 1 or 4 : 1
D. Flutter waves are saw tooth waves

20. PSVT, patient has bronchospasm on theophylline, drug used:
A. Adenosine B. Verapamil
C. Esmolol D. Digoxin

21. SLE all *except*:
A. Pericarditis is most common
B. Epicardial arteries is seen
C. Rarely myocarditis can cause CHF
D. Libman sacks endocarditis most commonly involve TV

22. IE all *except*:
A. In neonates, TV most commonly involved
B. In HIV, no special prediction
C. Afebrile presentation in IE with Whipple's disease
D. Persistent anticoagulation is given in mycotic aneurysm

23. Worst tolerable lesion in pregnancy:
A. PPH
B. COA
C. MR

24. PDA not required in:
A. Pulmonary atresia
B. Tricuspid atresia
C. D–TGA
D. COA

25. Worst prognosis CMP:
A. Amyloidosis induced CMP
B. HIV induced CMP
C. Doxorubicin
D. Ischemic CMP

26. White coat HTN true:
A. Risk ↑ as compared to normotensive and chronic hypertension
B. Risk intermediate between normotensive and chronic hypertension
C. Risk ↓ as compared to both
D. None

27. QT ↑ all *except*:
A. Metformin
B. TCA
C. Phenothiazines
D. Sotalol

28. Lung function testing in HF all are reduced, *except*:
A. Vital capacity
B. Lung compliance
C. Residual volume
D. Diffusion capacity

29. Orthostatic hypotension - True:
A. ↓ is SBP > 20 mm Hg and ↓ is DBP > 10 mm Hg, on 3 minutes of standing
B. ↓ is SBP > 20 mm Hg or ↓ is DBP > 10 mm Hg, OR 3 minutes of standing
C. ↓ is SBP > 20 mm Hg or ↓ is DBP > 10 mm Hg, OR 1 minute of standing
D. ↓ is SBP > 20 mm Hg or ↓ is DBP > 10 mm Hg, OR 2 minutes of standing

30. Oral active direct renin inhibitors efficacy comparable to ACE-I is:
A. Aliskinrin
B. Vernakalant

31. β blocker all *except*:
A. ↓ infarct size
B. ↓ pain
C. Facilitates thrombolysis
D. Favorable O_2–HR relationship

32. Nitrates is MI all *except*:
A. Can be given as buccal spray
B. Dose 5–10 microgram/kg/min
C. Relative C/I BP < 100 mm Hg
D. C/I with sildenafil if taken in last 24 hours

33. Drug interaction all *except*:
A. Pravastatin–ketoconazole
B. Sildenafil–nitrates
C. Simvastatin–erythromycin
D. Digoxin–verapamil

34. Nuclear radiology–used agent with longest half-life active myocardial uptake:
A. Thallium–201 B. Sestamibi
C. Tetrofosmin D. Tebroxime

35. Regular cannon wave:
A. AF B. CHB
C. Junctional rhythm D. VT

36. False +ve troponin all *except*:
A. PE B. CHF
C. CRF D. Costochondritis

37. AR associated with all *except*:
A. Barlow syndrome
B. Ankylosing spondylitis
C. Membranous subaortic stenosis
D. Bicuspid aortic valve

38. **Acute MR is all *except*:**
A. HOCM B. Angina
C. Trauma D. IE

39. **Patient of OS secundum ASD, JVP–10 cm, what is LVEDP?**
A. 10 cm B. 20 cm
C. 15 cm D. 25 cm

40. **TOF all *except*:**
A. Cyanosis inversely proportional to murmur
B. Increased pulmonary vascularity
C. 25% has right aortic arch
D. ECG-RVH

41. **ASD all *except*:**
A. Wide and fixed S2
B. Mid systolic murmur at ULSB
C. Mid diastolic murmur at LLSB
D. Apical impulse hyperdynamic

42. **Critical pulmonary stenosis in newborn all *except*:**
A. Acute pulmonary edema
B. Cynosis
C. Tender hepatomegaly
D. Right–left left–PFO

43. **OSA all *except*:**
A. Daytime hypoxia
B. HTN
C. Catecholamines ↑ as like pheochromocytoma
D. Atrial fibrillation

44. **Pulses alternans, not ↑ by:**
A. Hypovolemia
B. HTN
C. AR
D. Paget's disease

45. **In resting stage, metabolite used by heart:**
A. FFA
B. Glucose
C. Ketones

46. **Ventricular paced, inhibited, atrial triggered, pacemaker is:**
A. DDD B. VDI
C. VVI D. VDD

47. **Parasite involved in pulmonary HTN:**
A. Schistosomiasis
B. Paragonimiasis

48. **Most common risk factor for venous thrombo-embolism:**
A. Activated protein C resistance
B. Prothrombin gene mutation
C. Protein S deficiency
D. Antithrombin III deficiency

MEDICINE

49. **Site of action of K^+ sparing drug:**
A. DCT + CD
B. PCT
C. Ascending loop of Henle

50. **Ketones not used by:**
A. Brain B. Liver
C. Skeletal muscle D. Cardiac muscle

51. **Ca^{++} channels:**
A. Ryanodine receptor
B. Calsequestrin
C. Junctin
D. Triadin

52. **Max cause of which ion in distal part of PCT:**
A. Na^+ B. Cl^-
C. K^T D. HCO_3–

53. **Bronchodilation by:**
A. NE β_1 recep B. Ach M_1 recep
C. VIP (neurons) D. Exercise

54. **Corticosteroids all *except*:**
A. Osteonecrosis
B. Cataract
C. Prox. myopathy
D. Hyperkalemic alkalosis

55. **Anterior hypothalamic nuclei all *except*:**
A. Suprachiasmatic
B. Preoptic
C. Paraventricular
D. Arcuate

56. **HTN bleed most common site is:**
A. Pons
B. Putamen

57. **Anatomy of kidney all true *except*:**
A. DCT contains eosinophilia as compared to PCT
B. Gut epithelium has anterior relations of kidney
C. Macula densa cell and granular cell adjoint to PCT
D. Perirenal fat separated by fascia

58. **Acute pancreatitis:**
A. Infection of necrosis is ominous sign
B. +nt with acute upper abdominal pain with localized peritonitis
C. Alcohol and trauma on most common cause
D. Leads to pancreatic cancer

59. **18 years old man with anteriorolateral compartment of leg swelling pain false:**
A. Dorsalis pedis not palpable
B. Anterior fasciotomy to be done
C. Dorsiflexion cause pain
D. Loss of sensation between 1st space

60. Galactorrhoea + amenorrhea + visual disturbance:
A. Hyperprolactinemia
B. ↓ TSH

61. Multiple sclerosis:
A. Option n + cerebellar + spinal cord involved
B. Relapsing disease of PNS

62. Anatomy of heart all *except*:
A. Both MV/TV are in vertical axis to septum
B. Anterior superior leaflet is largest and attached with 2 papillary m.
C. Ventricles are inferior and left to respective atria
D. Supraventricular crest is connection between RV outflow and RV inflow

63. DIC all *except*:
A. ↑ sed PT
B. ↑sed apTT
C. ↑ sed D–Dimers
D. Clot lysis time

64. Zoonotic viral do not uncommon in India all *except*:
A. Hanta
B. West nile
C. Nipah
D. Marburg

65. True all *except*:
A. Radio immunoassay is most sensitive
B. Agglutination more sensitive than potation
C. Immunofluorescence assay more sensitive than Elisa
D. Inhibiting agglutination is more sensitive than agglutination

66. Fat soluble Vitamin C /Anti-oxidant with chain breaking property:
A. Vitamin E
B. Vitamin A
C. Bile salts
D. Vitamin C

67. 2 ordinal variables with pair values test to be used:
A. Pair t test
B. Chi-square
C. Sign test
D. Wisconsin test

68. Membrane carbohydrates digestion at mucosal level:
A. Isomaltose
B. Sucrase
C. Glucoamylase
D. Amylase

69. K^+ sparing diuretic not given with:
A. ACE inhibitor

70. NO present in:
A. Endothelial cell + Platelet (EC) + Macrophage
B. EC + CNS + Macrophage
C. EC + CNS + Plasma
D. EC + Plasma + Platelets

71. Type 2 DM insulin secretion:
A. Initial Phase Normal Delayed Phase ↓
B. Initial/Delayed Phase ↓
C. Both Phase Normal
D. Initial Phase ↓ Delayed Phase N

72. Black colored bag disposal:
A. Chemical disinfectants
B. Incinerations
C. Landfill
D. Segregations

73. WHO anemia 6–14 years:
A. < 13
B. < 12
C. < 11
D. None

74. DNA repairing enzyme:
A. Demethylased

75. Anti-epileptic all *except*:
A. Paraldehyde DOC for status epilepticus
B. Carbamazepine / valproic DOC for major epileptic
C. Ethosuccimide DOC for absence

76. Jaggery Rich source:
A. Zinc + Fe
B. Fe + Carotene
C. Carotene + Vitamin B_1

77. HDL true:
A. Reverse cholesterol transport
B. ABCA-1 transparent cholesterol effects
C. APOB-100 mediated endocytosis
D. Scavenger mediated cholesterol sequestration

ANSWERS

1	A	2	B	3		4	A	5	C	6	C	7	C
8		9	C	10	B	11		12		13	A	14	B
15		16		17		18	B	19	A	20		21	
22		23	A	24		25	B	26		27	A	28	C
29		30	A	31		32		33	A	34		35	
36	D	37		38		39		40		41	D	42	
43		44		45	A	46		47	A	48	A	49	
50		51		52		53		54		55		56	B
57		58		59		60	A	61	A	62		63	
64		65		66		67		68		69		70	
71		72	C	73		74		75		76	A	77	C

32

KOLKATA 2010

1. **Fibrates target:**
   A. TG B. LDL
   C. ApO (a) D. HDL
2. **Hibernating myocardium:**
   A. Parallel reduction in blood flow and metabolism
   B. Prolonged decreased perfusion at rest
   C. Transient decrease
   D. Reperfusion therapy
3. **Functional assessment of intermediate coronary lesion all *except*:**
   A. FFR
   B. Coronary flow reserve
   C. Quantitative coronary angiography
   D. IVUS
4. **Catheters in coronary angio all *except*:**
   A. Judkins B. Amplatz
   C. Sones D. Cournard
5. **BNP – True is:**
   A. Represents volume and/wall stretch
   B. Independent of renal function
   C. Always elevated in HF
   D. Elevated in systolic but not in diastolic HF
6. **Heparin S/E all *except*:**
   A. Alopecia
   B. Osteoporosis
   C. Hyperaldosteronism
   D. Rash
7. **Stress TMT – ST elevation in non-Q wave MI suggests:**
   A. Subendocardial severe ischemia
   B. Specific for coronary artery localization
   C. Normal in 10%
   D. Always due to vasopressin
8. **Free wall rupture AMI all *except*:**
   A. Elderly B. HTN
   C. Previous MI D. LV more common
9. **Absolute C/I of fibrmonolysis:**
   A. Embolic CVA 6 months back
   B. Severe dementia
   C. Duodenal ulcer with bleed × 4 weeks back
   D. Incidentally detected remote cerebral aneurysm (unruptured)
10. **MI – 4 days – autopsy shows:**
    A. Granulomatous inflammation
    B. Neutrophils + muscle necrosis
    C. Macrophages + collagen deposition
    D. Granulation tissue
11. **Epidemiology about CAD in India all *except*:**
    A. Stroke 3 times more common than CAD
    B. CAD accounts of 75% of CV death
    C. CA disease accounts for 24% of total death
    D. Fat intake in Indian diet is more
12. **Continuous murmur all *except*:**
    A. PDA + PR
    B. TOF + Pulmonary atresia
    C. CoA
13. **Non-pulmonary hypertensive:**
    A. Holosystolic B. Medium frequency
    C. Late systolic D. Midsystolic
14. **Acute severe AR associated with all *except*:**
    A. Loud S1
    B. Austin Flint murmur
    C. S3
    D. S4
15. **Apical HOCM associated with all *except*:**
    A. T wave inversion
    B. Spade appearance on angiography
    C. Severe MR common
    D. No intraventricular gradient
16. **Increase risk of I.E. with type of VSD:**
    A. Small restrictive VSD
    B. VSD + PS

C. VSD + AR
D. LV → RA

17. **Variable S1 seen in all *except*:**
A. AF B. VT
C. 2 : 1 AV block D. CHB

18. **Dicrotic pulse absent in:**
A. Cardiac tamponade
B. Severe cardiac failure
C. Hypovolemia
D. Nonobstructive HOCM

19. **IE prophylaxis is to be given in:**
A. Ostium secundum ASD + Dental extraction
B. Ligated PDA + Cystoscopy
C. CoA + Catheterization
D. AVR + Dental cleaning and scaling

20. **Rapid 'Y' descent is not seen in:**
A. TR
B. CCP
C. Endomyocardial fibrosis
D. RA myxoma

21. **Dynamic LVOT obst. all *except*:**
A. Amyloid
B. Hypereosinophilic syndrome
C. Post op AS
D. Anteroapical MI with posterobasal hypertrophy

22. **Left atrial appendage enlargement in:**
A. MS B. DORV
C. ECD D. AS

23. **PCWP not raised in:**
A. MS
B. Pulmonary vein stenosis
C. Cortriatrium
D. PPH

24. **Cardiogenic shock all *except*:**
A. CI < 1.0 B. BP < 80
C. PCWP >18 D. CVP < 3

25. **Native valve endocarditis + MRSA 1st line of treatment:**
A. Ceftriaxone
B. Vancomycin
C. Naficillin/Oxacillin + Gentamycin

26. **70 years female had 3 episodes of syncope in last 2 weeks. Sputum produce breathlessness × 2 days. Afebrile. Cholesterol = 170, X-ray prominent left heart border ano no, increase in any other chamber size with pulmonary edema BP = 130/90°. Most likely cause:**
A. Calcific AS B. IE
C. MS D. MVP

27. **AR common with all *except*:**
A. Subaortic VSD B. TOF
C. BAV D. Truncus arteriosus

28. **Pulmonary artery dilation are all *except*:**
A. Idiopathic pulmonary artery dilatation
B. Dysplastic pulmonary artery
C. TOF + absent pulmonary valve
D. DORV

29. **AV discordance:**
A. Single ventricle
B. TGA
C. Congenital CHB

30. **Factors which doesn't decrease in cyanotic HD:**
A. V
B. VI
C. VII
D. VIII

31. **Cyanotic disease with increased PBF:**
A. Eisenmenger
B. Ebstein's anomaly
C. Pulmonary atresia
D. Taussig bing anomaly

32. **13 years webbed neck, short stature, decreased perfusion of lower extemities, rib notching likely cause:**
A. Post ductal CoA
B. Preductal CoA
C. Down syndrome

33. **Max. pulmonary a pressure is seen in:**
A. ASD + Eisenmenger
B. Ebstein's anomaly

34. **AR common with all *except*:**
A. Subaortic VSD
B. TOF
C. BAV
D. Truncus arteriosus

35. **Low voltage ECG all *except*:**
A. Normal variant B. Myocarditis
C. Pericarditis D. COPD

36. **ββ – with additional alpha blocking action all *except*:**
A. Bisoprolol B. Bucindolol
C. Labetalol D. Carvedilol

37. **ββ - with additional vasodilatation due to calcium channel blocking at high dose:**
A. Carvedilol
B. Esmolol
C. Propranolol
D. Nadolol

38. 30 years male presents with history of transient loss of consciousness and palpitations ECG shows VT. Drug to be avoided:

A. Adenosine **B.** Verapamil
C. DC shock **D.** Amiodarone

39. At high dose β blocker having CCB effect causing vasodilatation:

A. Nadolol **B.** Carvidilol
C. Propranolol **D.** Esmolol

40. Hyperkalemia ECG all *except*:

A. Increase PR **B.** Increase QRS
C. Increase QT **D.** Asystole

41. Niacin side effect all *except*:

A. Hyperuricemia
B. Hyperglycemia
C. Hypercalcemia
D. Hepatotoxicity

42. Regarding anatomy of kidney true are all *except*:

A. DCT cell more eosinophilic than PCT
B. Macula densa cell are non-striated muscle
C. Since supplied symp N the renal disease may present as large bowl obstruction

43. Carpal Tunnel syndrome all *except*:

A. Adductor following paralysis
B. Opponens policis, palsy
C. Lateral 3 finger sensory palsy
D. 1st and 2nd lumbrical palsy

44. Regarding hand true all *except*:

A. Both radial/ulnar bursa above 2.5 cm in flexor retinaculum
B. Sensory supply – C7
C. C8-T1 for small m/s
D. Art and nerve cross superficial to metacarpal ligament

45. Thyroid anatomy:

A. Isthmus opposite to 4-6 ring
B. Lateral lobe derived from 4th branchial arch
C. Thyrocalcitonin release cause hype Ca++
D. L drainage to Jugulo digastric nodes

46. Pro drug:

A. Gemifloxacin
B. Prulifloxacin
C. Pancuronium
D. Lisinopril

47. A-V shunt of skin:

A. Not sensitive to circulating epinephrine
B. Depends on metabolic need
C. Respond to autoregulation
D. Cholinergic

48. Drug causing latent T.B. reactivation:

A. Nitozoxinide **B.** Tomoxifen
C. Leflunomide **D.** Cedofovir

49. Most common site for cerebral haemorrhage:

A. Ext. capsule / Putamen
B. Pons
C. Ventricle

50. True about multiple sclerosis:

A. Disease of Grey matter
B. Disease of PNS (chronic remitting) relapsing disease
C. Infectious disease
D. Optic N. cerebellum are most common site

51. Gibbus at T6 spinal cord segment compress:

A. T6 **B.** T7
C. T8 **D.** T9

52. CSF storage in pyogenic meningitis for few hours:

A. – 20°C **B.** 4
C. 10 **D.** 37°C

53. Most common side effect of lithium:

A. DI **B.** Tremor
C. Odema **D.** Sick sinus syndrome

54. Purine synthesis' substrate required:

A. Ribose PO_4 **B.** PPRP
C. Thymidine **D.** Arc b

55. Apoptosis mediated:

A. GMP **B.** AMP
C. Cyt c. **D.** No synthetase

56. Cytogentic abnormality in leukemia all *except*:

A. CML 9 : 22 **B.** AML 15 : 17
C. ALL 9 : 20 **D.** Burkitt 18 : 14

57. Swine Flu (Influenza A):

A. All 16 H cause swine infection
B. All 9 N cause bird infector
C. Genetic ressortment cause pandemic
D. RT PCR is diagnostic

58. MOTT true:

A. Not cause pulmonary disease immunocompetent individual
B. Rifampicin usually active
C. Sensitive to clarithromycin

59. Leptospira diagnostic test (most sensitive):

A. CFT
B. ELISA
C. MAT

60. REM sleep is due to:

A. Adrinergic
B. Cholinergic
C. Serotonergic
D. PGE2

61. **Prevalence increase by:**
A. In migration of susceptible
B. Moving out causes decrease incidence
C. Decrease incidence
D. Migration of healthy individual

62. **In well fed state the enzyme increased in fatty tissue:**
A. Glycerol kinase
B. Glycogen synthase
C. G PO_4ase
D. Glycogen phosphorylase

63. **Causal relation best determined by:**
A. RCT
B. Prospective cohort
C. Retrospective cohort
D. Case control

64. **HbA1C at:**
A. 6-12 weeks
B. 8-12 weeks
C. 6-8 weeks

65. **New drug in India after license takes:**
A. 3 years
B. 5 years
C. 10 years
D. 7 years

66. **Dobutamine stress echo in hibernating myocardium gives:**
A. Biphasic response
B. Continuous increase
C. Interrupted response

67. **Most common cause of embolic CVA:**
A. AF
B. Prosthetic valve
C. DCMP
D. IE

68. **S2 splitting:**
A. Increase venous return right side
B. Decrease VR lest side
C. Increase pulmonary valve hang out interval
D. All

69. **Pulmonary stenosis – all *except*:**
A. Pulmonary Ej. click increases on expiration
B. Severity increases, murmur becomes longer and early peaking
C. With non-restrictive VSD, murmur becomes shorter with increasing severity
D. Soft P2

70. **Most common cause of embolic CVA:**
A. AF
B. Prosthetic valve
C. DCMP
D. IE

71. **Mycotic aneurysm:**
A. IE
B. Atherosclerosis
C. Marfan's
D. None of the above

72. **True about anatomy all *except*:**
A. IVS 45 to sagittal plane
B. Right AV valve almost vertical axis
C. RA is ant, inf to right of LA
D. Anterosuperior leaflet of tricuspid valve is largest and attached to IVS through anterior and papillary muscles

73. **CCP echo feature:**
A. Thickened pericardium
B. Multi-phasic hepatic vein flow
C. Excessive respiratory variation in AV inflow velocities
D. Notching in pulmonary valve in M mode in systole

ANSWERS

1	A	2	A	3	D	4	D	5	A	6	C	7	B
8	C	9	D	10	B	11	A	12	A	13	B	14	A
15	C	16	C	17	C	18	D	19	D	20	D	21	B
22	A	23	D	24	D	25	C	26	A	27	B	28	B
29	A	30	B	31	D	32	A	33	A	34	B	35	C
36	A	37	A	38	B	39	B	40	C	41	C	42	A
43	A	44	A	45		46	B	47		48	C	49	A
50	D	51	C	52	B	53	B	54	A	55	C	56	D
57	D	58	C	59	C	60	B	61	A	62	B	63	A
64	B	65	B	66	A	67	A	68	D	69	B	70	A
71	A	72	B	73	C								

33

PGI 2011

CARDIOLOGY

1. **Causes of pulsus paradoxus:**
   A. CCP
   B. RCMP
   C. Massive pulmonary embolism
   D. LV failure

2. **True about EMF:**
   A. 80% LV involvement
   B. Eosinophilia present in most cases
   C. Systolic function is normal
   D. Seen in tropical and subtropical countries
   E. Commonly seen in middle aged and elderly

3. **Wide QRS tachy are:**
   A. Antidromic tachycardia
   B. Orthodromic tachycardia with aberrancy
   C. SVT with accessing conduction
   D. AT with functional RBBB
   E. AVNRT with nodoventricular conduction with antegrade conduction

4. **Rheumatic arthritis:**
   A. Seen in 2/3rd of cases with rheumatic fever
   B. Monoarthritis is most common
   C. Most cases recover within 3 to 4 weeks
   D. Jaccouds arthritis involve small joints
   E. Caused by α–hemolytic streptococcus

5. **Rheumatic carditis:**
   A. It is pancarditis
   B. New onset cardiomegaly significance myocarditis
   C. More common in older age
   D. Lifelong prophylaxis is required
   E. 70–75% cases have neutral involvement

6. **Mitral stenosis causes of chest pain:**
   A. Bronchitis
   B. Pericarditis
   C. Pulmonary embolism
   D. RV ischemia
   E. Coronary embolism

7. **MDM of MS:**
   A. OS and murmur ↓on inspiration and ↑ on expiration
   B. ↑ in strain phase of valsalva
   C. Intensity does not denote severity
   D. Severe RV dilatation is the cause of silent MS
   E. Murmur persist as long as gradient between LV and LA is > 10 mm

8. **Murmur of AS:**
   A. In severe AS intensity of murmur is $\geq 3/6$
   B. AVA 1.5–2 cm^2 is considered as moderate AS
   C. Mean gradient > 60 mm Hg denotes severe AS
   D. Velocity > 4 m/sec 13 severe AS
   E. AVA < 0.4 cm^2/m^2 in continuity equation denotes severe AS

9. **Regarding murmurs:**
   A. Murmur of MR is not affected by post extra-systolic accentuate
   B. Squatting ↓es murmur of AS

10. **MS with AF:**
    A. ↑es LV end diastolic volume
    B. LV fraction is supranormal
    C. Regional hypokinesia is common
    D. LVEDP is normal

11. **True/False:**
    A. 30–40% filling of LV occurs in early diastole
    B. Diastasis contributes 5%
    C. E/E < 15 normal
    D. PV systolic / PV diastolic ↓ means diastolic dysfunction

12. **Cardiac examination:**
    A. Double apical impulse is commonly due to palpable a wave
    B. Absent pericardium and thoracic abnormality

may cause precordial pulsations lateral to mid clavicular line

C. Right supraclavicular pulsations not commonly due to kinked and tortoms right carotid

D. Carotid and left apical impulse on examination appear synchronous

13. **Regarding thrombolytics:**

A. STK is as indirect activator of plasminogen

B. Less fibrin in specific

C. Longer t ½ than TNK

D. TIMI–3 flow with TNK is better than STK

14. **PCI preferred over thrombolysis:**

A. IWMI with RWMZ

B. Extensive anterior wall ML

C. Cardiogenic shock

D. PCI centre (Door to balloon) is 90 ms

E. < 1 hour presentation

15. **ARVD:**

A. It is acquired disease

B. MRI gold standard

C. ICD P_X of choice

D. Fibrofatty infiltration of RV occurs

16. **Absolute C/I to thrombolysis:**

A. Traumatic and prolonged CPR > 10 mins

B. Ischemic stroke > 2 years

C. Prior hemorrhagic stroke

D. BP > 180 mns / > 110 mns

E. Peptic ulcer history

17. **Periprocedural MI reduced in:**

A. Prasugrel before elective PCI

B. Statins before PCI

C. IV verapamil in venous graft

D. Intracoronary urokinase

E. PTFE covered stent

18. **High risk TMT:**

A. Symptoms < 6 METS

B. BP rise not more than 120 mns or fall of 10 mns

C. Typical angina

D. ST ↑ other than OVR

E. Reproducible sustained VT

19. **C/I of TMT:**

A. Acute MI < 7 days

B. High risk CIA

C. WPW syndrome

D. High grade AV block

E. Age > 75 years

20. **Following present absolutely in neonatal period:**

A. TOF

B. Severe PS

C. PDA

D. CHB with bradycardia

E. Massive AV fistula

21. **SLE with cardiac involvement:**

A. Pericarditis in 60%

B. Valvular involvement > 50%

C. Tamponade rax

D. Coronary arteritis most common cause of ischemic heart disease

E. Babies born to mother with SLE have ↑ed risk of CHB

22. **Mediterranean diet:**

A. High fat (35–40%)

B. Red meat and eggs allowed

C. Modifed wine allowed

D. Sunflower oil is most common source of fat

E. Poor compliance

23. **Cause of long QT:**

A. Digoxin

B. Quinidine

C. Hypomagnesemia

D. Hypokalemia

E. Liquid protein diet

24. **Mechanism of arrhythmia:**

A. Digoxin → DAD

B. Long QT → EAD

C. EAD is due to ↓ of membrane potential in phase III and IV

D. Overdrive atrial pacing ↓es amplitude

E. Post repolarization refractoriness is due to tachycardia dependent block

25. **Antiarrhythmic:**

A. Class IA ↓es Vmax and prolonged action potential duration

B. APD ↓es Vmax ↑ by Ib

C. IC ↓es and Vmax and ↑es refractoriness

D. Out of I_a I_b I_c ; I_e has slowest onset of action

26. **HCM:**

A. Risk of SCD ↑es as LU thickness ↑es

B. SCV MR is due to intrinsic heart disease rather SAM

27. **Balloon atrial septostomy:**

A. Neonates > 1 month old are suitable for surgery

B. Can be donc in TAPVC to coronary sinus with restrictive ASD

C. Critical PS with HF

D. Umbilical vein can be used

E. In … PAH it is done to ↓ cyanosis

28. **BMV:**

A. CMV better than BMV in long term

B. IJV approach best

C. BMV produce $\downarrow$es need for 2° prophylaxis
D. Contraindicated in suprasystemic PAH
E. Best results are seen when care is less and no MR

29. Percutaneous intervention are useful in:
A. Calcific MS
B. Calcific AS
C. Supra mitral ring
D. Degenerated prostolic aortic valve
E. Subaortic membrane

30. Difference between PCWP and LVEOP is seen in:
A. Parachute mitral valve
B. Cor-triatriatum
C. Pulmonary vein stenosis
D. Submitral aneurysm
E. PAH

31. Takayasu arteritis:
A. Subclavian in 90%
B. In India HTN is commoner than Japanese
C. Pulmonary arteritis in ½
D. Aortic involvement is not seen

32. Bicuspid aortic valve:
A. Inherently stenotic
B. Associated with $\uparrow$ed risk of aortic dissection
C. 50% associated with CoA
D. Incidence > 2%
E. Male: female: 4:/

33. Rhabdomyoma:
A. Common in atria
B. 80% in < 1 year
C. Disappears by 6 years
D. Can be associated with tuberous sclerosis
E. Male: Female: 4:/

34. Regarding pulmonary valvotomy:
A. Contraindication in Noorani
B. Should be diagnosed if gradient > 40 mm Hg
C. If cyanosis present contraindication
D. Gradient can $\uparrow$ after valvoline
E. Restenosis not seen

35. DES:
A. $\downarrow$es acute thrombosis
B. Drey between stent and balloon
C. Requires special catheter and technique for drug delivery
D. Biodegradable under clinical investigation
E. No need to monitor for side effects of antimitotic drugs used

36. FFR:
A. Estimated one catheter in coronary sinus and another beyond the obstruction
B. < 0.9 is abnormal
C. Adenosine is used
D. Instantaneously measured in cath. lab.
E. Should not be done in tortuous vessels

37. True:
A. Palpography measures temperature of unstable plaque
B. OCT is best to osseous healing of vascular injury
C. FFR is used to osseous effectiveness of stent deployment
D. CAG is best to osseous mechanism of restenosis
E. Temperature FFR is used to micro vascular resistance

38. AF cardiovision:
A. Oral ibutilide is DOC for pharmacologic cardio-version
B. Amiodarone can be used in AF with accessory pathway
C. Propafenone contraindicated in patients with structural heart disease
D. If AF of > 48 hours duration of anticoagulation after cardioversion 4 weeks
E. IV digoxin is mildly effective in controlling AV nodal conduction

39. JVP:
A. Normally < 3 cm rise in HJ reflux
B. Normally < 15 seconds in HJ reflux
C. Prominent X–decent produces systolic car lobe movement
D. Steep Y decent is seen in any HF

40. Pregnancy changes:
A. Volume risk at 10 weeks
B. Plasma volume $\uparrow$ at 2nd trimester
C. CO $\uparrow$es 40-50% from 3rd trimester
D. Post delivery $\uparrow$ in venous return

41. Fetal circulation:
A. RV contributes 55% of CO
B. Pulmonary flow is 7 to 8% of CO
C. Ductus arteriosus anatomically closes at birth
D. If weight is < 1500 gm then PDA is most common cause of CHF

42. $\uparrow$ed size of pulmonary artery on CXR in ToF seen in:
A. Absent pulmonary valve
B. Pink ToF
C. PDA
D. Severe RVOT obstruction
E. AV septal defect

43. ToF with HF causes:
A. Severe anemia
B. HTN
C. Prolonged survival
D. PR
E. Severe PS

44. Blood supply of heart:
A. Conus A. supplies RVOT
B. Acute marginal A. is branch of LCX
C. AV mide mostly supplied by RCA
D. Posteromedial papillary muscle has dual supplied
E. IVS is supplied by KCA and LAD

45. Thallium:
A. Myocardium with ↑ed activity has fast washout and vice-versa
B. Sestamibi is better than thallium
C. Thallium t½ 13 is shortest F
D. Tc and testofen has minimal redistribution
E. 0 to 4 is grading myocardial perfusion

46. Causes of ↓S_1:
A. Short PR
B. Premature mitral closure
C. ↓dp/dt of LV?
D. ↑ed flow through valve
E. Classified mitral valve

47. Regarding vasodilation and constrictions T/F:
A. NO can act on denuded endothelium
B. Endothelium is most potent vasodilator known
C. NO has antiplatelet effect
D. Adenosine causes endothelium independent nasodilatic

48. Shunts:
A. Pott's is ascending AO to PA
B. Glen's SYC to right PA
C. Waterstones
D. Modified BT subclavion artery to PA
E. Classical BT can be done in either side of arch of AO

49. True:
A. ANREP effect is tachycardia induced ↑ contractility
B. Treppe cause ↑ of contractility on sudden ↑ of aortic impedance
C. Aortic impedance is equal to pressure flow

50. PVR:
A. Hypoxia ↑es PVR
B. Total PVR = 80 dynes
C. SVR = PVR is normally 2.0
D. Expressed as resistance along arterioles and capillaries
E. PVR = mean pressure / flow

51. Pulmonary hypertension:
A. Obliterative bronchiolitis is a cause post long transpirant
B. Pulmonary HTN ↓es dyspnoea in MS
C. Fibrinoid necrosis and plexopathy is found in histology in MS
D. Chronic alveolar hypoventilation with N parenchyma is a mechanism

52. Exercise testing:
A. Super exercise cause ↑ of CO due to ↑ of HR + strike volume
B. HR = 220–Age underestimates HR in female
C. In bicycle ergometry 1 W = 6 kpm
D. Vagal reactivation is main mechanism in post exercise decentral response
E. Lactic acid accumulate @ 50–60% of aerobic activity

53. Carotid sinus:
A. Either terminates or no effect on AVNRT
B. Gradually slow sinus tachycardia
C. PAT slowly rate ↓es and then stop
D. In AFI ventricular rate is slumped

54. True:
A. Atropine worsens AV nodel block
B. Isoproterenol and exercise improves AV nodal block
C. Isoproterenol worsens his Purkinje block

55. Risk factors for CIN:
A. LV dysfunction
B. Prolonged procedure
C. DM_2
D. Dose
E. CAD stenosis > 70%

56. Framingham criteria:
A. HR > 120 is minor
B. ↑ HJR is major
C. Basal rales minor
D. PND minor
E. Night cough minor

57. Bioprosthetic valve v/s mechanical:
A. Lifelong anticoagulant regd.
B. Better than material
C. Stan Edwards ball cage is inherently stone
D. Thermlock is highest at risk
E. If thrombosis occurs then target INR is 2 to 3

58. PVE T/F:
A. For mechanical valve endocarditis duck's criteria is not useful
B. Early endocarditis is < 90 days
C. Fever is not seen in early endocarditis
D. Before fibroptic rigid bronchoscopy antibiotics prophylaxis is need
E. In late endocarditis streptococcus is common

59. True all *except*:
A. Ezetimibe acts by PPAR–α
B. Bile–acid sequestrants ↑es TG
C. Resins useful with statins to further ↓ LDL

D. Acanthosis nigricans is a major side effect of nicotinic acid
E. Fish oil contain monounsaturated fatty acids

60. **Fabry's disease:**
A. Dominant is X-linked
B. Enzyme difference
C. Angiokeratoma
D. HTN
E. CAD

MEDICINE

61. **Diagnostic criteria for hepatorenal syndrome–all *except*:**
A. Low GFR
B. Proteinuria > 500
C. Absence of shock
D. Urine RBC < 50

62. **Good prognostic sign in idiopathic pulmonary fibrosis all *except*:**
A. Male sex
B. Young age
C. Predominant cellular histology
D. Current smoking

63. **Hypogonadism A comorbid illnesses:**
A. ↑worst-hip ratio net A/W erectile dysfunction
B. Inverse association between sex hormone and Mitsubishi syndrome statistically significant in all race/ethnics
C. MI and worst circumference significant –ve correlate testosterone in men type 2DM associates in stronger for BMS
D. Love testosterone nor risk factor for CAD

64. **Differential diagnosis of heat stroke all *except*:**
A. Benign intracranial hypertension
B. Viral encephalitis
C. Valproate toxicity
D. Intracranial bleed

65. **Anti-convulsant drugs associated with depression:**
A. Phenobarbitone
B. Valproic acid
C. Phenytoin
D. Carbamazepine

66. **Treatment of acute gout of all *except*:**
A. Probenecid
B. ACTH
C. Colchicine
D. Steroid

67. **Acute presentation of sarcoidosis, uveitis, arthritis, erythema nodosum:**
A. Lofgren syndrome
B. Loffler
C. Heerfort
D. Fowler

68. **Activated protein C:**
A. APCHE > 25

69. **Most common organism in shunt infection:**
A. Staph aureus
B. Streptococcus pneumonia
C. Pseudomonas
D. E. coli

70. **Drug not used in RA:**
A. INF–α
B. Abatacept
C. Methotrexate
D. Etanercept

71. **Wegener granulomatosis all *except*:**
A. C-ANCA
B. P-ANCA

72. **Microcytic hypochromic anemia all *except*:**
A. An. of ch. do.
B. Sideroblastic anemia
C. Thalassemia
D. Celiac disease

73. **Anti-centromere antibody:**
A. Limited systemic sclerosis
B. Different systemic sclerosis
C. MCTD

74. **All are risk factors NSAIM induced mucosal injury *except*:**
A. Old age
B. Male sex
C. Severe infection
D. Steroid

75. **Good clinical practice guideline all *except*:**
A. Review board permission not required

76. **True about heat stroke:**
A. Classical heat stroke affect healthy young man
B. Exertional heat stroke common in acclimated athletics
C. Exertional heat stroke due to excess heat production/classical heat stroke defect in dissipation
D. EHS defective heat dissipation/classical heat stroke due to excess heat production

77. **Proteases inhibition all *except*:**
A. Tenofovir
B. Indinavir
C. Nelfinavir

78. **Polymorphism commonly seen in:**
A. SLC–2A9
B. SAD. 2BX
C. SLR. 202
D. SDA. 2PX

79. **High incidence of calcification all *except*:**
A. Craniopharyngioma
B. Ependymoma
C. Meningioma
D. Oligodendroglioma

80. **PEP rabies vaccine given all *except*:**
A. Rat B. Bat
C. Raccoon D. Fox

81. **Height of Raynauds all *except*:**
A. ARB B. ACE inhibitor
C. CAB D. Sildenafil

82. **Anti-epileptic not interact with OCP:**
A. Carbamazepine B. Oxcarbazepine
C. Valproate D. Topiramate

83. **Colistin effective in all *except*:**
A. Acinetobacter B. Staph aureus
C. Pseudoanemia D. E. coli

84. **Daptomycin effective in all *except*:**
A. Skin
B. Lung
C. Subculture tissue
D. Septicemia

85. **Post-transplant infection after 6 months all *except*:**
A. Nocardia B. Aspergillus
C. PCP D. CNV

86. **Guideline for weaning all *except*:**
A. $P_a O_2 > 60$ with $FiO_2 < 50$
B. PEEF < 5
C. Vital capacity > 10 w/m
D. Static compliance > 30 ml/H_2O

87. **Most likely trigger for status epilepticus:**
A. Sertraline
B. Pantoprazole
C. Imipenem cilastatin
D. Hydrochlorothiazide lisinopril

88. **False regarding HCV:**
A. Genotype II less responsive to treatment
B. G–III t/t 6 m
C. G–II t/t 6 m
D. G–I t/t 6 m

89. **Drug for $H_5 N_1$:**
A. Zanamivir B. Zidovudine
C. Indinavir D. Entecavir

90. **Stroke causing arrhythmia:**
A. Right insular B. Right mid brain
C. Occipital lobe D. Frontal lobe

91. **True TSS all *except*:**
A. Fever
B. True blood culture
C. Desquamating enytheme (macular)
D. Renal failure

92. **IgA nephropathy associated with:**
A. Gluten enteropathy
B. Cirrhosis
C. Dermatitis herpetiformis
D. Punpun fulminans

93. **Recovery of platelets dysfunction most prolonged with:**
A. Abciximab B. Eptifibatide
C. Infliximab D. Tirofiban

94. **Motor neuropathy all *except*:**
A. Lead
B. Dapsone
C. Hypoglycemia
D. Pyridoxine excess

95. **Physical sign show secondary polycythemia:**
A. Splenomegaly B. Cyanosis
C. Pruritus D. Easy bruising

96. **30 years male fever massive splenomegaly pancytopenia not used treatment all *except*:**
A. Paromomycin B. Miltefosine
C. Ciprofloxacin D. Amphotericin B

97. **MRI best for stroke:**
A. Grad echo MRI
B. T_2
C. T_2
D. Diffusion weighted

98. **20 years male Hb 5 gml, TLC 9000, P_2% lymphoblast 96%:**
A. IV ciprofloxacin
B. Oral ciprofloxacin
C. Packed cell RBC
D. GCSt Adv

99. **Drug induced lupus all *except*:**
A. Renal inv.
B. Anti histone
C. Anti disease DNA
D. Serositis

100. **All an early sign of infarct *except*:**
A. Loss of gravy white diffuser
B. Sulcus effacement
C. Insular ribbon sign
D. Hypodensity

ANSWERS

1		2		3		4	A,C	5	A	6		7	
8		9		10		11		12		13		14	
15		16		17		18		19		20		21	
22		23		24		25		26		27		28	
29		30		31		32		33		34		35	
36		37		38		39		40		41		42	
43		44		45		46		47		48		49	
50		51		52		53		54		55		56	
57		58		59		60		61		62		63	
64	A	65	A	66		67	A	68	A	69		70	A
71		72		73	A	74		75		76		77	A
78		79		80		81		82		83		84	
85		86		87		88		89		90		91	
92		93		94		95		96		97		98	
99		100											

34

PGI 2010

1. **Risk factors in Indians as composed to western:**
   A. Have more LP (a) levels
   B. Homocysteine levels are low
   C. Metabolic syndrome is less common
   D. Diffuse disease is more common
   E. Early age of onset

2. **False about increase TG:**
   A. Risk factor for CAD
   B. Tamoxifen increases TG
   C. Estrogen containing OCP decreases TG
   D. Very high levels – Retinal vessel occlusion
   E. Niacin decreases TG

3. **58 years male with DM2 with CAD with TVD with LVD has to undergo CABG after 3 months. Drugs to be avoided:**
   A. Cilostazol **B.** Ranolazine
   C. Ivabradine **D.** Tximetazidine
   E. Sildenafil

4. **Emerging CAD risk factors are all *except*:**
   A. Small dense HDL
   B. RA factor
   C. Hyper fibrinogenemia
   D. Lp (a)

5. **Risk factors for SCD in HOCM:**
   A. Wall thickness more than 20 mm
   B. Family history
   C. LVOTO
   D. Hypertensive response on TMT
   E. NSVT on 48 hours of Holter

6. **In HOCM, false is:**
   A. Tropin-T is associated with marked LVH
   B. Tropin-I is associated with restrictive physiology
   C. Flat response in BP is risk factor for SCD
   D. RV dilatation has good prognosis
   E. > 30 mm of LV thickness is a risk factor

7. **DIP and Plateau pattern in RV pressure tracing is not seen:**
   A. Chronic TR
   B. HCM
   C. Restrictive cardiomyopathy
   D. CCP
   E. Inf + RVMI

8. **Kussmaul's sign most common cause is:**
   A. CCP
   B. RVF irrespective of cause
   C. RCMP
   D. TS

9. **True in restrictive physiology:**
   A. Biatrial enlargement
   B. LVEDP increased
   C. Mean RA pressure
   D. RVEDP decreased
   E. LA pressure increased

10. **LVEDP increased in:**
    A. MS
    B. Pulmonary veno-occlusive disease
    C. Acute MR
    D. Cardiac temponade

11. **RV dilatation is seen in:**
    A. ASD
    B. Acute pulmonary embolism
    C. ARVD
    D. Severe PR

12. **Patient with MS, NYHA class - II, LA thrombus (small Focus) correct management is:**
    A. BMV
    B. Closed mitral commissurotomy
    C. Open mitral commissurotomy
    D. Mitral valve replacement
    E. Anticoagulant followed by TEE after 3 months If clot absent – BMV

13. **Continuous murmur:**
A. RSOV to RA
B. Coronary A-V fistula
C. PDA with PAH
D. AP window in 1 day neonate

14. **Wide splitting seen in:**
A. RBBB
B. Ebstein
C. LAHB
D. PDA with Eisenmenger
E. LPHB

15. **MSCT likely use:**
A. Coronary artery anomalies
B. Complex congenital heart disease
C. R/o CAD in new onset HF
D. To diagnosis CAD in obese patient with BMI > 40
E. Alternative to conventional CAG prior to CABG

16. **Reversibility in PAH is seen by:**
A. 100% O_2
B. 4.5% O_2
C. 40-80 ppm of NO
D. 40-80 ppm of N_2O
E. Prostacyclin infusion

17. **Mortality decreasing drug in CHF:**
A. Furosemide B. Spironolactone
C. Valsartan D. Nevibolol
E. Digoxin

18. **Beta-blocker in HF:**
A. Metoprolol is better than carvedilol in DCMP
B. β-blocker decrease mortality in diastolic HF
C. Should not be given in DCMP NYHA-II
D. Should not be given with ramipril
E. Carvedilol is useful in ICMP

19. **Takotsubo CMP true is:**
A. Occurs in a young male
B. Associated with emotional stress
C. Apices involved
D. CAG shows TVD
E. ECG is normal

20. **Severity of MS is indicated by:**
A. Loudness of OS proportional to severity
B. Presystolic accentuation is directly proportional to severity
C. Warfarin should be given if AF develops
D. Loud S1 indicates severity

21. **C-TGA all with:**
A. VSD is most commonly associated anomaly
B. In autopsy abnormal morphology of tricuspid valve is seen in all cases
C. Coarctation is rare association
D. Subpulmonary obstruction in 50% at LV
E. Progressive TR and CHB increases with age

22. **A patient with small VSD with IE with qp/qs, <1.5: 1. False is:**
A. Incidence of IE in VSD is 1-2/1000 patient occurred years
B. Mortality (lifetime) of IE is 6-7%
C. Surgery is indicated if previous IE
D. Size of VSD is related to incidence of IE
E. On closure of VSD risk of IE disappears

23. **True statement:**
A. Eisenmenger in ASD occurs early than VSD
B. Left parasternal heave more common with ASD with Eisenmenger
C. Reverse splitting can be seen with ASD with Eisenmenger
D. Closure of VSD should be done early in VSD with Eisenmenger

24. **PDA true is:**
A. Increase incidence of PDA is seen in 1st trimester Rubella
B. Holt-Oram syndrome
C. Down's syndrome
D. Fetal valproate syndrome
E. Incontinentia pigmenti

25. **AVSD:**
A. Associated with Trisomy 21
B. Closure should be done @ 3-4 years
C. Associated with LVOT obstruction
D. Early onset of Eisenmenger

26. **Fabry's disease:**
A. Auto recessive
B. Angiokeratoma most commonly on face
C. Deficiency of α-glucosidase
D. Renal involvement is common
E. Associated with LVH

27. **Visceral artery aneurysm seen in:**
A. Behcet's disease
B. Takayasu arteritis
C. Dermatomyositis
D. Polymyositis
E. PAN

28. **Mid aortic aneurysm seen in:**
A. Takayasu type I
B. Behcet's disease
C. Wegener's granulomatosis
D. SLE
E. GCA

29. **Most common cause of RAS in children:**
A. Takayasu B. FMD

C. Arteriosclerosis D. PAN
E. None

30. **CPR in pregnancy:**
A. DC shock is contraindicated
B. Cricoid pressure during positive pressure ventilation
C. ET size 1-2 mm higher required then usual.
D. CPR should be done in right lateral position
E. Hysterotomy indicated if < 20 weeks of gestation

31. **Trisomy 21 true is:**
A. PAH occurs early
B. AVSD should be operated normally
C. Increased risk of infective endocarditis

32. **HOCM, useful drugs (obstruction in case of HOCM):**
A. Disopyramide B. Metoprolol
C. Quinidine D. Digoxin
E. Nifedipine

33. **Not a K+ channelopathy is:**
A. LQT_1
B. LQT_3
C. Anderson Tarwail
D. Brugada
E. SQTS

34. **A football had sudden collapse while playing and was revived by CPR. ECG was done in hospital. Show T invention in V_1-V_4 slurring of S in V_1. QRS was 110 ms. Which is correct?**
A. δ is Brugada
B. δ is ARVD
C. ICD implantation is required
D. Quinidine is helpful to prevent electric storms
E. Next step is EPS followed by RFA

35. **ARVD mutation gene are:**
A. Plakoglobin
B. Desmorplakin
C. Plakophilin
D. Titiplatin
E. Troponin

36. **CHB is seen in:**
A. cTGA
B. dTGA
C. Maternal lupus
D. Tricuspid atresia
E. DORV

37. **Exercise induced VT seen in:**
A. ARVD B. Fasicule VT
C. CPVT D. Idopathic vF
E. RVOT-VT

38. **QT prolongation seen in all *except*:**
A. Sotalol B. Digoxin
C. Disopyramide D. Amiodarone
E. Quinidine

39. **LBBB:**
A. 3% incidence in general population
B. 20% incidence in MI
C. More incidence of HF on follow-up
D. Acute LBBB has better prognosis than pre-existing LBBB

40. **EMF true:**
A. Recent incidence in India increased
B. Steroid is causative in most cause
C. Outflow tract involvement occurs
D. Endocardial calcification can be present
E. Age of onset 60 years

41. **Increased risk of cholelithiasis seen with:**
A. Obesity
B. Chronic hemolytic anemia
C. Pregnancy
D. High protein

42. **Absolute indication of surgery in IE:**
A. >10 mm vegetation
B. Relapsed prosthetic valve IE
C. Myocardial abscess
D. Moderate to severe HF

43. **Hypercalcemia causes all *except*:**
A. Diarrhoea B. Polyuria
C. Confusion D. Nephrolithiasis

44. **LGBS in HIV seen in:**
A. Early stage
B. Late stage
C. Irrespective of stage
D. After virological failure of therapy

45. **DNA RNA both seen in organism:**
A. Bacteria B. Virus
C. Prions D. Plasmid

46. **IgM production without activation of TH cells seen with:**
A. Tetanus toxin
B. TSS toxin
C. Bact. LPS
D. Bovine penicillin
E. Albumin complexes

47. **Not an inclusion criteria for diagnosis of RA:**
A. AntioCCP Ab
B. Rheumatoid factor
C. Morning stiffness >1hour
D. Rheumatoid nodules

48. **Not used in RA:**
A. Abatacept B. IFN-α
C. Methotrexate D. Rituximab

49. **Not used in acute goat:**
A. Colchicine B. Probenicid
C. ACTH D. Steroids

50. **Uveitis + Arthritis + Sarcoidosis + Erythema nodosum:**
A. Lofgren's syndrome
B. Loffler's syndrome
C. Heerfordt syndrome
D. Fowler's syndrome

51. **Left upper lobe lung lesion in centre with hypercalcemia 16 mg/dl, phosphate 2.5 mg/dl. Likely morphology at autopsy:**
A. Small cell carcinoma
B. Suamous cell carcinoma
C. Adenocarcinoma
D. Bronchoalveolar

52. **Patient with myaesthenia gravis. Findings in PFT:**
A. TLC decrease, RV decrease, FEV_1/FVC normal
B. TLC decrease, RV increase, MIP decrease
C. TLC decrease, VC decrease, increase FEV_1/FVC, MIP normal

53. **Extracorpuscular defect is seen in:**
A. TTP
B. Sickle cells
C. PNH
D. Elliptocytosis

54. **Microcytic hypochromic anemia not seen in:**
A. Celiac disease
B. Thalassemia
C. Anemia of chronic disease
D. Sideroblastic anemia

55. **Relapsing polychondritis all *except*:**
A. Nose involvement
B. Aortic dilatation
C. ILD
D. Ear involvement

56. **Renin increase seen in all *except*:**
A. β-blocker B. AT_1 blocker
C. ACE blocker D. ECF

57. **Patient with RF with CHF with anemia with polyneuropathy with severe proteinuria. What should be done for diagnosis?**
A. Renal USG
B. Fat pad biopsy
C. Right heart catheterisation
D. Bone marrow biopsy

58. **Anti-centromere antibody seen in:**
A. Diffuse cutaneous SS
B. Limited cutaneous SS
C. MCTD

59. **Cause of hemoptysis in MS all *except*:**
A. PVH
B. PAH
C. Resolving pneumonitis
D. Pulmonary edema

60. **Finding according to Keith. Wegener classification in stage III:**
A. Flame shaped hemorrhage
B. Silver wiring
C. AV-nipping
D. Papilloedema

61. **Large fibre polyneuropathy seen with:**
A. Cisplatin B. Taxol
C. Pyridoxine D. All

62. **73 years female with progressive right knee pain especially on walking. Regarding osteoarthritis which is most important risk factor?**
A. Previous joint injury
B. Age
C. Gender
D. Obesity

63. **A patient with limited UC limited to mucose. Colonoscopy showed crypt abscess. Unlikely to be found:**
A. Current smoker
B. Age 15-30
C. Fraternal twin incidence not increase
D. Intact appendix

64. **Brainstem herniation through F. magnum. Classical finding:**
A. Miotic pupils
B. Ipsilateral facial N. palsy with pupil dilatation
C. Respiratory arrest
D. Locked-in state

65. **Not a cause of Vitamin D associated hypercalcemia:**
A. Vitamin D intoxication
B. Sarcoidosis
C. Hyperthyroidism
D. Idiopathic hypocalcemia of pregnancy

66. **True about hypogonadism:**
A. Decreased testosterone not associated with loss of libido and ED
B. C/P are decreased bone mass, fatigue, osteoporosis increased fat
C. Primary testicular failure is not associated with increased gonadotropin

D. Secondary testicular failure is associated with increase gonadotropin

67. **Protease inhibitors all *except*:**
A. Tenofovir
B. Indinavir
C. Nelfinavin
D. Lopinavir

68. **NSAID induced mucosal injury. All are R/F *except*:**
A. Male gender
B. Age (Elderly)
C. Sense infection
D. Steroid use associated with NSAID

69. **Subacute thyroditis. True finding is:**
A. With 2 weeks history of pain in thyroid with increase radio I_2 uptake, increase T_3, increase T4, decrease TSH
B. With painless thyroid history with increase radio I_2, uptake with decrease T_3, increase T_4, increase TSH
C. With 4 months history of neck pain T_3 decrease T_4 decrease increase TSH
D. With painful thyroid with USG mass

70. **DTRs all are involved *except*:**
A. Gamma motor
B. α motor neurons
C. Pyramidal neurons
D. Afferent muscle spindle

71. **Which is most characteristic function of MHC-I and II protein?**
A. Activation of complement
B. Presentation of antigens non-specifically to macrophages and granulocytes
C. Antibody production by B-cells
D. T-cell activation for phagocytosis

72. **How to differentiate SVC obstruction from cirrhosis?**
A. Dilated veins with downward flow
B. Increases fullness of flanks
C. Pulsating liver
D. Venous hum at umbilicus

73. **Guidelines for good clinical practice:**
A. Informed consent from all subjects participating in trial
B. Clearance from IRB/ethical committee not mandatory
C. Right of patient important than interest of science

74. **Mechanism of frequent change of bacter virulence in trypansoma and Neisseria:**
A. By plasmid through transduction
B. Frequent mutation at hotspots
C. Conjugation

75. **Anorexia nervosa. Not seen is:**
A. Avoidance of food related jobs
B. Distorted body image
C. Excessive exercise
D. Do not show hunger

76. **Pancreatic CA:**
A. 5% survival after 5 years
B. Most common site is tail
C. Mean age of presentation 48 years
D. Usually localized and responds to surgical resection

77. **Correctation coefficent 0.8:**
A. 64% variance is due to other variable
B. 64% value fall on the regression line
C. 80% variance is due to other variable
D. 80% value fall on the regression line

ANSWERS

1	A,D,E	2	B,D,E	3	A,E	4	A	5	B,E	6	A,D	7	A,B
8	A	9	A,B,C,E	10	C,D	11	A,B,C,D	12	E	13	A,B	14	A,B
15	A,B,C	16	E	17	B,C,D	18	E	19	B,C	20	C	21	A,D,E
22	B	23	C	24	A,C	25	A,C,D	26	D,E	27	B,E	28	B,C,D,E
29	A	30	B	31	A,B,C	32	A,B	33	B,D	34	B,C	35	A,B,C
36	A,C	37	A,B,C,E	38	B	39	B,C	40	A,D	41	D	42	A
43	A	44	A	45	A	46	C	47	C	48	B	49	B
50	A	51	B	52	B	53	A	54	C	55	C	56	A
57	B	58	B	59	B	60	A	61	D	62	B	63	A
64		65	C	66		67	A	68	A	69	C	70	C
71	B	72		73	B	74	A	75	A	76	A	77	B

35

PGI JUNE 2009

CARDIOLOGY

1. **AIVR:**
   - A. Seen in 20% of acute STEMI
   - B. Specific sign of reperfusion (specific)
   - C. More common in anterior wall MI
   - D. A/w worse prognosis
   - E. Amiodarone used to treat
2. **CABG:**
   - A. 8-12% of venous grafts get blocked by time of discharge
   - B. 30% of venous grafts get blocked by 1 year
   - C. 85% patency rate of LIMA at 10 years
   - D. SVG patency is better than radial artery
   - E. 5% rate of blockage after 1st year
3. **Obligatory myocardial ischemia is seen in:**
   - A. ALCAPA
   - B. Myocardial bridging
   - C. LCA from RC sinus with inter arterial course
   - D. Split RCA
   - E. AV fistula (coronary)
4. **Abciximab:**
   - A. Monoclonal antibody
   - B. Used in complicated PTCA
   - C. Inhibits Gp IIb / IIIa receptor thereby inhibiting its final pathway
   - D. Inhibits ADP receptor
   - E. Active orally
5. **Atrial infarction:**
   - A. RA > LA
   - B. Free wall > Appendage
   - C. A/w decrease in ANP
   - D. Isolated atrial infarction occurs in 15% of STEMI
   - E. Rupture never occurs
6. **Usual contraindication to thrombolysis with STK:**
   - A. Recurrent M.I. within 24 hours of acute M.I.
   - B. Aortic dissection
   - C. Atraumatic CPR
   - D. Internal bleed
   - E. Uncontrolled HTN
7. **Tall R in V1:**
   - A. Inferior wall MI
   - B. Posterior wall MI
   - C. RVH
   - D. Duchenne's
   - E. Apical MI
8. **Lipid profile:**
   - A. HDL <35 is a positive risk factor
   - B. HDL >35 is a negative risk factor
   - C. Cholesterol (total) less than 200 mg is target in CAD
   - D. In CAD, LDL goal is < 160
9. **Absolute contraindication to thrombolysis does not include:**
   - A. Acute pericarditis
   - B. Active internal bleeding (Peptic ulcer)
   - C. Aortic dissection
   - D. Head trauma < 3 months
10. **Recovery of platelet function is most delayed with:**
    - A. Abciximab
    - B. Eptifibatide
    - C. Tirofiban
    - D. All
11. **Contraindication to TMT are all *except*:**
    - A. Asymptomatic AS
    - B. MI < 2 days
    - C. UA
    - D. Acute myocarditis
12. **70 years male highest cardiovascular risk.**
    - A. 150/70
    - B. 110/90
    - C. 120/96
    - D. 140/80
13. **Pulsus paradoxus not seen in:**
    - A. Pericardial effusion
    - B. CCP

C. COPD
D. Tamponade

14. **Wide split S2 seen in:**
A. MR
B. LBBB
C. VSD
D. MS
E. ASD

15. **Reverse split S2 seen in:**
A. LBBB
B. RBBB
C. RV pacing
D. MS
E. Hypertensive heart disease

16. **Cervical venous hum:**
A. Most common in elderly
B. Typically louder in diastole
C. Decrease in anemia
D. Can be harsh and noisy
E. Disappears in pregnancy

17. **NYHA is useful in grading for all *except*:**
A. Cyanosis
B. Syncope
C. Fatigue
D. Palpation
E. Dyspnea

18. **Clonidine:**
A. Long $t_{1/2}$ in weeks
B. Centrally acting antihypertensive
C. May cause tachycardia on stopping
D. Rebound HTN on stopping
E. Sedation is a side effect

19. **RCMP vs CCP (in favor of RCMP):**
A. Pulmonary artery systolic increase
B. Septal bounce
C. Pulsus paradoxus
D. Square root sign
E. Raised JVP

20. **Coronary AV fistula:**
A. Large shunt
B. Most common in RCA
C. Most common in LV
D. Most commonly present with dyspnea and chest pain
E. I.E. never occurs

21. **I.E.:**
A. Most cases of patients present within 2 weeks of bacteremia
B. Splenomegaly is most common in acute than subacute IE
C. 5% patients have ICH
D. Most common embolic infarct involve MCA territory
E. Embolism is more common after 2 weeks of therapy

22. **Acute rheumatic fever:**
A. Is a streptococcal infection
B. Chorea
C. Carey Coomb's murmur may be seen
D. Pancarditis is seen
E. Has residual deformity after arthritis

23. **Thoracic artery aneurysm:**
A. A/w atherosclerosis
B. Syphilis
C. Cystic medial degeneration
D. Periarteritis nodosa
E. SLE

24. **Pulsus paradoxus:**
A. Obesity (Morbid)
B. Pregnancy
C. Cardiac tamponade
D. A.R.
E. M.R.

25. **ECG changes in acute pericarditis:**
A. P.R. depression
B. ST elevation more in aVR
C. Tall P wave
D. RBBB
E. LBBB

26. **Valsalva maneuver:**
A. Square wave in MS
B. Square wave in CHF
C. SBP decrease in stage I
D. Reflex bradycardia in phase II
E. Right sided murmur increase in phase III

27. **Hand grip (Isometric) exercise:**
A. Murmur of AS increase
B. Murmur of HOCM decrease
C. MR decrease
D. AR decrease
E. LVS3 decreases

28. **I.E. prophylaxis is indicated in (Valvular heart disease):**
A. Tonsillectomy
B. Tooth extraction
C. Gallbladder surgery
D. Endotracheal intubation
E. Cardiac catheterization

29. **Which is 1st treatment in SVC obstruction before definitive diagnosis?**
A. Endovascular stenting
B. Chemotherapy
C. Radio
D. CT + Radiotherapy

30. **cc TGA a/w:**
 A. VSD – 75%
 B. q wave absent in right precordial leads and present in its sided leads
 C. Subpulmic PS
 D. Congenital CHB
 E. Left side AV valve abnormality in 10%

31. **Anomalous pulmonary venous drainage:**
 A. Loud P2
 B. S2-narrow split
 C. Subdiaphragmatic is most common
 D. Left axis deviation in ECG
 E. 80% untreated die in 1st year

32. **ECG changes in athletic heart syndrome:**
 A. Sinus bradycardia
 B. Sinus tachycardia
 C. AF
 D. AFL

33. **Long QT syndrome:**
 A. Most commonly caused by Na channel mutation
 B. LQT 1 SCD occurs at rest > exercise
 C. LQT 2 SCD occurs on arousal
 D. LQT 3 SCD occurs during exercise > rest
 E. Most common cause of SCD in young athletes

34. **ECG changes in hyperkalemia:**
 A. Tall tented T wave
 B. Narrow QRS
 C. PR prolonged
 D. Decrease in P wave amplitude
 E. Disappearance of T wave

35. **Sjögren's syndrome – following is not seen:**
 A. Thrombocytopenis
 B. Vasculitis
 C. Arthritis
 D. Segments

36. **MET:**
 A. 3.5 ml O_2 /min/kg
 B. 5 ml O_2 /min/kg
 C. Refers to 70 kg man of 40 years
 D. Estimates working capacity in multiples
 E. Useful in exercise programmes (rehabilitation)

37. **Primary tumors of heart:**
 A. 75% malignant
 B. In adults, most common malignant tumor is angiosarcoma
 C. Valve tumor, most common is lipoma
 D. Myxoma most common in RA
 E. Sporadic atrial myxoma presents at a mean age of 10 years

38. **Autosomal dominant are:**
 A. Noonan's
 B. MVP
 C. HOCM
 D. Holt-Oram syndrome
 E. Fabry's disease

39. **Cyanosis:**
 A. A/w reduced Hb > 4.0 gm/dL
 B. Meth Hb > 0.5 gm/dL
 C. Reduced Hb > 4.0
 D. Saturation of O_2 <85%
 E. Saturation of O_2 <90%

40. **Disease spectrum of Marfan's syndrome:**
 A. AS **B.** Aortic dissection
 C. MVP **D.** Myopia
 E. Splenomegaly

41. **Most common cause of venous thrombosis:**
 A. Factor V deficiency
 B. Prothrombin gene mutation
 C. Protein C deficiency
 D. Protein S deficiency

42. **Arterial thrombosis caused by:**
 A. APLA
 B. Protein C deficiency
 C. Protein S deficiency

43. **Young male – Iron loss for every 1 unit donated:**
 A. 100-150 mg **B.** 150-200 mg
 C. 200-250 mg **D.** 250-300 mg

44. **Roth spots seen in all *except*:**
 A. Polycythemia rubra vera
 B. Severe anemia
 C. IE
 D. SLE

45. **Prazosin:**
 A. α adrenergic receptor antagonist and selective against α receptor
 B. Has bad effect on lipid profile
 C. Arterial + venous dilator
 D. Contraindicated in BPH
 E. Used as an antihypertensive

46. **Familial hypercholesterolemia, false is/are:**
 A. Autosomal dominant
 B. Heterozygous individual 700-900 mg/dL
 C. LDL apheresis is an option
 D. Homozygous individual have poor response to drugs
 E. Tendon xanthomas are seen

47. **RV vs LV:**
 A. Trabeculation (Apical)
 B. Moderator band

C. Septal papillary muscle attachment
D. Basal attachment of AV valves
E. Elleptical shape

48. **HELLP:**
A. Hepatitis, elevated live enzymes, low platelet
B. Hemolysis, elevated liver enzymes, low platelet
C. May be seen in gestation HTN
D. May be seen in obstructive jaundice
E. Has worse prognosis

49. **Which are PDE inhibitors?**
A. Theophyline B. Amrinone
C. Sildenafil D. Losartan
E. Clonidine

50. **Kussmaul's sign seen in all *except*:**
A. CCP B. Heart failure
C. TS D. VSD
E. MR

51. **True about ARB:**
A. Equivalent to ACEI in treatment of HTN
B. Acts on AT 1 receptor
C. Does not increase bradykinin
D. Incidence of cough is equal to ACEI
E. Indicated in gestational HTN

52. **Which is not used in acute gout?**
A. Probenecid B. ACTH
C. Corticosteroids D. Colchicine

53. **Paclitaxel causes most commonly:**
A. Sensory neuropathy
B. Motor neuropathy
C. Encephalopathy
D. Multifocal myoclonus

54. **APC is given in sepsis with:**
A. APACHE > 25
B. APACHE < 25
C. None of the above

55. **Which drug is not used in rheumatoid arthritis?**
A. Abatacept B. Rituximab
C. IFN-α D. Methotrexate

56. **Most common antibody associated with Wegener's:**
A. P-ANCA
B. C-ANCA
C. ANA

57. **Small vessel vasculitis:**
A. PAN B. Churg-Strauss
C. TA D. Giant cell

58. **Pulmonary A HTN defined as:**
A. PAP > 25 at rest and > 30 exercise
B. PAP > 25 both at rest and exercise
C. PAP > 30 both at rest and exercise
D. PAP > 20 at rest > 25 at exercise

59. **Non-cardiogenic pulmonary oedema all *except*:**
A. Re expansion pulmonary oedema
B. Sepsis
C. Pneumonia
D. Aspiration

60. **True about ARF:**
A. Renal function does not recover in 5% of cases
B. Oliguric prognosis bad than non-oliguric
C. Over last 25 years, there has been 25% decrease in mortality
D. Sepsis is not a usual cause of death

61. **Overflow protein were seen in:**
A. Amyloidosis
B. MCD
C. Multiple myeloma
D. Fanconi syndrome

62. **Angiotensinogen gene mutation is HTN best responds to:**
A. Sotalol B. Amlodipine
C. Ramipril D. Clonidine

63. **Bilateral trigeminal neuralgia most common cause:**
A. Idiopathic
B. Schwannoma
C. Multiple sclerosis
D. Vascular malformation

64. **CSF shunt infection most commonly caused by:**
A. Pseudomonas B. E. coli
C. Staph. aureus D. S. pneumoniae

65. **Sea-saw nystagmus seen in:**
A. CV junctional anomaly
B. 3rd ventricle tumor
C. Cerebellar lesion

66. **Which MRI modality best for ICH?**
A. Proton density imaging
B. Gradient recall echo
C. Diffusion weighted imaging
D. MR spectroscopy

67. **Non-modulating HTN all *except*:**
A. Low renin
B. Insulin resistance
C. More common in post menopausal female
D. Responds to ACE - I

68. **Acute leukemia with counts 200 × 109 which is not done?**
A. BM examination B. Hydroxy urea
C. Cyt. arabinoside D. Leucopheresis

69. **Increased T3, increased T4, decrease TSH, decrease radio uptake:**
A. Sub-acute thyroiditis
B. Hashimoto's

C. Graves
D. Toxic-nodular goiter

70. (A – a) O_2 calculation for pH 7.36, PO_2 60, PCO_2 50 HCO_3 – 30:
A. 20 B. 28
C. 40 D. 10

71. Usually pH of blood ranges between:
A. 7.36-7.44 B. 7.38-7.44
C. 7.44-7.56 D. 7.56-7.66

72. Inhalation anthrax characterized by:
A. Mediastinal widening with pleural effusion
B. Interstitial infiltrate with pleural effusion
C. Consolidation with contralateral effusion

73. Nephrolithiasis is caused by:
A. Nelfinavir B. Indinavir
C. Saquinavir D. Ritonavir

74. What is true about ataxia telangectasia?
A. Ovarian agenesis
B. Normal thymus
C. Pulmmonary infection are uncommon
D. Good response to live vaccine

75. A patient of HIV, RX of CMV is indicated when:
A. IgG to CMV
B. Early antigen of CMV on BAL
C. On transbronchial biopsy intracytoplasmic inclusion pulmonary infiltrates on CT

76. Ulcerative colitis in female in pregnancy:
A. Disease flare up
B. Increase chances of extracolonic manifestation
C. Increase risk of abortion
D. No change

77. Patient develops cyanosis and breathlessness after ingestion of aniline dye – treatment is:
A. Methylene blue
B. Hemodialysis
C. Forced alkaline diuresis
D. High flow O_2

78. What is false about TSS (Toxic Shock Syndrome):
A. Fever
B. Blood culture positive
C. Macular desquamative rash
D. Renal failure

79. Not true about endotoxin:
A. Seen in Gram positive
B. Seen in Gram negative
C. Important for viability of bacteria
D. Lipopolysaccharide

80. What is not true about tumor lysis syndrome?
A. Hypocalcemia
B. Hypercalcemia
C. Hyperphosphatemia
D. Hyperkalemia

81. D-Dimer true is:
A. Has Got high negative predictive value
B. Useful in hospitalized patients with PE
C. In acute MI level decreased
D. Done by PCR

82. Wide split of S2 seen in:
A. Mod MR
B. LBBB
C. LV diastolic function
D. CCF

83. Patient of sarcoidosis with acute presentation with inflammatory arthritis, uveitis and lymphadenopathy, erythema nodosum:
A. Lofgren syndrome
B. Heerfordt syndrome
C. Loffler's syndrome

MEDICINE

84. Bilateral cervical α axillary LNT, 90 years old female, DM, HTN with CAD came with fatigue on investigation CT Abd/thorax/..... LN↑ CD 20+, CD 23+, CD 5t. Next line of treatment:
A. Observation
B. BMT
C. Chlorambucil + ...

85. Hemophagocytosis all *except*:
A. ↑ed ferritin B. ↑ed TG
C. Splenomegaly D. Pancytopenia

86. Heat stroke all *except*:
A. Core king > 40°C B. Piloerection
C. Anhidrosis D. Coagulopathy

87. Heat stroke all *except*:
A. Thrombocytopenia
B. DIC
C. Leukocytosis
D. Hemophagocytosis

88. RA all *except*:
A. Abatacept B. IFN α
C. Rituximab D. Mt_x

89. RA patient on Mt_x + NSAID swelling over elbow since 4 days worsening pain + fever (98.8°F), not able to move elbow, all features of RA in hands. Treatment:
A. Add oral prednisolone long to treatment
B. Leflunomide due to worsening of RA
C. Give intra articular steroid and ↑se NSAID dose
D. Aspirated joint fluid and look for Gout + Infection

90. Not an endogenous nephrotoxin:
- A. Myoglobin
- B. Aristolochic acid
- C. Uric acid
- D. Doalate

91. Uveitis + Arthrosis + Erythema .... in sarcoidosis.
- A. Lofgren
- B. Heerfordt
- C. Fowler's syndrome

92. Pseudomonas gene responsible for drug resistance:
- A. Amp C–β lactamase
- B. SHV– β lactamase
- C. CTX– β lactamase
- D. TEMI– β lactamase

93. Earthquake victim best treatment for ↓ing mortality:
- A. Give ½ saline while patient in rubble seen
- B. ½ mannitol
- C. ½ soda bicarb
- D. Prophylactic hemodialysis

94. Patient with DKA, Na^+–149; HCO_3–12 mg K^+–5.2; S. Cr–2.1; B. urea–56:
- A. N/2 Saline + Insulin
- B. N Saline + Insulin
- C. N Saline + Insulin + Na bicarb
- D. Oral free water + Insulin

95. Peritoneal dialysis not effective for:
- A. Uremic encephalopathy
- B. Fluid overload
- C. Hyperkalemia
- D. Met acidosis

96. Most effective treatment for rhabdomyolysis:
- A. Large vol. of ½ crystalloids
- B. ½ Soda bicarb →
- C. ½ Dextrose + Insulin
- D. ½ Calcium chloride

97. Patient of chemical burns with intubation done. Now tracheal aspiration done what level of CFU will differentiate infection from colonization:
- A. 10^2 CFO/ml
- B. 10^3 CFO/ml
- C. 10^4 CFO/ml
- D. 10^5 CFO/ml

98. A patient with diagnosed gastrinoma on octreotide sean. Now which other most sensitive test for gastrinoma?
- A. EUS
- B. PET
- C. Abdominal USG
- D. CT abdomen

99. Severity of pancreatitis by all *except*:
- A. S. amylase
- B. CRP
- C. Urine trypsinogen degradation peptide
- D. CT abdomen

100. Microcytic hypochromic anemia all *except*:
- A. Sideroblastic
- B. Celiac disease
- C. Ythalassemia
- D. Anemia of chronic disease

101. Patient with hypogonadism. Next step:
- A. Do evening total testosterone levels
- B. First do PSA + Penn rectal exam before starting testosterone
- C. Equilibrium dialysis for free testosterone not used now
- D. Most circulating testosterone is unbound (free)

102. Causes of gastric ulcer all *except*:
- A. Treponema pallidum
- B. Cryptosporidium
- C. CMV
- D. H. pylori

103. 60 years patient with dyspepsia + anaemia abdominal USG N. Now what?
- A. UGI endoscopy
- B. Stool for OCB
- C. PP for 1 month then reevaluate

104. Vitamin B_{12} serum level ↓ses in all *except*:
- A. 10 days of oral antibiotic
- B. Ileal resection
- C. Strict vegetarians

105. CJD true is:
- A. Can be familial
- B. Caused by retro virus
- C. Confined to north American and European nations
- D. Respond to IFN–α in refractory cases

106. H_1N_1 all *except*:
- A. It to a paramyxovirus
- B. Resistant to amantadine
- C. Pregnant females poor outcome
- D. Spread by droplet infection

107. APC given in:
- A. APACHE > 25
- B. APACHE < 25
- C. Single organ involvement
- D. None

108. Known patient with CHF +inted with 3 days Tachypnea. Traces of pedal edema + JVP N + P_2 loud–Best next management. No tenderness in lower limb:
- A. Pulm angio
- B. CT pulm angio + contrast
- C. D–Dimer
- D. Duplex lower limb USG

109. CHF NYHA III patient on diuretic which does not use mortality:
A. ACEI
B. Spironolactone
C. Digoxin
D. Carvedilol

110. All favour pulmonary embolism all *except*:
A. Hemoptysis B. Tachypnea
C. RVS_3 D. Bibasilar rales

111. AVRT, true is:
A. AF with WPW mandates verapamil
B. +ve of bypass tract makes ablation impossible
C. May be associated with SCD dft vf
D. AVRT improves in pregnancy

112. 60 years patient mild asthma hypothyroid on thyroxine refered to emergency because of Na+–120 meg/L Cl–100 meg/L U. Na–48 mg; S. osmol–268, Urine osmol–300. What treatment?
A. 3% NaCl
B. Diuretics
C. N saline
D. Restriction of fluid

113. 60 years O+ with DM + HTN +inted chronic fatigue + Cervical and inguinal and abdominal LN with splenomegaly CD 5 +ve : CD 20 +ve + CD 25 +ve. Treatment TLC–98,000 → P_{45} L_{50}:
A. Deoxyadenosine
B. Chlorambucil + Prednisone
C. BMT
D. Observation

114. Criteria for severe malaria all *except*:
A. Splenomegaly
B. Lactic acidosis
C. Renal failure
D. Thrombocytopenia

115. Imipenem + Cilastatin due to:
A. Cilastatin degrades carbepenemase
B. Cilastatin degrades end with degrades imipenem in PCT
C. Combination better against Gr –ve bacilli

116. ARF true:
A. 5% land in CRF
B. Oliguria worse prognosis than non-oliguric
C. Mortality improved 25% over 25 years
D. Septicemia not the most common cause of mortality in ARF

117. Anti-centromere Abdomin in:
A. Limited cutaneous systemic sclerosis
B. Diffuse systemic sclerosis
C. MCTD
D. Overlap syndrome

118. Which does not rule out possibility of prerenal ARF?
A. U. Na > 20 meg/L
B. Absence of oliguria
C. Urine osmol < 200
D. RBC cast

119. Leptospirosis true:
A. Meningoencephalitis uncommon testation
B. Common in dry winters
C. Organism easily visible on biopsy
D. Case fatality 40–50%

120. OSA treatment of choices:
A. Intranasal CPAP
B. Tracheostomy with Bi pap
C. O_2 by nasal canmia
D. Medroxy progesterone acetate

121. Patient with COPD +inted with recent onset dyspnea. Definite feature of dysfunction:
A. Pulsus alternans
B. Gr IV apical systolic murmur rod to axilla
C. Recumbent dyspnea
D. Persistent split S_2

122. Urinary catheter infection correct statin:
A. …… after 2 weeks of catheterization
B. Periurethral povidone iodine
C. Prophylactic ciprofloxacin started always
D. Infection is always asymptomatic

ANSWERS

1	A	2	A,B,C	3	A	4	A,B,C	5	A,C	6	B,D	7	B,C
8	A,C	9	A	10	A	11	A	12	A	13	A	14	A,E
15	A,C,E	16	B,D	17	A,D	18	B,C,D,E	19	A	20	B	21	A,C,D
22	B,C,D	23		24	A,B,C	25	A	26	A,B	27	B	28	A,B
29	A	30	A,C,D	31	A	32	A	33	A,C	34	A,C,D	35	
36	A,C	37	B	38	A,B,C,D	39	C,D	40	B,C,D	41	A	42	A
43	C	44	A	45	A,C,E	46	A,C,D,E	47	A,B,C	48	B,C,E	49	
50	B,C	51	A,B,C	52	A	53	A	54	A	55	C	56	B
57	B	58	A	59	A	60	B	61	C	62	C	63	C
64	C	65	B	66	B	67	A	68	A	69	A	70	B
71	A	72	A	73	B	74	A	75	B	76	A	77	A
78	B	79	A	80	B	81	A	82	A,B,C,D	83	A	84	
85		86		87		88		89		90		91	
92		93		94		95		96		97		98	
99		100		101		102		103		104		105	
106		107		108		109		110		111		112	
113		114		115		116		117		118		119	
120		121		122									

36

PGI 2008

1. **Panayiotopoulos syndrome all *except*:**
   A. Autonomic disturbances, visual symptoms follow and/or not
   B. Normal brain imaging
   C. CNS exam s/o homonymous hemianopia
   D. Occipital and pre-occipital EEG s/o spikes

2. **Foix Chavany Marie syndrome:**
   A. Spastic paraplegia
   B. Pseudobulbar palsy
   C. Peripheral neuropathy
   D. Quadriparesis

3. **12 years old boy with bilateral Genu-valgum with muscular weakness 61 FR N, MCU s/o bilateral VUR. True:**
   A. $\downarrow K^+$, $\downarrow Cl$; N Urine PH N S PH
   B. $\downarrow K^+$, N Cl; $\uparrow\downarrow$
   C. $\uparrow K^+$, $\downarrow Cl^-$; $\downarrow$ Urine PH $\downarrow$ S PH
   D. $\uparrow K+$, $\uparrow Cl$; $\uparrow \downarrow$ S PH

4. **MRI better than CT in all *except*:**
   A. Calcification B. Dysplasia
   C. Infarct D. Demyelination

5. **Radiation plexopathy EMG, true:**
   A. Myokymia B. Normal
   C. Fasciculation D. Myotonia

6. **Tumour lysis all *except*:**
   A. $\uparrow Ca^{++}$ B. $\downarrow Ca^{++}$
   C. $\uparrow K^+$ D. $\uparrow PO_4$

7. **Intramedullary lesion most specific, true:**
   A. B/B early involvement
   B. Saddle anesthesia
   C. Asymmetric involvement
   D. Radicular pain

8. **Alcoholic male in emergencies in pH = 7.05, HCO_3 = 8 mcg (local alcohol):**
   A. Forced alkaline diuresis
   B. Hemodialysis
   C. PD
   D. Venovenous hemofiltration

9. **Acute leukaemia with TLC = 20 × 10^9/l early management all *except*:**
   A. Bone marrow aspiration
   B. IV hydroxyurea
   C. IV cytarabine
   D. Hemiparesis

10. **D.O.C. for idiopathic generalized seizure:**
    A. Sodium valproate
    B. Vigabatrin
    C. Carbamazepine
    D. Phenytoin

11. **Anti-epileptics causing depression:**
    A. Phenytoin
    B. Carbamazepine
    C. Phenobarbital
    D. Sodium valproate

12. **Most teratogenic period for antiepileptics:**
    A. I trimester
    B. II trimester
    C. Early III trimester
    D. Late III trimester

13. **Feature of complex partial seizures all *except*:**
    A. Automatism
    B. Behavioural arrest
    C. Coma
    D. Dissolution from surrounding

14. **Hemochromatosis all *except*:**
    A. DM
    B. Gonadal failure
    C. Depigmentation
    D. Transferrin saturation<40%

15. **Most specific indication of iron deficiency:**
    A. Low ferritin
    B. $\downarrow$ MCV
    C. $\downarrow$ S. iron
    D. Microc.

16. **TPN most serious complication:**
A. Cholestasis with hepatic cell necrosis
B. Cholestasis with hepatic all fibrosis
C. Cholestasis with partial vein thrombosis
D. Cholestasis with bridging necrosis

17. **Plasma dissolved O_2 without erythrocytes:**
A. 2.5 ml B. S
C. 7.5 D. 10

18. **Chronic PPI R_x complication all *except*:**
A. Hypergastrinemia
B. Bacterial overgrowth in small bowel
C. ↓ Vitamin B_{12} absorption
D. ↓ Sens. of IF

19. **Pernicious anemia all *except*:**
A. ↑ Gastrin
B. Na H^+ atpase
C. Life long B_{12} treatment
D. ↑ risk of gastric cancer

20. **RPGN with PMN infiltrates with cellular crescent in renal R_x:**
A. Anti-GBM
B. IgA
C. Post infectious GN – II
D. ANCA a/w + type III pauci immune

21. **Renal glycosuria C aminoaciduria with nephritic syndrome:**
A. Cystinosis B. Amyloid
C. IgA D. DM

22. **Sjögren's syndrome renal involement:**
A. FSGS
B. MCD
C. MPGN
D. Distal RTA

23. **Refsum disease all *except*:**
A. ↓ phytanic acid
B. Cerebellar ataxia
C. Symmetric sensorimotor polyneuropathy

24. **Tracheobronchial aspiration without swallowing all *except*:**
A. Globus hystericus
B. Achalasia cardia
C. GERO
D. Zenker's diverticulum

25. **Coeliac disease all *except*:**
A. Anti gliadin Ab
B. Anti endomysial Ab
C. Anti glutamin Ab
D. TTG Ab

26. **Vitamin B_{12} deficiency all *except*:**
A. Nitrous oxide uses
B. Methotrexate
C. Blind loop syndrome
D. ZES

27. **CAD with counterclockwise volation all *except*:**
A. Endocardial cushion defect
B. Tricuspid atresia
C. TGA
D. DORV VSD

28. **MR A/W:**
A. Congenital MS
B. ALCAPA
C. Ebstein
D. SVC into LA

29. **R_x of choice for acute SVC thrombosis:**
A. Radio R_x
B. Chemo R_x
C. Stenting
D. Chemo + Radia

30. **Fetal circulation physiology affected by:**
A. PDA
B. Mitral atresia
C. Tricuspid atresia with restrictive VSD
D. Pulmonary atresia with restrictive VSD

31. **Immediate change in fetal circulation:**
A. ↑ SVR
B. ↓ PBF
C. Anatomic closure of PDA
D. Anatomic closure of PFO

32. **Patient of CAD on ACE; Aspirin, β-blocks, ticlopidine present renal dysfunction with fever with fragmented RBC. Drug involved:**
A. Ticlopidine B. ACE
C. Aspirin D. β-blocks

33. **Childhood survival exceptional in:**
A. Ebstein
B. Interrupted aortic arch
C. TGA
D. PA

34. **$PAO_2 - PO_2$:**
A. 10 B. 28
C. 20 D. 50

35. **Max mixed venous SO_2 in:**
A. Septic shock
B. Cardiogenic shock
C. Neurogenic
D. Hypovolemic

36. $\uparrow T_3 \uparrow T_4 \downarrow$ TSH $\downarrow$ uptake of radioactive:
A. Hashimoto's **B.** Subacute thyroditis
C. Graves **D.** TNG

37. Relapsing polychondritis characteristics:
A. Sparing of ear lobe

38. Migratory motor complex 'MMC':
A. Occurs in fasting
B. Lasts < 1 min
C. Colonic sweeping
D. Mixing of gastric juice with food

39. Most common of venous thromboisis:
A. Factor V leiden deficiency
B. Protein with deficiency
C. Protein S deficiency
D. GP2021 A mutation

40. D-dimmer true:
A. Very high negative productive value
B. Useful in diagnosis of PE in hospitalized patient

ANSWERS

1	C	2	B	3	D	4	A	5	A	6	A	7	A
8	B	9	A	10	A	11	C	12	A	13	C	14	C
15	A	16	B	17	A	18	D	19	B	20	C	21	A
22	D	23	A	24	A	25	C	26	D	27	C	28	B
29	C	30		31		32	A	33	A	34	B	35	A
36	B	37	A	38	A	39	A	40	A				

37

PGI 2007

CARDIOLOGY

1. **Rituximab is most useful in:**
   A. Diffuse large B cell
   B. Burkitt's
   C. Precursor T-cell lymphoma
   D. Mycosis fungoides

2. **I_x for status of hematopoietic tissue in bone marrow best is:**
   A. MRI B. CT
   C. 3D USG D. 4D USG

3. **Lipodystrophy is seen with:**
   A. Membranous
   B. MPGN-II
   C. Mesangioproliferative
   D. FSGS

4. **ATN characterized by:**
   A. Muddy brown casts
   B. Failure index < 1
   C. Fe Na < 1
   D. Urine Na < 10

5. **Non-modulator essential HTN by all *except*:**
   A. Low renin
   B. Pathophysiology corrected by ACEI
   C. Most common in post menopausal
   D. More than 50% of NPRA are non-modulators

6. **Most predictive for CAD is:**
   A. Homocysteine
   B. Fibrinogen
   C. hsCRP

7. **Most common of febrile neutropenia on chemo for leukemia is 15 years child with no provisions of infection:**
   A. Aspergillus
   B. Candida
   C. Gram -ve organism
   D. HSV

8. **ACEI, BB, Aspirin, Ticlopidine after PTCA developed febrile renal dysfunction with pigmented RBC cause:**
   A. Ticlopidine B. BB
   C. ACE D. Aspirin

9. **Aztreonam all *except*:**
   A. Cross sensitivity with penicillin
   B. Not effective against anaemia
   C. Not effective again gram +ve
   D. Effective in gram –ve

10. **Actinomycosis all are given *except*:**
   A. Tetracycline B. Penicillin
   C. Oxacillin D. Amoxy

11. **GVHD can be seen in all *except*:**
   A. Autologous
   B. Allogenic
   C. Blood transfer
   D. Umbilical stem cell

12. **PO_2 60 PCO_2 50 PH 7.36:**
   A. Normal serum air oxygen Arkrial Alvet oradent is
   B. 10 C. 20
   D. 28 E. 35

13. **Highest mixed venous O_2 saturation is seen in:**
   A. Septic shock B. Hypovolemic
   C. Cardiogenic D. Neurogenic

14. **Hematopoietic growth factors are:**
   A. Glycoproteins B. Protein
   C. Carbohydrates D. Carboprotein

15. **Most successful for persistent stem cell growth:**
   A. CD 34+, 38– B. CD 34 CD 38+
   C. CD 34+ 138+ D. CD 34+ 138–

16. **Causes for thrombocytopenia in:**
   A. Hepatorenal
   B. Hypersplenism
   C. Thromboplastin deficiency
   D. DIC

17. **One unit of blood transfusion donation leads to loss of:**
A. 100 – 150 B. 150 – 200
C. 200 – 250 D. No loss

18. **Inhalation anthrax:**
A. Mediastinal widening with pleural effusion
B. Pulmonary infiltrate with pleural effusion
C. Consolidation on one side with C/L pleural effusion
D. B/c consolidate

19. **Extramedullary hematopoiesis means:**
A. RBC product in liver and spleen
B. In BM, liver and spleen
C. In BM

20. **Diagnosis of hepatitis C HCV type II:**
A. IFN peg– + ribavirin = 48 weeks
B. IFN peg– + ribavirin = 24 weeks
C. Peg IFN – 48 weeks
D. Peg IFN – 24 weeks

21. **D Dimer:**
A. Highest negative predictive value
B. PE diagnosis in hospitalized patient
C. Not ↓ in MI
D. Detected by PCR

22. **Relapsing polychondritis characteristics:**
A. Sparing of ear lobe
B. Bronchitis obliterans
C. Involvement of eye
D. Rapidly progressive RF

23. **Fundus finding of takayasu:**
A. Venous dilation
B. Hard exudates
C. Papilledema
D. A-V shunting

24. **NHL classification prognostic all *except*:**
A. Stage III, IV
B. Age > 60 years
C. Pg microglobulin
D. Extranodal involvement

MEDICINE

25. **Long term hematopoiesis stem cells:**
A. CD 34+ and CD 38–
B. CD 34+ and CD 38+
C. CD 34+ and CD 138+
D. CD 34+ and CD 138–

26. **Friedreich's ataxia:**
A. DM B. ILD
C. Diabetes insipidus

27. **Ataxia telangiectasia feature:**
A. Pulmonary infections uncommon
B. Ovarian agenesis
C. Thymus normal development

28. **Imaging of hematopoietic system:**
A. 3–D USG B. 4–D USG
C. CT D. MRI

29. **Insulin resistance true all *except*:**
A. Central obesity
B. Acne
C. Moon facies
D. Hirsutism

30. **L + B caries all *except*:**
A. O_2 B. CO_2
C. Nitric oxide D. Sulfur dioxide

31. **Extramedullary hematopoiesis:**
A. Development of bone marrow and spleen
B. Development of bone marrow and liver
C. Development of bone marrow
D. Spleen and liver

32. **Not true of aztreonam:**
A. Gram negative enteric bacilli active
B. No response of anaerobes
C. No response on Gram positive
D. Hypersensitivity in Pn sensitive

33. **Fundus takayasu all *except*:**
A. Dilated venous B. A-V shunt
C. Papilledema D. Hard exudate

34. **Hematopoietic growth factors:**
A. Glycoprotein B. Protein
C. Carbohydrate D. Carboprotein

35. **Not true for bile and acid diarrhea:**
A. Bile acid pool is reduced
B. Ideal disease is limited
C. Bile acid absorption reduced

36. **HCV-2 genotype R_x:**
A. IFN peg – + ribavirin = 48 weeks
B. IFN peg – + ribavirin = 24 weeks
C. Peg IFN – 48 weeks
D. Peg IFN – 24 weeks

37. **Rituximab most used:**
A. Burkitt's
B. Mycosis fungoides
C. Diffuse large B-cell
D. Premature T cell lymphoma

38. **Paraneoplastic cerebellar degeneration breast cancer associated with:**
A. Anti–HY B. Anti–YO
C. Anti–TR D. ACKR

39. **ATN:**
A. Muddy brown granular
B. Drug Nephrolithiasis → Indinavir

40. **Stored blood 48 hours which is not damaged:**
A. Platelet B. WBC
C. Factor V D. Factor VII

41. **Arterial thrombosis:**
A. APLA
B. Factor V leiden mutation
C. Protein C deficiency
D. Prothrombin gene mutation

42. **Thrombocytopenia in cirrhosis all *except*:**
A. Hypersplenism
B. Thrombopoietin deficiency
C. DIC
D. Hepatorenal syndrome

43. **↑T_4, T_3↑; TSH↓; RAIU↓:**
A. Hashimoto's
B. Subacute
C. Toxic nodular goiter
D. Graves' disease

44. **40 years old boy WBC = 200 × 10^9/L with acute leukemia, all can be initial management *except*:**
A. Hydroxyurea
B. Cytarabine
C. Leukapheresis
D. BM examination

45. **Undiagnosed SVC thrombosis without knowing etiology can be treated:**
A. Stenting B. CT + RT
C. C therapy D. R therapy

46. **Pulmonary alveolar proteinosis all *except*:**
A. LDH ↑
B. S level surfactant ↑
C. Bat wing appearance
D. BAL may be useful in same point

47. **Inhalational anthrax CXR:**
A. Interstitial with Ph effusion
B. Mediastinal widening with pleural effusion
C. Bilateral consolidation
D. Unilateral consolidation with C/L pleural effusion

48. **IV blood donateed leads to iron loss:**
A. 200–250 B. 150–200
C. No loss D. 100–150

49. **51 years diabetic on beta blocker, aspirin, ACOM, ticlopidine presents with dysmorphic RBC:**
A. Ticlopidine

50. **Best marker for CAD:**
A. hs–CRP B. Fibrinogen
C. Homocysteine D. Lipoprotein (a)

51. **Lipodystrophy:**
A. MCD
B. MPGN
C. Focal segmental glomerulosclerosis
D. Membranous

52. **pH=7.36; HCO_3=30; PO_2=60; PCO_2=50; Age 30 years:**
A. 10 B. 28
C. 35 D. 20

53. **Relapsing polychondritis:**
A. Earlobe spared
B. Lung involvement
C. Rapidly progressive renal failure
D. Early eye involvement

54. **Dimer true:**
A. High negative predictive value
B. Dx of PE in hospitalized patients
C. ↓ in MI

55. **Not true for non-modulating primary HTN:**
A. Low plasma renin
B. ACE–1 improve pathophysiology
C. ↑ risk post-menopausal
D. Insulin resistance

56. **High venous O_2 saturation:**
A. Septic shock
B. Cardiogenic
C. Neurogenesis
D. Hypovolemic

57. **Diagnosis of actinomyces all *except*:**
A. Pn B. Amoxicillin
C. Oxacillin D. Tetracycline

58. **Prognostic indicator NHL all *except*:**
A. Age >60
B. Ann-Arber III and IV
C. > 1 extranodal
D. B_2 microglobulin

59. **Febrile neutropenia – most commom:**
A. Gram positive B. Aspergillus
C. HSV D. Oral candidiasis

60. **B.P. goal, DM goal:**
A. < 120 B. < 85
C. < 130 D. < 80

ANSWERS

1		2		3	B	4	A	5	A	6	C	7	
8		9	A	10	C	11	A	12		13		14	A
15		16		17	C	18	A	19		20		21	A
22		23		24		25		26	A	27	B	28	
29		30		31		32	D	33		34	A	35	
36		37		38		39	A	40		41	A	42	
43		44		45		46		47	B	48	A	49	
50	A	51	B	52		53	A	54	A	55	A	56	
57	C	58		59		60							

38

PGI JUNE 2006

1. **α-coma seen in:**
   A. Hepatic coma
   B. Sedative
   C. Pontine haemorrhage
   D. Hyponatremia

2. **Acute tubular necrosis seen with:**
   A. Urine $Na^+ < 10$ meq/l
   B. Urine creatinine / S. creatinine
   C. Specific gravity > 1.020
   D. Muddy brown ratio > 40

3. **Botrezomib used commonly in:**
   A. NHL B. ALL
   C. HD D. Myeloma

4. **Proximal RTA all *except*:**
   A. $HCO_3 < 15\%$
   B. Anion gap
   C. Positive urine anion gap
   D. Urine ph < 5,5

5. **Sjögren's syndrome associated with:**
   A. MGN
   B. MPGN
   C. Tubulointerstitial
   D. Amyloidosis

6. **Marrow iron stores in a patient on dialysis best assessed by:**
   A. S. ferritin
   B. S. erythropoietin
   C. MCHC
   D. Transferring cone

7. **All vasculitis are infection associated *except*:**
   A. PAN hepatitis B
   B. Wegener's
   C. Macrocryoglobulinemia
   D. Hypersensitivity vasculitis

8. **Carcinoma pyrophosphate dehydrate deposit in knee joint all *except*:**
   A. Hyperparathyroidism
   B. Haemochromatosis
   C. Hypermagnesemia
   D. Post meniscectomy

9. **A 25 years old man presents with history of recurrent anemia and jaundice since childhood + splenomegaly. History of gallstones diagnosis:**
   A. Thalassemia trait
   B. Hereditary spherocytosis
   C. Heterozygous β thalassemia
   D. G6PD

10. **A young primigravida 25 years female with PPH on 2nd day with aptt ↑sed and VIII factor 10% of normal, PT and TT is normal. Diagnosis is:**
    A. Hereditary hemophilia
    B. Acquired haemophilia
    C. Lupus anticoagulant
    D. Anticardiolipin syndrome

11. **A 40 years present with acute breathlessness with ST ↓ in ant. leads with echo showing normal, LV function and RV dilated and dysfunction with BP 80/60. What will you give?**
    A. IV propranolol B. IV Stk
    C. IV NTG D. IV heparin

12. **Pure red cell aplasia seen in cases of multi-transfusion recipient due to:**
    A. Parvovirus B_{19}
    B. HCV
    C. HIV

13. **Most common cause of PVO in India:**
    A. Malaria
    B. TB
    C. Enteric fever

14. **Infective endocarditis large mobile vegetation with culture negative is:**
    A. Strep viridans B. E. coli
    C. Strep pneumonia D. H parainfluenzae

15. **Least likely infection in neutropenia:**
A. Aspergillus fumigates
B. Staph. aureus
C. Pneumocystis carinii
D. Klebsiella

16. **HLA-B27 associated with all *except*:**
A. Ankylosing spondylitis
B. Reiter's
C. Psoriasis vulgaris
D. Anti-uveitis

17. **Skin manifestation in CRF:**
A. Ecchymosis
B. Calciphylaxis

18. **Akathisia:**
A. Restlessness

19. **Pseudobulbar fibres are:**
A. Corticobulbar fibers
B. Dentatorubro fibers
C. U fibers
D. Mammillo-thalamic fibers

20. **80 years old female asymptomatic with M spike in electrophoresis with IgG 1.5 gm/dl; 8% myeloma cells in bone marrow likely disease diagnosis:**
A. Indolent myeloma B. MGUS
C. Waldenstrom D. TB

21. **4 years old child with 10 tablet of $FeSO_4$ present with all *except*:**
A. Meta alkalosis B. Hypoglycemia
C. Hypotension D. Hematemesis

22. **Fasting hypoglycemia all *except*:**
A. Glucagonoma
B. Insulinoma
C. Endotoxic shock
D. Addison's

23. **For DVT 4 mg warfarin given for 10 days shows PT 16 sec. and test control 12 sec with ISI = 1 reagent is:**
A. Normally controlled
B. Undercontrolled
C. Mildy overcontrolled
D. Severely overcontrolled

24. **Multiple sclerosis least commonly presents:**
A. Ataxia
B. Blindness in one eye
C. Headache
D. Diplopia

25. **TEE more useful than TTE:**
A. Severity of MS B. Emphysema
C. LA thrombus D. Poor window

26. **Dumping can be best managed by:**
A. Lying down immediately after food
B. Reoperation
C. Ondansetron
D. ↑ starch in diet

27. **Intrinsic factor release not disturbed in taking:**
A. Cimetidine B. Misoprostol
C. Omeprazole D. Somatostatin

28. **Dementia all drugs given *except*:**
A. Donepezil B. Selegiline
C. α-tocopherol D. γ-interferon

29. **Tick bone diseases:**
A. Leptospira icterohaemorrhagica
B. L-donovani
C. Rickettsia rickettsii
D. Spirillum minus

30. **Methanol toxicity late manifestation:**
A. Peripheral neuropathy
B. Convulsion
C. Retinal injury
D. Abdominal pain

31. **Ulcerative colitis in pregnancy:**
A. Flare up

32. **Inhibitory neurotransmitters:**
A. Aspartate
B. Ach
C. GABA

33. **Pulmonary embolism is suggested by:**
A. Lobar perfusion defect
B. Multiple segmental defect
C. Multiple matched sub-segmental defect with ventilation

34. **GFR fall by 25% when hyperkalemia appears:**
A. 50% B. 40%
C. 15% D. 25%

35. **Mycobacterium TB will not be clinically manifested as infection:**
A. Previous mycobacterium infection
B. Live virus vaccinations
C. BCG vaccination
D. Multiple tuberculosis testing

36. **Macro hepatosteatosis all *except*:**
A. Alcohol B. TPN
C. Lipodystrophy D. Rye syndrome

37. **Safest drug in pregnancy:**
A. Isoniazid
B. Ethambutol
C. Thiacetazone
D. Streptomycin

ANSWERS

1	C	2	D	3	D	4	A	5	C	6	A	7	D
8	C	9	B	10	B	11	B	12	A	13	B	14	D
15	C	16	D	17	A	18	A	19	A	20	B	21	A
22	A	23	B	24	C	25	C	26	C	27	B	28	D
29	C	30	C	31	A	32	C	33		34	D	35	C
36	D	37	A										

39

PGI 2005

MEDICINE

1. **M spike of 1.5 g/dL with bone marrow plasma cytosis <8% absence are:**
   A. MGUS
   B. Multiple myeloma
   C. Solitary myeloma
2. **Anemia, osteopenia, neutropenia, depigmentation of hair, hypothermia. Mental retardation, growth retardation due to deficiency of:**
   A. Zinc B. Chromium
   C. Selenium D. Copper
3. **Anemia with jaundice all *except*:**
   A. ↑ Haptoglobin
   B. ↑ Hemosiderin in urine
   C. Cooms +ve
4. **Microangiopathic anemia +ve in:**
   A. HSP
   B. Malignant HTN
   C. HUS and TTP
5. **Renal vein thrombosis increased incidence found in:**
   A. MCD
   B. Membranous GN
   C. Lupus nephritis
   D. Diabetic nephropathy
6. **Cold sore seen in:**
   A. TB
   B. T pallidum
   C. Leishmaniasis
   D. Herpes simplex
7. **Post delivery primi, PPH, ↓ Factor VIII<10%:**
   A. Inherited hemophilia A
   B. Acquired hemophilia A
8. **MND all *except*:**
   A. Numbness B. Atrophy
   C. Weakness
9. **Akathesia is:**
   A. Inner restlessness
   B. ↓ movement
   C. Extreme rigidity
10. **Wilson's disease inherited as:**
    A. Ch 21 B. Ch 10
    C. Ch 13 D. Ch 20
11. **Scorpions sting treatment:**
    A. Prazosin B. Lignocaine
    C. Bretylium
12. **Oxidative stress induced CMP:**
    A. Mitochondria
    B. Cisplatinum
    C. 5 FU
13. **HbA 2 > 40% anemia Hb 9.2:**
    A. α thalassemia
    B. β thalassemia major
    C. β thalassemia trait
14. **Eye movement upward and by left:**
    A. Left inf oblique
    B. Right inf oblique
    C. Left sup oblique
    D. Right sup oblique
15. **Culture negative, indolent, without fever, persistent infection endocarditis:**
    A. Coxilla burnetti
    B. HACEK
    C. T Whippeli
16. **Neutropenia increases infections of all *except*:**
    A. Staphylococcus
    B. P. carinii
    C. K. pneumonia
    D. Aspergillus
17. **Pitressin resistant diabetes insipidus:**
    A. Nephrogenic DI

18. **Acanthocytosis:**
A. Refsums
B. Ataxia telangectesia
C. Tangiers
D. A beta lipoproteinemia

19. **Lead toxicity all *except*:**
A. ↑ protoporphyrin
B. Microcytic hypochromic
C. Macroagtic anemia

20. **Thymoma in mysthenia gravis found in:**
A. <10%   B. 10-15%
C. 15-25%   D. >40%

21. **GMCSF used in:**
A. Afebrile neutropenia
B. Post bone marrow transplantation
C. Before BMT
D. To increase the dose of chemotherapy

22. **Thallidomide treatment:**
A. M-myeloma
B. Hairy cell leukemia
C. CML
D. AML

23. **Promyelocytic leukemia treatment:**
A. ATRA
B. AML – type 6
C. Hairy cell leukemia
D. Mantle cell lumphoma

24. **A patient with leukemia with CD 19 + 10 + 13 + 33 + ve:**
A. ALL-L2   B. AML M2
C. AML M_0 D. Biphenotypic

25. **Anaplastic large cell true all except:**
A. Survival 5 years > 80%
B. Simulate Hodgkin's
C. High grade
D. Survival >70%

26. **Physiological vasodilator:**
A. Prostacyclin   B. Endothelin
C. Renin   D. Norepinephrine

27. **Angiogenesis inhibitors:**
A. Leptin   B. TNF α
C. Endostatin   D. IL-8

28. **Tamponade true:**
A. Prominent x, y negative

29. **Antioxidant all *except*:**
A. β carotene
B. α tocopherol
C. Ascorbic acid
D. Pentothenic acid

30. **In plague antibiotic ineffective is:**
A. Zentamycin
B. Cefotaxim
C. Chloramphenicol
D. Tetracyclin

31. **Prion protein causes:**
A. SSPE
B. FFI
C. PMLE

32. **1st trimmest ATT given:**
A. Streptomycin
B. INH
C. Ethambutol
D. Thiacetazone

33. **HIV vaccine not be given:**
A. Oral polio   B. Influenza
C. Pneumococcal   D. BCG

34. **TB response decreases:**
A. BCG
B. Live attenuated measles
C. Tuberculin test
D. Previous mycobacterial infection

35. **High anion gap all *except*:**
A. CO
B. Ethylene glycol
C. Distal RTA-IV
D. Chr RF

36. **High probability lung scan:**
A. Multiple segmental defect with normal ventilation
B. Large lobar with normal ventilation
C. Large wedge shaped defect
D. Multiple segmental with matched ventilation defect

37. **Meningoencephalitis:**
A. E-histologica
B. Acanthomoeba
C. Cysticercosis

38. **Trans pulmonary pressure depends on:**
A. Chest wall   B. Alveola
C. Pleural space   D. Airway

39. **Asterixis all *except*:**
A. Metabolic encephalopathy
B. Hypoxic
C. Upper midbrain
D. Organophosphorous

40. **Metabolic alkalosis is caused by:**
A. Hypoxemia   B. ↓ K^+
C. ARF   D. Acetazolamide

CARDIOLOGY

41. **Wide splitting of S2:**
A. RBBB
B. PS
C. Cardiac tamponade
D. VSD
E. PHT

42. **Soft S1:**
A. 1° HB
B. Ac AR
C. AS
D. Rheumatic MR
E. PPH

43. **Post MI TMT indicated in:**
A. 1 week
B. 3 weeks
C. VT
D. Persistent ST
E. Angina

44. **HOCM murmur increases:**
A. Post NTG
B. Valsalva phase IV
C. Inotropes
D. Leg rising
E. Standing

45. **Non rheumatic MR increases by:**
A. Expiration
B. Squatting
C. Standing
D. Leg rising
E. Hand grip

46. **Chronic stable angina avoid:**
A. Push up
B. Sexual activity
C. Jogging
D. Cycling
E. Pushing static vehicle

47. **Feature of mild HTN:**
A. No sp. symptoms
B. Tachycardia
C. Loss of circadian rhythm
D. ↑ Pulse pressure
E. ↑ Stroke

48. **High risk markers in essential HTN:**
A. Glycosuria
B. Grade II retinopathy
C. Alcohol
D. LVH
E. Labile HTN

49. **Acute MI treatment all *except*:**
A. I/V metolar
B. I/V streptokinase
C. Oral ACE I
D. Oral CCB
E. Ecosprin

50. **Nitrates mechanism in MI:**
A. Antioxidant
B. ↓ Blood volume
C. Venodilatation
D. Arterial dilatation
E. Cerebral vasodilatation

51. **Nitrates in MI:**
A. CHF
B. Angina
C. Upto 3 months
D. Upto 6 months
E. Prior to CABG

52. **Hypotension in MI is caused by:**
A. Sweating
B. Chest pain
C. Tachycardia
D. Morphine
E. Nitrate

53. **Central chest pain with hemodynamic compromise:**
A. Pulmonary embolism
B. Oesophageal spasm
C. Myocarditis
D. MI

54. **PSVT:**
A. LAD
B. RBBB
C. Visible P wave
D. Capture beat
E. Carotid sinus massage

55. **Drug acting on metabolism of myocardium in angina:**
A. Trimetazidine
B. L-carnitine
C. Nitrates
D. β blocker

56. **Early CAG after MI (1st week):**
A. Pericarditis
B. CHF
C. Angina
D. Embolism
E. PSVT

57. **Max reperfusion after MI by:**
A. Primary PTCA
B. Streptokinase
C. Streptokinase + aspirin
D. tPA
E. Eurokinase

58. **Volume of infarct is assessed by:**
A. ECG
B. CPK-MB
C. Echo
D. Troponin
E. SGOT

59. **Antioxidant all *except*:**
A. Pentothenic acid
B. Flavinods
C. α tocopherol
D. β carotene
E. Vitamin C

60. **HAPE all *except*:**
A. ↑ PCWP
B. ↑ Pulmonary artery pressure
C. Hypoxia
D. ↓ diffusion capacity
E. Tachycardia

61. **Diastolic murmur at mitral valve in all *except*:**
A. ASD
B. VSD
C. AR
D. Rheumatic activity at MV
E. MR

62. **High first month mortality in CHD:**
A. TA
B. TGA
C. TOF
D. Truncus arteriosus
E. TAPVC

63. **CHF with NSR drug to be avoided on long term use:**
A. Digoxin
B. Aminophyllin
C. Salbutamol
D. β blocker
E. Lithium

64. **Drug used in CHF with NSR:**
A. LMWH
B. Digoxin
C. ACEI
D. Amiodarone

65. **Drug interaction of M dopa:**
A. Halloperidol
B. Lithium
C. Levodopa
D. Amlodipine

66. **Drug interaction with statin:**
A. Gemfibrozil
B. Erythromycin
C. Warfarrin
D. Digoxin

67. **HTN is most common cause of:**
A. CRF
B. CVD
C. Stroke
D. Sacular artery aneurysm

68. **In primary myocardial disease, heart failure increases by:**
A. AV asynergy
B. Chest infection
C. Anemia
D. Myxodema
E. Persistent apoptosis

69. **Mechanism of peripheral edema in CHF:**
A. ↑ Catecholamine
B. Venoconstriction
C. ↑ hydrostatic pressure
D. ↑ ANP

70. **Restenosis is significantly decreased by:**
A. DCA
B. Stenting
C. Laser
D. Aspirin + Dipyradamole
E. Anticoagulant

71. **Indication of thrombolytic therapy:**
A. Reinfarction within 1st week
B. Only after establishing - enzyme
C. Hyper acute ECG changes without chest pain
D. Typical chest pain without ECG changes
E. Non Q MI

72. **Mechanism of fatigue in CHF:**
A. Activation of J receptors in muscle
B. Decreased CO
C. ↓ PaO_2
D. ↓ Metab of muscle

73. **Aortoarteritis typically involves:**
A. Subclavian artery
B. Renal artery
C. Axillary artery
D. Femoral artery
E. Internal carotid artery

74. **β blockers with ISA:**
A. Pindolol
B. Acebutalol
C. Sotalol
D. Attenolol
E. Propanolol

75. **High incidence of SCD:**
A. MVP
B. Romanoward syndrome
C. Pulmonary embolism
D. Rapid weight ↓ protocol
E. HTN

76. **Central cyanosis with pulmonary edema due to:**
A. ↓ diffusion capacity
B. ↑ Hb concentration
C. V/Q shunt
D. Hyperventilation
E. ↑ Circulation time in pulmonary circulation

77. **ACE – I C/I in:**
A. Dehydration
B. COPD
C. L renal art stenosis
D. Disease of aorta
E. AS

ANSWERS

1	A	2	D	3	A	4	B	5	B	6	A	7	B
8	A	9	A	10	C	11	A	12	A	13	C	14	A
15	C	16	B	17	A	18	C	19	B	20	D	21	A
22	A	23	A	24	D	25	D	26	A	27	C	28	A
29		30	B	31	B	32	B	33	A	34	D	35	C
36	A	37	B	38	C	39	D	40	B	41	A,B,C	42	A,B,D
43	A,B	44	A,C,E	45		46	A,E	47	A,E	48	A,B,D	49	D
50	B	51	A,B	52		53	A,C,D	54	E	55	A	56	C
57	A	58	A,B,C	59	A	60	A	61	A	62	D,E	63	A,E
64	C	65	A,C	66	A	67	C	68	A,B,C,E	69	A,B,C	70	B
71	A,C	72	B,D	73	A,B	74	B	75	D	76	B,C	77	A,E

40

RML 2011

1. **Stain least protein binding:**
   A. Pravastatin **B.** Simvastatin
   C. Fluvastatin **D.** Lovastatin

2. **Drug causing pedal edema all *except*:**
   A. Methyldopa **B.** Cyclosporine
   C. OKT_3 **D.** Sulfonamides

3. **Drug causing CMP all *except*:**
   A. Lithium **B.** Emetine
   C. Quinidine **D.** Sulfonamides

4. **Drug causing pericarditis all *except*:**
   A. Levodopa **B.** Emetine
   C. Methysergide **D.** Procainamide

5. **Anti-arrhythmic–not excreted through liver:**
   A. Procainamide **B.** Lignocaine
   C. Phenytoin **D.** Quinidine

6. **All drugs removed by hemodialysis *except*:**
   A. Captopril **B.** Nitroprusside
   C. Furosemide **D.** Hydrazine

7. **CHADS score for all *except*:**
   A. DM_1 **B.** Female gender
   C. HTN_1 **D.** CHF

8. **Severity of PE all *except*:**
   A. Age > 20
   B. CHF
   C. Bradycardia
   D. Chronic lung disease

9. **LCX and branches, best surg:**
   A. RAO caudal **B.** RAO cranial
   C. LAD caudal **D.** LAO cranial

10. **Least common branch of RCA:**
    A. SA nodal **B.** Canal
    C. PDA **D.** Acuta marginal

11. **All are end holes *except*:**
    A. Berman **B.** Counard
    C. Goodlelubin **D.** Angulated

12. **All are both end and side holes *except*:**
    A. NIH **B.** Sanes
    C. Multipurpose **D.** Pigtail

13. **All are used for selective left coronary angiography *except*:**
    A. Judikins **B.** Amplate
    C. Multipurpose **D.** Goodler lebin

14. **Highest fiber specific:**
    A. TNK
    B. STK
    C. TPA
    D. Staphylokinase

15. **Not true for TNK:**
    A. Mutant of TPA
    B. More fibrin specific than STK
    C. Less plasma clearance than TPA
    D. More sensitive to PAI-1

16. **Heparin all *except*:**
    A. Direct inhibitor of Xa
    B. Equal acting against Xax
    C. During PCI kept at 250-350
    D. NTG reduces the effect

17. **Rheumatic subcutaneous nodules all *except*:**
    A. Late manifestation
    B. Non tender, painless
    C. Seen in 1–21% of cases
    D. Disappear in 4–6 weeks

18. **Rheumatic MR severity all *except*:**
    A. Diastolic rhumble
    B. S_3
    C. Duration of murmur
    D. Thrill

19. **Rheumatic fever all *except*:**
    A. Fibrinous pericarditis is seen
    B. Myocyte necrosis
    C. Pinhead vegetation on vulvar surface
    D. Fibrinoid necrosis of vulvar neovascularization

20. **Early systolic murmur seen in:**
A. Mold rheumatic MR
B. MVP
C. Non restrictive VSD with PAH
D. TR hypertensive

21. **TR:**
A. Circumference 10–12 cm
B. Septal papillary muscle is absent or rudimentary
C. Anterior septal leaflet attaches to large anterior papillary muscle
D. Post and septal leaflets are attached to posterior papillary muscle

22. **Pulmonary values cusp absent:**
A. Anterior B. Post
C. Left D. Right

23. **NADAS criteria for child with murmur:**
A. ECG major changes
B. Cyanosis
C. CHF
D. Distolic murmur

24. **2 years old child recurrent pulmonary infection, with VSD gradient 40 mm Hg, best M_x:**
A. Early VSD closure
B. Pre OP cath to assess reversibility of PAH
C. ACE–I for H.F.
D. PA bonding

25. **ADH antagonist–tolvaptan. Largest trail of aspirin in MI:**
A. ISIS–1 B. ISIS–2
C. GISSI–1 D. GISSI–3

26. **Highest protein boundary:**
A. Sustained release metoprolol
B. Propranolol
C. Atenolol
D. Bisoprolol

27. **Acute MI, mortality not effected by:**
A. Baseline EF
B. Presentation as acute HF
C. Residual ischemia
D. Susceptibility of life threatening arrhythmia

28. **High risk finding of stress ... all *except*:**
A. LV dilation on exercise
B. Lung uptake
C. Large fix
D. Multiple ... ultiple territory

29. **Lowest speci...**
A. Exercise ...
B. Exercise SP...
C. Dobutamine st...
D. Pharmacolog...

30. **Type C lesion all *except*:**
A. Occlusion > 3 month's
B. Moderate to heavy calcification
C. Excessive tortuosity
D. Inability to protect major side branch

31. **Acute stent thrombosis all *except*:**
A. Overlapping of stent
B. Crush technique
C. Polymer coating
D. Direct stunting

32. **Predictors of restenosis:**
A. Proximal LAD
B. SVG graft
C. Excessive tortuosity
D. CTO

33. **High risk factor of or UA all *except*:**
A. DM B. HTN
C. Post MI angina D. Previous PAD

34. **LV non-compaction all *except*:**
A. Absence of co-existing cardiac defect
B. Clordy visible trabeculation
C. Blood flow is direct to trabeculation on doppler
D. Non-compaction to compaction ratio vs 4:1

35. **ABI:**
A. N > 1
B. Mild – 0.6 – 0.9
C. Moderate – 0.4 – 0.8
D. Severe < 0.4

36. **ECG R/F USA:**
A. T wave inversion > 0.3 MV
B. STE > 0.5
C. LBBB
D. AVB

37. **Most specific for RVH:**
A. RAD > 90
B. R/S > 1 in V_1 with > 0.5
C. $S_1Q_3T_3$
D. P. pulmonale

38. **Which is not of one patient in romhilt criteria?**
A. LAD
B. ST–T on digitalis
C. Intrinsicoid deflection > 50 ms in V_5/V_6
D. PTF > 4

39. **P waves may be absent in:**
A. SA block B. AF
C. WPW type A D. Hyperkalemia

40. **Safe S_1 all *except*:**
A. RBBB
B. ↑ PR interval

C. Severe LV dysfunction
D. Acute AR

41. **Paradoxical split S_2 seen in:**
A. Tamponade
B. Complete RBBB
C. PS
D. Right sided accessory pathway

42. **Very prominent X descent in all *except*:**
A. TR
B. Tamponade
C. ASD
D. RV volume overload

43. **Post capillary pulmonary HTN:**
A. Supravalvular AS in child
B. Acute MR
C. Truncus without stenosis or regurgitation
D. Obstructed TAPVC

44. **Pregnancy maximum blood volume and CO at:**
A. 12 – 14 weeks B. 25 – 27 weeks
C. 32 – 34 weeks D. Full term

45. **In pregnancy all murmur dec. *except*:**
A. Rheumatic mitral stenosis
B. AR
C. MR
D. VSD

46. **Morality in pregnancy between 25 – 50% with all *except*:**
A. Marfan with aortic root involve
B. Primary pulmonary HTN
C. Complicated CoA
D. MS with NYHA III

47. **NYHA grade III cannot do:**
A. Roller skate
B. Walk at 2.5 mph
C. Golf
D. Shower without stopping

48. **Hereditary hemorrhagic telangiectasia all *except*:**
A. Central cyanosis
B. PHT
C. GI hemorrhage
D. Capillary hemangioma

49. **Which of the following is true about PCWP?**
A. PCWP is slightly higher than LVEDP
B. PCWP is equal to mean PAP
C. During MR, V mane is equal to LV is DP

50. **Pericardial knock all *except*:**
A. Occurs after 0.8–1.2 msec after A_2
B. Low pitch sound
C. Snapping and clicking sound
D. Occurs earlier than S_3

51. **LV – S_4:**
A. Seen only at apex
B. Low pitch sound
C. Does not change with respiration
D. Attenuates when bell is hard pressed

52. **Fontan indicated all *except*:**
A. HLHS
B. DICN
C. TA
D. cTGA with VSD with PS

53. **↓ PBF seen is all *except*:**
A. TA – type Ic
B. DORV with PS
C. Single ventricle with PS
D. cTGA with VSD with PS

54. **Severity of tricuspid atresia depends on:**
A. Size of ASD
B. Size of VSD
C. Size of PDA
D. Presence of TGA or not

55. **Heart failure in first week all *except*:**
A. HLHS
B. Large VSD
C. Interrupted aortic arch
D. TGA with PS

56. **Balloon atrial septostomy all *except*:**
A. Restrictive PFO with TA
B. Restrictive PFO with PA
C. VSD with PS

57. **Polysplenia all *except*:**
A. ASD
B. TAPVC
C. Left pulmonary isomerism
D. Absent IVC

58. **Asplenia all *except*:**
A. PS B. LVOT obs.
C. TGA D. AV canal defect

59. **Klinefelter's all *except*:**
A. ASD
B. VSD
C. PDA
D. PS

60. **Ellis-Van Creveld true:**
A. ASD

61. **Rubella all *except*:**
A. CoA
B. ASD
C. Pulmonary artery stenosis
D. PDA

62. **Iridodonesis seen in:**
A. Marfan
B. Dawn
C. Ehlers-Danlos
D. Osteogenesis imperfecta

63. **Osteogenesis imperfecta all *except*:**
A. Defect is type III collagen
B. 50% scoliosis
C. Cardiac involvement – AR
D. Fractures with mild injury

64. **Friedreich ataxia:**
A. Autosomal recessive
B. Chr. 6 defect
C. Frataxin gene
D. Frataxin gene is a mitochondrial gene of iron homeostasis in respiratory chain

65. **Right heart border all *except*:**
A. RA
B. RV
C. Aortic knuckle
D. PA

66. **Type III hyperlipoproteinemia seen in:**
A. LDL
B. IDL
C. VLDL
D. LDL+VLDL

67. **Xanthoma all *except*:**
A. Eruptive xanthoma in Type I
B. Palmar xanthoma in Type IV
C. Tenden xanthoma in Type II
D. Tuberoeruptive xanthoma in Type III

68. **Rhabdomyoma all *except*:**
A. Most common in childhood
B. > 50% associated with tuberous sclerosis
C. Presence is multiple location
D. Present commonly at RV free wall

69. **Spinal muscular atrophy:**
A. Most common defect – VSD
B. DCMP in Type III
C. Cardiac involvement in I Q 3
D. AF, AFl and supraventricular arrhythmia and atrial standstill

70. **Amyl nitrate ↓ all *except*:**
A. Valvular AS
B. TOF
C. PDA
D. VSD

71. **Amyl nitrate all *except*:**
A. S_1 – loud
B. A_2 – soft
C. A_2 – OS gap narrow
D. OS – Soft

72. **RVOT – VT all *except*:**
A. LBBB is V_1
B. Sup. A
C. Adenosine terminates
D. Exercise, stress ppt

73. **Triggered activity is all *except*:**
A. RVOT – VT
B. Torsades
C. Digitalis
D. AIVR

74. **Sudden death in HCM:**
A. Hypotension during exercise
B. Syncope on exertion
C. Wall thickness > 20 mm
D. Sustained VT

75. **TR murmur - all *except*:**
A. Squatting
B. Leg elevation
C. Valsalva phase III
D. Muller's murmur

76. **MDM seen is all *except*:**
A. Grahm Steel murmur
B. Large VSD
C. Rheumatic TS
D. Severe AR

77. **Early systolic murmur:**
A. VSD with pulmonary HTN
B. TR with pulmonary HTN
C. MVP with MR

78. **Severe AR with normal LV function all murmur are seen *except*:**
A. PSM_1
B. EDM
C. MDM_1
D. ESM

79. **M_1 QT_1 gap:**
A. 20 msec
B. 30 msec
C. 60 msec
D. 56 msec

80. **Cilostazol all *except*:**
A. Quinoline derivative
B. PDE-5 inhibitor
C. ↓ stent restenosis post PCI
D. Symptomatic improvement is PAD

81. **Ergonomics proactive test C/I:**
A. PDA
B. Severe HTN
C. AS
D. Severe dysfunction

82. **All are coronary vasoconstrictor *except*:**
A. Cold water
B. Cholinergic stimulation
C. Mental stress
D. Cocaine

83. **Post MI – VSD all *except*:**
A. Incidence 0.2% all to recent trial
B. Thrombolysis dec. incidence
C. ↑ Age, AWMI, HTN are risk factor
D. Inferior wall MI–VSD is associated with worse prognosis

84. **Contrast reaction Type 3 all *except*:**
A. Repeated vomiting
B. Laryngospasm
C. Hypotension
D. HTN

85. **Atropine dose in pediatric heart block:**
A. 0.01-0.03 mg/kg
B. 0.05-0.1

86. **Side effect of PGEI all *except*:**
A. Fever
B. Hypotension
C. Apnea
D. Hypoglycemia

87. **MDM is not normally seen is:**
A. Star-Edwards
B. Carpentier-Edwards

88. **All are bioprosthetic *except*:**
A. Carpentier-Edwards
B. Inance-Shelley
C. Harlock
D. Bjork-Shelley

89. **BMS is POBA, ↓ is favour of BMS *except*:**
A. Abrupt vessel closure
B. ↓ required CABG
C. ↓ slow flow
D. Restenosis

90. **All are long term continuous flow LVAD *except*:**
A. Jaruk
B. Tandem
C. Heart mate II
D. Micro Debekay

91. **ATP – III oriental 0–1 risk factor, goal:**
A. < 100 B. < 130
C. < 160 D. < 200

92. **INC – 7 criteria all *except*:**
A. N < 120
B. DM – 138/82 = drug should be started
C. BP – 150/98 Thiazide directive is enough
D. Stage II > 160/100

93. **Severe AS all *except*:**
A. N area > 2 cm^2
B. Severe > 0.8 cm^2
C. Mild to moderate 1.5-2
D. Progresses from mixed to severe AS in 3 years

94. **Endocarditis prophylaxis required in:**
A. Urethral catheterization
B. Cardiac catheterization
C. Caesarean section
D. Intrauterine device

95. **Relative contraindication of thrombolysis all *except*:**
A. INR – 2-3 on anticoagulation
B. Noncompressible vascular punctuation
C. Internal bleeding 2-4 weeks
D. Surgery < 6 weeks

96. **Pulsus bisferiens all *except*:**
A. AR1
B. AS with AR
C. Severe AS with LV dysfunction
D. High cardiac output state

97. **Gorlin formulae in MS with MR:**
A. Over estimate
B. Under estimate
C. Overestimate with tachycardia
D. No change

98. **Least common branch of RCA:**
A. PDA
B. SA node artery
C. Acute marginal
D. Conus

99. **Pulmonary valve (Tricuspid) all *except*:**
A. Anterior
B. Posterior
C. Left
D. Right

ANSWERS

1		2	A	3	C	4		5	A	6		7	B
8	C	9		10		11		12	A	13		14	A
15		16	A	17	A	18	C	19	B	20	C	21	
22	A	23	A	24		25	B	26	B	27		28	
29	A	30	B	31		32		33		34		35	
36		37		38		39		40	A	41	D	42	
43		44	B	45	A	46		47	A	48		49	
50	B	51		52		53		54		55		56	
57		58		59		60	A	61		62		63	A
64	A	65	B	66		67	B	68	D	69		70	
71		72	B	73	D	74	C	75		76	A	77	A
78	A	79		80	B	81	A	82		83		84	
85	B	86		87	A	88		89		90	B	91	
92	C	93		94	A	95	D	96	C	97		98	
99		100											

41

RML 2010

1. **Variables a/w with acute thrombosis all *except*:**
   A. Long lesion B. Small vessel
   C. Ostial D. Bifurcation

2. **Stent thrombosis defined by all *except*:**
   A. Acute < 24 hours
   B. Subacute 24 hours-7 days
   C. Late 30 days- 1 year
   D. Very late > 1year

3. **Stent thrombosis increased by all *except*:**
   A. Under expansion of stent
   B. Crush technique
   C. High pressure post dilation
   D. Margin dissection

4. **ST resolution 50% seen after STK ——— in AMI.**
   A. 1 hour B. 2 hours
   C. 6 hours D. 3 hours

5. **High risk for UA/NSTEMI all *except*:**
   A. DM
   B. Prior CVA
   C. Advanced age
   D. Obesity (BMI > 28)

6. **LAD distal during bifurcation to D1 can be visualized by all *except*:**
   A. Lateral B. LAO caudal
   C. RAO caudal D. LAO cranial

7. **Dominant RCA with distal bifurcation best seen in:**
   A. RAD caudal B. AP cranial
   C. RAO cranial D. LAO

8. **Branch of RCA are all *except*:**
   A. Acute marginal B. Obtuse marginal
   C. Conus D. RV branch

9. **ECG in pulmonary embolism all *except*:**
   A. QRS axis 0-90° B. AF/AFl
   C. Sinus tachycardia D. RBBB

10. **End + side hole are all *except*:**
    A. Pigtail
    B. NIH catheter
    C. Multipurpose catheter
    D. Jones catheter

11. **True about Swan-Ganz all *except*:**
    A. Balloon at distal end
    B. End hole present
    C. Thermistor at distal end
    D. Injector pant at 30 cm proximal to distal end

12. **All *except* in RV angiography:**
    A. Eppendorf B. Grellman pigtail
    C. Berman D. Cournard

13. **Evaluation of significant ischaemia producing coronary artery lesion done best by:**
    A. FFR B. Thermography
    C. CAG D. IVUS

14. **Fibrous cap and lipid core are best delineated by:**
    A. IVUS B. OCT
    C. Angioscopy D. CAG

15. **MDCT better over angio in all *except*:**
    A. Instent restenosis
    B. Coronary artery fistula
    C. Coronary anomalies
    D. CABG graft

16. **Ranolazine all *except*:**
    A. Decrease calcium overload by blocking late Na+ current
    B. Half life of sustained release is 7 hours
    C. Significant mortality benefit at 1 years and in UA/ NSTEMI/UA in MERLIN - TMI36
    D. QT prolongation

17. **Ticagreolar all *except*:**
    A. Oral reversible ADP antagonist
    B. Plato trial showed mortality benefits over clopidogrel

C. Dose 90 mg OD against clopidogrel - 75 mg OD
D. Causes dyspnea > clopidogrel

18. **Fondaparinaux all *except*:**
A. Selective factor -Xa inhibitor
B. Small compound synthetic
C. Inhibits ADP receptor
D. Useful in UA/NSTEMI as shown in Oasis-5 in 20,000 patients

19. **Direct thrombin inhibitor all *except*:**
A. Ximelofiban B. Ximelagatran
C. Argatroban D. Bivalivudin

20. **Warfarin inhibits all factor all *except*:**
A. II B. V
C. IX D. VII

21. **Protamine antagonises heparin:**
A. 1 mg for 100 U B. 1 ml for 100 U
C. 1 mg for 1000 U D. 1 ml for 1000 U

22. **Framingham major all *except*:**
A. Hepatomegaly
B. Cardiomegaly
C. CVP > 16 cm H_2O
D. PND

23. **Inotrope which is not a vasodilator?**
A. Amrinone B. Dopamine
C. Norepinephrine D. Epinephrine

24. **Not an inotrope:**
A. Nesiritide B. Enoximone
C. Levosimendan D. Milrinone

25. **Highest O_2 saturation:**
A. Renal vein B. IVC
C. Internal jugular D. Coronary sinus

26. **High dose Atorvastatin all *except*:**
A. MIRACL
B. TNT
C. Prove - IT - TIMI 22
D. ASCOT - LLA

27. **Free wall rupture all *except*:**
A. More in women
B. Ruptures at centre
C. 1-4 days of MI
D. In patients without prior MI

28. **Episodic ischaemia all *except*:**
A. ACAOS
B. Ectopic RCA from right cusp.
C. Fistula
D. Bridging

29. **Systemic → PA arterial shunt all *except*:**
A. Glenn shunt B. Waterston
C. Central D. Potts

30. **Triangle of Koch boundaries all *except*:**
A. Mouth of coronary sinus makes base
B. Tendon of Todaro superiorly
C. Inferiorly septal leaflet attachment of Tricuspid valve
D. Opening of IVC medially

31. **Kerley lines all *except*:**
A. Kerley A from periphery to hila
B. Kerley C at base
C. Kerley B due to fluid in interlobular septa
D. Kerley A is due to small pulmonary vein dilatation

32. **All *except* in balloon septostomy:**
A. Fogartly catheter
B. Lehman catheter
C. Rashkind catheter
D. Miller catheter

33. **Balloon atrial septostomy in all *except*:**
A. 5 mm primembranous VSD with pulmonary atresia
B. Tricuspid atresia
C. PA with intact ventricular septum with restrictive PFO
D. HLHS with restrictive PFO

34. **a = V are all *except*:**
A. Hypervolemia B. Tamponade
C. CCP D. RV failure

35. **Prominent X-descent in all *except*:**
A. Tamponade
B. Severe TR
C. ASD
D. RV overload states

36. **Tamponade without pulsus paradous in all *except*:**
A. Hypovolemia
B. AR
C. Aortic root dissection
D. Severe emphysema

37. **Soft S1 all *except*:**
A. Long PR interval
B. RBBB
C. Severe COPD
D. Decreased LV contractility

38. **Low aortic pulse pressure in all *except*:**
A. CHF B. RSOV
C. AS D. Tamponade

39. **Handgrip increases murmur of all *except*:**
A. AR B. MR
C. VSD D. HOCM

40. **All *except* cause wide split of S2 not due to decreased Q-A2 interval:**
A. LBBB B. MR
C. VSD D. LA myxoma

41. **Severe TR echo findings are all *except*:**
A. Jet occupying > 30% RA area
B. Late systolic hepatic vein flow reversal
C. Vena contracta 6.5
D. Regurgitant vol 30 ml

42. **Mild AR echo shows all *except*:**
A. Vena contracta < 5 mm
B. Central jet < 4 cm
C. Regurgitant fraction < 30%
D. Regurgitant jet occupying < 20% of LA area

43. **Asymptomatic severe MR surgery indication:**
A. LVEF < 60%
B. LVESD > 45 mm ESD > 40 mm
C. LVEDD > 65 mm
D. Pulmonary HTN

44. **Abnormal low pressure MDM in:**
A. Bjork-Shelly
B. Star Edwards
C. St Jude
D. Carpenter Edward

45. **Tilting disc valve:**
A. St Jude
B. Medotronic hall
C. Carbomedics
D. Star Edward

46. **Early prosthetic valve IE most common:**
A. Coagulase –ve staph
B. Staph. aureus
C. Streptococcus
D. Klebsiella

47. **Major symptom of HF all *except*:**
A. Pleural effusion
B. Hypotension
C. Tachycardia
D. Rales

48. **Athlete's heart all *except*:**
A. LVH by TGF-b and Angiotensin II
B. Systolic function normal to increased
C. Increased early diastolic filling
D. Sinus bradycardia

49. **Which increases gradient in HOCM all *except*?**
A. Muller's maneuver
B. Strain phase of valsalva
C. Isoproterenol
D. Amyl nitrite

50. **About pulse – all are correct *except*:**
A. Bisfireins seen commonly in severe AR
B. Alternans best in femoral artery
C. Bifid in HOCM
D. Dicrotic in DCMP with HF in young patients

51. **Auscultation frequencies:**
A. Cardiac frequencies 1500-3000 Hz
B. Low frequencies 25-150 Hz
C. Human ear can hear 16-18,000 Hz
D. Very low frequency (<25 Hz) are not audible but often palpable

52. **JVP all *except*:**
A. A wave corresponds to S2
B. X descent wave prominent than Y
C. A descent wave prominent than V
D. V starts in late systole and continues in diastole

53. **Rheumatic fever all *except*:**
A. Arthritis is most common manifestation
B. Arthritis self limiting
C. Arthritis earliest to manifest after streptococcal pharyngitis
D. Individual joint involvement resolves in 6-8 weeks

54. **Most common presentation in neonate with Ebstein:**
A. Cyanosis
B. Heart failure
C. Arrhythmia
D. Murmur

55. **Reverse differential cyanosis:**
A. TGA with PDA with high PVR
B. PDA with reversal
C. L-TGA with reversal
D. TGA with VSD with PS with PDA

56. **PCWP not more than LVEDP in:**
A. Cor triatriatum
B. LA myxoma
C. Chronic pulmonary thromboembolism
D. Pulmonary venous obstructive disease

57. **Peripheral pulmonary artery stenosis with intact IVS all *except*:**
A. Alagille syndrome
B. William syndrome
C. Turner's syndrome
D. Rubella syndrome

58. **Blue sclera in all *except*:**
A. Turner's syndrome
B. Ehler-Danlos syndrome
C. Marfan syndrome
D. Osteogenesis imperfecta

59. **Choussat's criteria for fontan all *except*:**
A. PVR ≤ 8 units/m^2
B. PA pressure < 15 mmHg
C. Competent mitral valve
D. Pulmonary artery: Aorta > 0.75

60. **Congenital MS diagnostic:**
A. MVA < 1 cm^2

B. MVA < 0.6 cm^2/m^2
C. Transmitral gradient 12-15 mmHg
D. LA pressure > 18 mmHg

61. **TOF treatment not given in cyanotic spell:**
A. Morphine B. I/V beta blocker
C. Phenylephrine D. Adrenaline

62. **CYP 3A4 all *except*:**
A. Pravastatin B. Atorvastatin
C. Rosuvastatin D. Simvastatin

63. **Univentricular correction surgery done in all *except*:**
A. HLHS
B. Double inlet ventricle with PS
C. Tricuspid atresia
D. VSD and pulmonary atresia

64. **ST elevation in V_1 V_2 associated with all *except*:**
A. Hypocalcemia
B. Hyperkalemia
C. IC antiarrythmics
D. Brugada

65. **ERP increased in both AV node and accessory pathway:**
A. IA B. IC
C. II D. IV

66. **Most common arrhythmia after fontan surgery:**
A. AF/AFl B. VT
C. AV block D. VF

67. **Class IA:**
A. Ajmaline B. Azimilide
C. Flecanide D. Sotalol

68. **SVT vs VT suggests VT in all scenario *except*:**
A. RBBB with superior axis
B. LBBB with inferior axis
C. QRS during tachycardia narrow than sinus rythm
D. Onset of R to nadir of S <60 m sec

69. **A patient with SVT with RBBB > 0.14 sec; LBBB > 0.16 sec. In which of following conditions above condition cannot occur?**
A. Patient on flecainide
B. Given I/V beta blocker during tachycardia
C. Patient is elderly having fibrosis of bundle branches
D. When anterograde conduction occurs through accessory pathway

70. **Typical atrial flutter all *except*:**
A. Positive P waves in inferior leads
B. Circuit confined to RA
C. Ablation of tissue between IVC and tricuspid annulus

71. **Class I indication for pace maker in sick sinus syndrome all *except*:**
A. Documented symptomatic bradycardia with frequent symptomatic pause
B. Symptomatic chronotropic incompetence
C. Essential drug causing symptomatic bradycardia
D. Mildly symptomatic bradycardia with <40/min in awake patient

72. **Reentry all *except*:**
A. AF
B. Long QT
C. Brugada
D. Preexcitation syndrome

73. **All *except* in long QT syndrome:**
A. SCN 4B B. CAV
C. KCNJ2 D. GDPL – 1

74. **Cardio selective beta-blocker all *except*:**
A. Carvedilol B. Bisoprolol
C. Acebutalol D. Atenolol

75. **Renal excretion of β-blocker:**
A. Atenolol B. Propanolol
C. Metoprolol D. Isoprolol

76. **Pregnancy not safe on routine use:**
A. Amiodarone B. Aspirin
C. Digoxin D. Hydralazine

77. **Intermediate risk surgery all *except*:**
A. Orthopedic surgery
B. Endoscopic procedure
C. Prostatectomy
D. Carotid endarterectomy

78. **Abdominal aortic aneurysm all *except*:**
A. < 5 cm rupture chance 1.5%
B. Chance of rupture less common in females and less chance in same
C. High risk in current smokers

79. **Arterial desaturation < 93% seen in all *except*:**
A. Pulmonary edema
B. Oversedation
C. VSD with gradient of 35 mmHg
D. DORV with VSD with severe PS gradient of 70 mmHg

80. **Enalapril all *except*:**
A. Save B. Consensus
C. V-HeF T 2 D. Solved

81. **Primary prevention trial of SCD all *except*:**
A. AVID B. MADIT - II
C. SCD - HeF D. DINAMIT

82. **Long term use artificial heart:**
A. Jarvik B. Hemopump
C. Impella D. Tandom heart

83. Fontaine classification all *except*:
A. I: Asymptomatic
B. IIa: Claudication > 500 metres
C. IIb: Claudication < 200 mts
D. III: Nocturnal and Rest. pain

84. All *except* about ABI:
A. > 1 is normal
B. Abnormal is < 0.9
C. Critical limb ischemia at < 0.75
D. Poor healing of skin ulcer associated with ankle venous pressure < 55 mmHg

85. CT Houston units all *except*:
A. Air - 1000
B. Acute thrombus + 20 to 90
C. Bone + 800 to 3000
D. Fat 20-250

86. Polysplenia all *except*:
A. TAPVC
B. Single atrium/ASD
C. Absent IVC
D. Left pulmonary isomerism

87. Scimitar syndrome all *except*:
A. Associated with dextrocardia with situs inversus
B. Right lung hypoplasia
C. Anomalous right lung supply by systemic arteries from aorta

88. Contrast agents all *except*:
A. Iodixonol has highest iodine content among non-ionic contrast
B. All contain iodine which absorbs X-ray
C. Maglumin ditriazoate is high osmolar agent
D. Iodixanal has lowest osmolarity of < 300

89. Hereditary hemorrhagic telangiectasia all *except*:
A. Autosomal recessive
B. Associated with hypoxia polycythemia
C. Recurrent epistaxis
D. Mucocutaneous telangiectasia around, lip, tongue 0.5-3 mm

90. Beautiful trial:
A. Ivabradine
B. Ranolazine
C. Prasugrel
D. Rosuvastatin

91. RV/LV favors RV all *except*:
A. Moderator band
B. Elleptical
C. Septal attachment
D. Trabeculated apex

ANSWERS

1	C	2	B	3	C	4		5	D	6	A	7	B
8	B	9	A	10	B	11	C	12		13	A	14	B
15	A	16	C	17	C	18	C	19	A	20	B	21	A
22	A	23	C	24	A	25	A	26	D	27	B	28	B
29	A	30	D	31	B	32	B	33	A	34	D	35	
36	A	37	B	38	B	39	D	40	A	41	D	42	A
43	A	44	B	45	B	46	A	47	B	48	A	49	A
50	C	51		52	A	53	D	54	B	55	A	56	C
57	C	58	A	59	A	60	B	61	D	62	A	63	B
64	A	65	B	66	A	67	A	68	D	69	D	70	A
71	D	72	B	73	D	74	A	75	A	76		77	B
78	B	79		80	A	81	A	82	A	83	B	84	C
85	D	86	A	87	A	88	A	89	A	90	A	91	B

42

RML 2009

1. **CRF triad of ECG includes all *except*:**
   A. AV blocks B. TQT
   C. LVH D. Tall T waves
2. **Carney complex all *except*:**
   A. Constitutional symptoms
   B. Spotty skin pigmentation
   C. Acromegaly
   D. Cardiac myxoma
3. **CCP like picture:**
   A. Acute LV dilatation
   B. RVMI – massive PE
   C. Early RCM
4. **Cardiac myxoma triad all *except*:**
   A. Pericardial effusion
   B. Intracardiac obstruction
   C. Systemic embolization
   D. Constitutional symptoms
5. **In AIDS least common policardial manifestation:**
   A. Acute pericarditis
   B. CCP
   C. Kaposi sarcoma
   D. Infective pericardial effusion
6. **Most common infective organism in HIV pericardial effusion:**
   A. MTB B. CMV
   C. M. Kansasi D. Cryptococcus
7. **Cardiac tamponade all *except*:**
   A. Pulsus paradoxus
   B. Electrical alternans
   C. RS with Y descent
8. **In a study of RCT 1000 patients treatment with A 13.5% event rate C/T placebo16.0% (p = 0.08). In other study treatment with B 14.5% event rate C/T placebo 15.0% true:**
   A. 2.5% ARR in A
   0.5% ARR in B
   A is superior to B
   B. B is superior to A
   C. NNT for B is 67
   D. NNT for A is 6
9. **Specificity is:**
   A. Patient with disease with abnormal result
   B. Patient without disease with normal result
   C. Patient with normal result with disease
   D. Patient with normal result without disease
10. **In world CVS death:**
    A. 20% B. 30%
    C. 40% D. 50%
11. **In India 2010 CVS deaths of all world:**
    A. 40 B. 50
    C. 60 D. 70
12. **Peripartum cardiomyopathy all *except*:**
    A. Disease in last month of pregnancy and 0 in 2 months
    B. No known cardiac disease
    C. LV dysfunction systolic on echo
    D. No precipitating factor
13. **Dallas criteria:**
    A. Endomyocardial biopsy
14. **Right sided accessory pathway ablation with persistent T ↓ in II, III, aVF:**
    A. RCA spasm B. Cardiac memory
    C. Pericarditis
15. **Hypertriglyceredemia TG 1620 in female 60 years with DM II, no history of CAD, TC 280, HDL 22, asymptomatic:**
    A. Type I hyperlipoproteinemia
    B. III
    C. V
    D. Familial hypercholesterolemia

16. **Brugada most common arrhythmia:**
A. AF
B. Monomorphic VT
C. Polymorphic VT
D. VF

17. **Brugada most specific diagnosis:**
A. Saddle back ECG
B. Cored ST
C. T ↓
D. None

18. **↓ QT:**
A. 300 B. 320
C. 310 D. 360

19. **Brugada diagnosis can be done by testing with which class of drug?**
A. Ia B. Ib
C. Ic D. III

20. **Patient with old Alwmi with non-sustained symptomic VT with syncope received ICD. Intolerant to amiodarone and placemia patient had 3 shocks in 1 hour with syncope on day of admission. Treatment:**
A. Metoprolol
B. Azonitide
C. Reprogram with defiltrating only rapid VT with stopping antibody cardia pacing
D. Remove ICD and no anti-arrhythmia

21. **A flutter converted to sinus rhythm. Most irrational treatment:**
A. Wait and watch to recurrent arrhythmia
B. Ablation
C. Continue with fluoride long-term
D. Continue with amiodarone

22. **Adenosine used all *except:***
A. Terminates AF
B. Terminates AVNRT
C. Acts on A_1 receptor
D. Activates K^+ channel

23. **Ivabradine all *except:***
A. Acts better at > 70/min
B. If in SA node
C. Beautiful trial showed benefit in all cases of CSA
D. ↓HR without affecting any cardiac function

24. **Reversed differential cyanosis:**
A. TGA with COA with PDA

25. **Einthovan triangle:**
A. I+III = II
B. I+II = III

26. **L-TGA:**
A. Systemic return to RA
B. AO origin from pulmonic ventricle
C. PA and right atria reversed
D. Mucosal cyanosis

27. **Fontan all *except*:**
A. DILV
B. Tricuspid atresia
C. HLHS
D. AV canal defect

28. **Least sensitive ECG criteria for LVH:**
A. Romhilt
B. Cornell voltage criteria
C. Cornell voltage measurement criteria

29. **Most important determinant of TOF:**
A. RVOT destruction
B. Site of VSD
C. Size of VSD

30. **Most common arrhythmia in post operative TOF:**
A. Atrial tachycardia
B. VT
C. Functional tachycardia

31. **Absolute contraindication of PFO closure:**
A. RV dysfunction with R → L shunt with PAH with arterial hypoxemia
B. Arterial hypoxemia after RV MI
C. Atrial septal aneurysm
D. Protein C/S deficiency with hypercoagular state

32. **Most common cause of HF with normal EF:**
A. HTN B. CAD
C. DM D. Obesity

33. **Most common cause of HF:**
A. CAD
B. HTN
C. DM
D. Valvular heart disease

34. **HF with normal EF:**
A. 30% B. 40-45%
C. 50-55% D. > 55%

35. **↓ BNP:**
A. Renal dysfunction
B. Early acute HF (< 1 hour)
C. ACS
D. High output state

36. **High output state all *except*:**
A. Systemic HTN
B. Fibrous dysplan dysplasia
C. Multiple myeloma
D. Beriberi

37. **IABP:**
A. ↓ Preload
B. ↓ HR
C. Both A/B and B
D. ↑ Preload

38. **Tumor of cardiac valves:**
A. P. fibroelastonia

39. **Fetal heart failure manifestion all *except*:**
A. Bradycardia
B. Scalp edema
C. ↓ fatal movements
D. Ascites

40. **Shone's complex all *except*:**
A. Valvular AS
B. Supraanular AS supravalvules
C. CoA
D. MS

41. **Coronary artery anomaly on CAG:**
A. Coronary from right sinus
B. RCA from left sinus
C. LAD from pulm trunk
D. Left main from right sinus

42. **B_2 lesion:**
A. 99% mid LAD obstruction concentric
B. LCX 60% angulation with mod. calcification
C. Diffuse degenerated venous graft
D. CTO > 3 months

43. **Long QT worse prognosis all *except:***
A. $QT_c > 500$
B. Female LQT3
C. Male LQT3
D. LQT 1

44. **Acoasery ......**
A. PWD
B. CWD
C. Tissue doppler
D. Any of above

45. **Tissue doppler is a modification of:**
A. PWD B. CWD
C. Both D. None

46. **Athlete's heart all *except*:**
A. LV cavity dimension
B. Symmetrical hypertrophy
C. Wall thickness rarely > 17 mm
D. Diastolic function normal

47. **IWMI on 3rd day SBP < 80 years P. edema, no auscultable murmur, normal JVP, normal ECG:**
A. VSD
B. RVMI
C. Massive PE
D. Papillary muscle rupture with severe MR

48. **Reperfusion injury all *except*:**
A. Lethal reperfusion injury
B. Vascular reperfusion injury
C. Reperfusion arrhythmia
D. Hibernation

49. **Treatment CPVT:**
A. β blocker
B. CCBS – verapamil, diltiazem
C. Mg

50. **Cardiogenic shock all *except*:**
A. SBP < 80 mmHg
B. CI < 1.8
C. PCWP < 18
D. Evidence of organ hypoperfusion

51. **Framingham's major criteria all *except*:**
A. PND
B. Radiographic cardiomegaly
C. Bilateral ankle edema
D. Rale with

52. **Highest specificity for HF:**
A. Resting HR
B. Orthopnea
C. Rales
D. S_3

53. **Major symptoms of HF all *except*:**
A. Dyspnea
B. Orthopnea
C. Peripheral cyanosis
D. Exercise intolerance

54. **Radiographic evidence of LA enlargement:**
A. Kerley B line
B. Double right heart shadow
C. Positively directly bulge on lateral view
D. Dilatation of LA appd.

55. **Bad prognostic marker in HF:**
A. ↓ Na^+ B. ↓ K^+
C. ↑ K^+ D. ↓ Mg^{2+}

56. **USA risk factor for death/non-fatal MI:**
A. Chest pain > 20 min
B. S_3 arth angina
C. Angina with new onset MR
D. New onset-exertional angina

57. **Beye's theorem:**
A. Exercise stress test
B. Stress echo
C. SPECT
D. All of above

58. Absolute contraindication of TMT are all *except*:
A. Uncontrolled HTN
B. MI < 2 days
C. USA
D. Severe symp. AS

59. High risk factor for I/E:
A. MR
B. PS
C. Degenerative valve in elderly
D. Corrected shunt with minimal/No haemodynamic abdomin

60. TMT interpretation altered by:
A. Vectopic
B. Ventricular paced beats
C. ST changers with MVP with severe anaemia
D. Digitalis

61. Surgery in IE:
A. Relapse of NVE after optimal treatment
B. Unstable prosthesis
C. Uncontrolled infection despite optimal therapy
D. Moderate to severe HT

62. Roth spots all *except:*
A. AIDS B. SLE
C. IE D. Anaemia

63. Immune mediated complications IE:
A. Osler nodes
B. Splenomegaly
C. Splinter hemorrhage
D. Petechiae

64. CHF ECG changes:
A. LVH
B. AV blocks
C. Tall T waves
D. Poor 'r' wave progression

65. Indication of angio in CCF:
A. Elderly patient with CCF of unknown etiology
B. Patient with past history of MI with CAD
C. Patient with CCF with severely dyskinetic myocardium
D. High risk TMT findings

66. $S_1 Q_3 T_3$ in IE:
A. 10% B. 15%
C. 20% D. 25%

67. Poor prognostic markar in TMT, all *except*:
A. < 6 MET
B. ST elevation except (AVR)
C. BP < 2 omity/fall more than 10
D. Angina at low workload

68. Diuretic lasix maximum dose:
A. 200 B. 400
C. 500 D. 600

69. Drugs acting on PCT:
A. Anuloride B. Frusemide
C. Acetazolamide D. AVP

70. Metabolic acidosis:
A. Acetazolamide
B. Frusemide
C. K^+ sparing
D. Of tricuspid aortic valve

71. Progression of calcification - in AS:
A. Male sex B. Plasma LDL
C. Age D. Uneven cusps

72. ECG changes of RV overload in PE indicate obstruction of:
A. 30% of palvascular bed
B. 50% of pulmonar vascular bed
C. 70% of palvascular bed

73. Pregnancy all *except*:
A. ↑ Plasma volume B. ↑ Hct
C. ↑ RBC mass D. ↑ Stroke volume

74. TOF with pregnancy high risk all *except*:
A. Syst. HTN B. $DpO_2 < 80\%$
C. Hct> 60%

75. Statins not metabolised by Puso:
A. Atorvastatin B. Pravastatin
C. Pituvastatin D. Ceruvastatin

76. E.C.F. required to produce ankle edema:
A. 3 lit B. 4 lit
C. 5 lit D. 6 lit

77. ↑ renin all *except*:
A. 2° Aldosteronism
B. Malignant HTN
C. 1° Aldosteronism
D. OC pills induced HTN

78. PE day 2, plate count 2.25 lakhs → 16,000, on heparin:
A. Stop heparin, start LMWH
B. Start lepuridin
C. Continue heparin as it is a transit phenomena

79. Not antithrombin III dependent:
A. Bivaluridin B. Enoxaparin
C. Fonda parinaux D. Heparin

80. Contraindication of thrombolysis:
A. CPR < 10 min B. DPB > 10 months
C. Pregnant

81. **Contraindication TEE all *except*:**
A. Dysphagia unknown cause
B. Active bleeding ulcers
C. Coumadine with INR 2
D. Osc. varices

82. **Marker of systolic CV dysfunction all *except*:**
A. Tei index
B. Cardiac index
C. Stroke volume index
D. Preload recruitment stroke volume index

83. **Diastolic function of LV depends on all *except*:**
A. HR
B. Myocardial relaxation
C. Elastic properties of LV
D. Ventricular filling

84. **BP measurement does not depend:**
A. Examiner
B. Patient position
C. Place of examination
D. All of the above
E. None of the above

85. **BP measurement depends all *except*:**
A. Rate of ↓ in Hg < 33 mmHg/sec
B. Cuff size
C. Width 70%/30%
D. Arm with respect to heart

86. **1 c cum of blood/water in JVP:**
A. 1.34 H_2O = 1 mmHg
B. 1.36 H_2O = 1 mmHg
C. 1.32 H_2O = 1 mmHg

87. **Symptoms of hypoperfusion in CHF all *except*:**
A. Altered mental status
B. Abdominal bloating/dyscomfort
C. Pre syncope
D. Fatigue

88. **Occlusion of subclavian arteritis occurs in all *except:***
A. Acute AO dissection
B. Thromboangitis obliterans
C. Spondyloarthropathy
D. Takayasu

89. **Pulmonary valvuloplasty true indicated:**
A. Asymptomatic with gradient > 40 mmHg
B. Asymptomatic with gradient > 50 mmHg
C. Asymptomatic with vavle area < 0.5 cm^2/m^2
D. Obstruction > 50% by 5 years

43

RML 2008

1. **1 mmHg equivalent to cm of water:**
A. 1.36 B. 1.34
C. 1.32 D. 1.33

2. **Changes in pregnant female are all *except*:**
A. Increase blood volume
B. Increase SV
C. Increase R.B.C. mass
D. Increase HCt

3. **Max dose of frusemide:**
A. 200 B. 400
C. 600 D. 800

4. **Drug active in PCT:**
A. CA inhibitor
B. Amiloride
C. Frusemide
D. AVP

5. **Diuretic causing metabolic acidosis:**
A. Lasix
B. Acetazolamide
C. Thiazide

6. **Percent of cardiac patient in India by 2010:**
A. 30% B. 60%
C. 40% D. 50%

7. **Specificity:**
A. Percent of patients with normal test who do not have disease
B. Percent of patients with disease with normal test
C. Percent of patients without disease with abnormal test
D. Percent of patients with disease with positive test

8. **CRF all true *except*:**
A. LVH
B. QT prolongation
C. Tall T wave
D. Decrease QRS voltage

9. **HIV least common cardiac presentation:**
A. CCP
B. Acute pericarditis
C. Kaposi's sarcoma pericardial involvement
D. Effusion of infective etiology

10. **HIV – most common cause of infective pericardial effusion:**
A. M. tuberculosis
B. CMV
C. M. kansasii
D. C. neoformans

11. **Roth spots are seen in all *except*:**
A. Anemia severe B. SLE
C. AIDS D. IE

12. **C/I to TEE are all *except*:**
A. INR of > 2
B. Undiagnosed dysphagia
C. Varices
D. Active bleeding ulcer

13. **Diagnostic criteria for CARNEY complex are all *except*:**
A. Constitutional symptom
B. Acromegaly
C. Spotty skin pigmentation
D. Cardiac myxoma

14. **Edema manifested when fluid accumulate >:**
A. 3 L B. 4 L
C. 5 L D. 6 L

15. **Brugada syndrome diagnostic:**
A. Coved ST elevation
B. Saddle ST elevation
C. T wave decrease
D. None

16. **Brugada arrhythmia present is:**
A. Monomorphic VT
B. Polymorphic VT

C. AF
D. VF

17. **Brugada ST-T change seen in:**
A. I_A B. I_B
C. I_C D. III

18. **CPVT DOC:**
A. Beta blocker
B. CCB
C. Mg

19. **Short QTc:**
A. <350 B. <320
C. <300 D. <310

20. **Lethal are all *except*:**
A. LQT3 male B. LQT3 female
C. QTc >500 D. LQT1

21. **AFl reverted to NSR least reasonable management:**
A. Long term flecainide
B. Long term amiodarone
C. Flutter ablation
D. No Rx and observation for recurrence

22. **Adenosine all *except*:**
A. Terminates AF
B. Causes APC + VPC
C. Acts on A, receptor + causes activation of K^+ channels
D. Terminates AVNRT

23. **Patient on ICD - for NSVT with provision of overdrive pacing. Patient intolerant to Flecainide + Amiodarone having multiple shocks for recurrent VT within 1 hour, 3 episodes of shock - cause, accelerated VT due to pacing management would be:**
A. Change programme and remove anti-tachycardia pacing and give shock for rapid sustained VT only
B. Remove ICD
C. I/V metoprolol
D. Start azimulide

24. **Ivabradine all *except*:**
A. Inhibits current in sinus node
B. Beautiful triad showed improved outcome in all patients of stable CAD
C. Controls sinus rate without effect on other cardiac function
D. Most benefited if HR > 70

25. **CYP 450 all *except*:**
A. Pitvastatin B. Lovastatin
C. Pravastatin D. Cerivastatin

26. **Tall R wave seen in all *except*:**
A. WPW syndrome
B. Hyperkalemia
C. Posteroinferior MI

27. **ECG (Triad) criteria of CHF all *except*:**
A. AV block B. LVH
C. QT prolonged D. Peak T wave

28. **Immunological manifestation of IE:**
A. Osler node
B. Splenomegaly
C. Petechiae
D. Splinter haemorrhage

29. **High risk (Relatively) for IE:**
A. PS
B. MR
C. Surgically corrected intracardiac shunt with minimal hemodynamic derangement
D. Degenerative valvular disease in elderly

30. **Absolute indication for surgery in IE in all *except*:**
A. Relapse of NVE after anti microbial therapy
B. Unstable prosthesis
C. Uncontrolled infection despite therapy
D. Moderate to severe CHF

31. **Dallas criteria for:**
A. Endomyocardial biopsy
B. MI
C. Myocarditis

32. **Myxoma triad are all *except*:**
A. Intracardiac obstruction
B. Pericardial effusion
C. Systemic embolization
D. Constitutional symptoms

33. **Most common tumor of cardiac valve:**
A. Fibroelastoma B. Hematoma
C. Lipoma D. Haemangioma

34. **NEF in how many percentages of patients with CHF?**
A. 50-55 B. 30-35
C. > 55 D. 40-45

35. **Most common cause HF with NEF (Normal ejection fraction):**
A. HTN B. CAD
C. Obesity D. Diabetes

36. **BNP decrease in:**
A. HF < 1 hr B. CRF
C. Acute MI D. High output HF

37. **Indication of coronary angiography in HF patients:**
A. Known CAD with prior MI
B. Age > 65 with unexplained HF
C. Positive TMT with risk factor
D. HF with severely dyskinetic myocardium

38. **Acute decomposition of HF all *except*:**
A. Excessive salt restriction
B. Worsening HTN
C. Inappropriate decrease in HF medication
D. Alcohol consumption

39. **Diastolic function depend on all *except*:**
A. Ventricular filling
B. HR
C. Active elastic property of ventricle
D. LV relaxation

40. **Peripartum cardiomyopathy diagnostic criteria are all *except*:**
A. Decrease LV systolic function
B. No prior cardiovascular disease before
C. < 2 months post delivery
D. Not known etiology

41. **Bad prognostic factor in heart failure:**
A. Hyponatremia
B. Hypokalemia
C. Hyperkalemia
D. Magnesium decrease

42. **Major Framingham criteria of HF are all *except*:**
A. PND
B. Bilateral ankle edema
C. Cardiomegaly
D. S3

43. **Major criteria of HF all *except*:**
A. Orthopnea
B. Dyspnea
C. Peripheral cyanosis
D. Excise intolerance

44. **Framingham major criteria all *except*:**
A. HR > 120
B. HJ reflux
C. Radiographic cardiomegaly

45. **Hepatojugular reflex:**
A. Decreased preload
B. Increase RV afterload
C. Imminent HF
D. Any of the above

46. **IABP major hemodynamic reflect:**
A. LV decrease preload
B. Decrease HR
C. Increase preload
D. A + B

47. **Most accurate for HF:**
A. S3
B. Rales
C. Orthopnea
D. Resting tachycardia

48. **Definition of cardiogenic shock includes all *except*:**
A. PCWP < 18
B. CI <1.8
C. BP <90
D. PCWP >18

49. **LV systolic function parameter are all *except*:**
A. Tei index
B. Cardiac index
C. Stroke volume index
D. Preload recruitable stroke volume

50. **LA enlargement radiographic sign are all *except*:**
A. LA enlargement
B. Double atrial shadow
C. Kerley B lines
D. None

51. **Aliasing seen in:**
A. Continuous doppler
B. Pulse wave

52. **Tissue doppler modification of:**
A. Pulsed doppler
B. Continuous
C. Both
D. None

53. **Doppler finding in patient of CCP seen in all *except*:**
A. Acute dilatation of heart
B. Early phase of restrictive CMP
C. Massive PTE
D. RVMI

54. **Fetal heart failure all *except*:**
A. Scalp edema
B. Bradycardia
C. Ascitis
D. Reduced fetal movements

55. **Newborn with HF all *except*:**
A. TGA
B. HLHS
C. Sustained tachycardia
D. Myocarditis

56. **High cardiac output all *except*:**
A. Fibrous dysplasia
B. Beri-Beri
C. Multiple myeloma
D. Syst. HTN

57. **Athlete's heart vs HOCM all *except*:**
A. Wall thickness > 15 mm
B. LV cavity dilatation
C. Symmetrical hypertrophy
D. Normal diastolic function

58. **PS - valvuloplasty indication:**
A. Asym with gradient > 40 mmHg
B. Asym with gradient > 50

C. Sym with valve area < 0.5 cm^2
D. This is a palliative modality

59. **Postmenopausal, T2 DM, 45 years, TG = 1620, T. cholesterol = 220, HDL = 22:**
A. Type I
B. Type III
C. Type V
D. Familial hypercholesterolemia

60. **Calcified tricuspid AS progression caused by all *except*:**
A. Age B. Size of cusps
C. Male D. LDL

61. **Subclavian artery occlusion possibility are all *except*:**
A. Aortic dissection B. Takayasu arteritis
C. Cranial arteritis D. TAO

62. **Least sensitive criteria for LVH:**
A. Romhilt
B. Coronell voltage
C. Coronell regression
D. All are same

63. **Most common condition causing HF:**
A. HTN
B. CAD
C. DM
D. Valvular heart disease

64. **Reversed differential cyanosis:**
A. Taussig bing with pulm HTN with shunt reversal
B. TGA with coarctation with PDA
C. ASD with coarctation with PDA
D. PDA with reversal

65. **Shone all *except*:**
A. Supravalvular AS
B. MS
C. Valvular AS
D. CoA

66. **Most common arrhythmia in surgically corrected TOF:**
A. AF B. VT
C. AT D. Junctional

67. **TOF in females bad prognosis in all *except*:**
A. Hypertension B. Saturation < 80%
C. HCt > 60% D. Syncope

68. **Fontan done in all *except*:**
A. TA
B. HLHS
C. Double inlet ventricle
D. AV septal defect

69. **Determinant of PHT in AV septal defect:**
A. Size of VSD
B. AV regurgitation
C. Down syndrome present or not
D. High altitude

70. **Physiology of TOF depends on:**
A. RVOT obstruction
B. Size of VSD
C. Location (site) of VSD
D. All

71. **PFO closure done in all *except*:**
A. Right to left shunt with pulm HTN
B. Right to left shunt with RV infarction with hypoxemia
C. Atrial septal aneurysm
D. Hyper coagulation state

72. **Most common coronary artery anomaly:**
A. Left coronary from right sinus
B. LCx from right sinus
C. ALCAPA
D. Right coronary artery from left sinus

73. **L-TGA characterised by:**
A. Reversal of anatomic atria
B. Systemic venous return to LA
C. Aorta from pulmonic vessel
D. Cyanosed mucous membrane

74. **BP measurement affected by all *except*:**
A. Examiner
B. Position
C. Place of measurement
D. None

75. **BP measurement all are correct *except*:**
A. Arm at the level of heart
B. 70/30 length/width
C. Deflation < 33 mm/sec
D. No talk between patient and observer

76. **World percent of death caused by CVD:**
A. 30% B. 40%
C. 20% D. 50%

77. **$S_1Q_3T_3$ found in PE in:**
A. 10% B. 15%
C. 20% D. 25%

78. **Massive PE with ECG change of RV overload pulmonary bed involved:**
A. 30% B. 70%
C. 50% D. No relation

79. **AT III binding not required for:**
A. Bivalirudin B. Fondaparinaux
C. LMWH D. Heparin

80. Patient of PE an heparin developed platelet from 2.2 lakh to 16,000 on day two. What to be done?
- **A.** Continue haparin as this is transient phenomenon
- **B.** LMWH
- **C.** Gp IIb /IIIa inhibitor
- **D.** Lepirudin

81. Patient of IWMI, JVP N, no murmur, acute breathlessness on 3rd day. Pulmonary oedema present BP <80:
- **A.** Acute MR
- **B.** V.S. rupture
- **C.** PE
- **D.** RVMI

82. B-2 lesion according to ACC:
- **A.** Degenerated vein graft to circumflex marginal
- **B.** Chronic total occlusion of RCA > 3 months
- **C.** Angulation LCx (60°) with mod. calcification
- **D.** Mid-LAD occlusion with 99% concentric with minimal calcification

83. TMT, ECG changes get obscured by all *except*:
- **A.** Digoxin
- **B.** MVP with severe anemia with ST-T changes
- **C.** Paired rhythm
- **D.** VPC with ST-T changes

84. Baye's theorem applicable in:
- **A.** TMT
- **B.** Stress echo
- **C.** Stress thallium
- **D.** All

85. Absolute contraindication of TMT are all *except*:
- **A.** AMI (< 2 days)
- **B.** USA
- **C.** Uncontrolled HTN
- **D.** Severe symptomatic AS

86. TMT-high risk criteria are all *except*:
- **A.** Symptom limited exercise < 6 MET
- **B.** Failure to increase SBP > 120 mmHg or > 10 mmHg fall
- **C.** ST increase (aVR excluded)
- **D.** Low workload angina

87. Reperfusion injury all true *except*:
- **A.** Vascular reperfusion injury
- **B.** Lethal
- **C.** Hibernation
- **D.** Reperfusion arrhythmia

88. Female with MI, all *except*, over males:
- **A.** DM
- **B.** CHF
- **C.** ST elevation
- **D.** HTN

89. Renin in HTN is increased in all *except*:
- **A.** Primary aldosteronism
- **B.** Secondary aldosteronism
- **C.** Malignant HTN
- **D.** O.C.P.

90. Least predictor of mortality:
- **A.** Angina with MR
- **B.** Angina with S3
- **C.** New onset exertional angina
- **D.** Pain > 20 min

91. Symptoms suggestive of systemic hypoperfusion:
- **A.** Abdominal bloating
- **B.** Fatigue
- **C.** Pre syncope
- **D.** Alt mental state

ANSWERS

1	A	2	D	3	C	4	A	5	B	6	B	7	A
8	D	9	C	10	A	11	C	12	C	13	A	14	A
15	A	16	B	17	C	18	A	19	B	20	B	21	D
22	A	23	A	24	B	25	C	26	B	27	A	28	A
29	C	30	A	31	A	32	B	33	A	34	A	35	A
36	A	37	B	38	A	39	C	40	C	41	A	42	B
43	C	44	A	45	C	46	C	47	A	48	A	49	A
50	D	51	B	52	A	53	B	54	B	55	A	56	D
57	A	58	B	59	A	60	B	61	D	62	A	63	B
64	A	65	A	66	A	67	A	68	D	69	C	70	A
71	A	72	A,D	73	D	74	D	75	B	76	A	77	A
78	C	79	A	80	D	81	A	82	C	83	C	84	A
85	B	86	A	87	C	88	C	89	A	90	C	91	C

44 SGPGI DECEMBER 2008

1. **CIN:**
   A. Typically occurs immediately after procedure and early peaking creatinine (T/F)
   B. Almost complete recovery within 1 week (T/F)
   C. Direct toxicity of contrast or vaso-constriction (T/F)
   D. Urine → active sediments with granular cast (T/F)
   E. Sometimes may require HD (T/F)
2. **DES T/F:**
   A. Polymer coating can be toxic (T/F)
   B. Radial force decrease after drug depletion (T/F)
   C. Paclitaxel polymerizes tubules (T/F)
   D. Sirolimus act on regulator genes in cells cycle (T/F)
   E. Allergic reaction unknown (T/F)
3. **Polymer coating in DES:**
   A. Potentially toxic (T/F)
   B. Act as reservoir (T/F)
   C. Sirolimus act later than paclitaxel on cell (T/F)
   D. Unavoidable for drug delivery (T/F)
   E. Extracelluar matrix deposition blocked (T/F)
4. **BMV:**
   A. Successful BMV > 1.5 cm^2 MVA with < 2 + MR (T/F)
   B. Dense spontaneous echo contrast is a relative contraindication (T/F)
   C. LA thrombus = relative contraindication (T/F)
   D. Metallic commissurotomy is more effective than in one balloon (T/F)
   E. Early successful BMV prevents recurrence (T/F)
5. **BAV (Balloon Aortic Valvuloplasty):**
   A. Mild AR is usual (T/F)
   B. Curative in neonatal AS (T/F)
   C. Femoral complication can occur in 1/3rd patients of congenital AS (T/F)
   D. Can be used as bridge in severe AS with CHF (T/F)
   E. Subvalvular membrane AS: BAV is better than surgery (T/F)
6. **Gp IIb-IIIa (B-2073):**
   A. Tirofiban most common cause of thrombocytopenia (T/F)
   B. Tirofiban can be used in associated renal failure (T/F)
   C. Tirofiban toxicity treatment with reduced dose by platelet transfusion (T/F)
   D. Abciximab longest t½ (T/F)
   E. Abciximab treatment is by any patient (T/F)
7. **Abciximab:**
   A. Is used for medical R_x in ACS→ (T/F)
   B. > 90 years age of patients with ACS→ should not be used (T/F)
   C. Cardiogenic shock with PIL → can be used (T/F)
   D. LMCA stenting can be used (T/F)
   E. Recent stroke → should not be used (T/F)
8. **HIT:**
   A. < 50% ↓ in platelet from baseline (T/F)
   B. < 1.5 lakh/cmm for diagnosis (T/F)
   C. LMWH can be used (T/F)
   D. After heparin use of > 4 days (T/F)
   E. All of the above (T/F)
9. **LMWH:**
   A. Anti Xa/IIa activity correlates with efficacy (T/F)
   B. Deltaparin = maximum IIa/Xa ratio (T/F)
   C. Lepirudin = reversible DTI (T/F)
   D. Dose is ↓ed in renal failure (T/F)

10. **Pacemaker:**
   A. Insulation failure ↑es impedance (T/F)
   B. Set screw loose ↓ threshold (T/F)
   C. Lead dislodgement ↓ threshold (T/F)
   D. Battery depletion ↑ impedance (T/F)
   E. Insulation failure ↓ threshold (T/F)

11. **ICD:**
   A. Maximum 24 Joule delivered (T/F)
   B. MI with EF < 30% reasonable indication (T/F)
   C. May itself cause arrhythmic storms sometimes (T/F)
   D. All long QT require ICD (T/F)
   E. Idiopathic VT with LBBB with inferior axis is an indication (T/F)

12. **Anterior wall MI, T/F:**
   A. Complete qRBBB is sensitive marker of proximal LAD before 1st septal (T/F)
   B. ST ↑aVR is specific for proximal LAD (T/F)
   C. V_5–V_6 ST ↓ is indicative of distal LAD (T/F)
   D. In proximal LAD →superior axis vector (T/F)
   E. ST ↑ in inferior leads is indicative of distal LAD (T/F)

13. **IWMI, T/F:**
   A. T ↓ in V_4R → is indicative of distal RCA (T/F)
   B. Vector directed to lead III →LCx (T/F)
   C. Ta segment in inferior lead →LCx (T/F)
   D. ST normal with T ↑ in V_4R →LCx (T/F)

14. **Echo used in all these condition as non-invasive investigation of choice. In which condition, there is a better alternative investigation for the assessment of these conditions?**
   A. MS (T/F)
   B. TGA (T/F)
   C. Cardiac tamponade (T/F)
   D. Aortic dissection (T/F)
   E. Cardiac contusion (T/F)

15. **True or False:**
   A. Myocardial stunning—normal lactate (T/F)
   B. Preserved flow—stunning (T/F)
   C. ↑ Lactate in hibernation (T/F)
   D. Ionotropes temporary ↑ed contraction in hibernation (T/F)
   E. Stunning may take 10 days to weeks to recover (T/F)

16. **CHF:**
   A. ↓β_1 and β_2 → both primarily (T/F)
   B. Spironolactone is class I indication in CHF (T/F)
   C. In neonates profuse diaphoresis is suggestive of CHF (T/F)
   D. Digitalis ↓es mortality in CHF (T/F)
   E. Cheyne-Stokes breathing is due to prolonged circulation (T/F)

17. **True or False:**
   A. LAO cranial view → visualization of cardiac chambers without superimposition (T/F)
   B. 50% diameter stenosis ↔ 70% ↓ in stenotic area (T/F)
   C. EDV normal is 150 ml/m² (T/F)
   D. LV output > RV output (T/F)
   E. Stoke volume is 75% of EDV (T/F)

18. **IABP with cardiogenic shock → drug given is:**
   A. Dopamine (T/F)
   B. Dobutamine (T/F)
   C. NE (T/F)
   D. NTG (T/F)
   E. Levosimendon (T/F)

19. **Endothelial dependent vasodilation:**
   A. NO (T/F)
   B. NTG (T/F)
   C. Verapamil (T/F)
   D. Adenosine (T/F)
   E. Serotonin (T/F)

20. **Balloon atrial septostomy:**
   A. Can be done upto 3 months of age (T/F)
   B. Umbilical vein can be used in neonates (T/F)
   C. 1/3 neonates develop femoral complication (T/F)
   D. Can be used in ASD dependent circulation (T/F)
   E. Can be used in TGA (T/F)

21. **Vasopressin v/s dopamine in cardiac arrest → vasopressin is superior because of:**
   A. Vasopressin induced bradycardia causes reflex vasoconstriction (T/F)
   B. Cerebral blood preserved (T/F)
   C. Dopamine is less chronotropic and ionotropic (T/F)
   D. Cerebral V_2→ causes vasodilation (T/F)
   E. Vasopressin causes vasoconstriction and dopamine-vasodilation (T/F)

22. **PFO → indication of surgery, all *except*:**
   A. Recurrent thromboembolism (T/F)
   B. Decompression sickness (T/F)
   C. Orthodeoxia and platypnea (T/F)
   D. Severe PAH (T/F)
   E. R → L shunt → leading to hypoxia (T/F)

23. **Phlebotomy: indication:**
   A. Non-cardiac surgery and Hct> 65% (T/F)
   B. Microcytosis with hyperviscosity→ phlebotomy with replacement isovolumic fluid is beneficial (T/F)

C. It ↓es pulmonary vascular resistance in cor pulmonale replacement is beneficial (T/F)
D. Acute cor pulmonale→ can be used (T/F)
E. Long term O_2 therapy ↑es polycythemia (T/F)

24. Carney complex:
A. Multicentric in heart (T/F)
B. Endocrine involvement (T/F)
C. Lentigenes (T/F)
D. Cardiac and mucocutaneous myxoma (T/F)
E. Cushing's (T/F)

25. Duchenne muscular dystrophy:
A. R in V_1 (T/F)
B. Q-long and deep in II, III <aVF (T/F)
C. MR is common in late stages (T/F)
D. Extensive septal fibrosis (T/F)
E. Primary ventricular arrhythmia common (T/F)

26. MD (Muscular dystrophy):
A. CHB common (T/F)
B. SVT uncommon (T/F)
C. Arrhythmia causes death in 1/3rd cases (T/F)
D. Barth syndrome is isolated noncompaction (T/F)
E. Friedreich's ataxia CMP and severe arrhythmias (T/F)

27. Marfan, all *except:*
A. Malar hypoplasia (T/F)
B. Arm span < 105% of height (T/F)
C. Pesplanus (T/F)
D. Pectush carinatum (T/F)
E. Wrist/thumb +ve (T/F)

28. Post streptococcal reactive arthritis:
A. Involves small joints of hand (T/F)
B. No response to salicylates (T/F)
C. Required secondary prophylaxis for RF (T/F)
D. Lasts longer than RF (T/F)
E. Occurs early (T/F)

29. Rheumatic fever:
A. In chorea → change in cerebellum and basal ganglia (T/F)
B. Aschoff nodules → s/o active carditis (T/F)
C. Mucoid strain more pathogenic (T/F)
D. 25 subtypes of GABHS based on M. protein (T/F)
E. Maximum recurrence in previous rheumatic fever patients (T/F)

30. Anti-arrythmic drugs:
A. IB — ↓ conduction velocity (T/F)
B. IA — ↓ conduction velocity (T/F)
C. IA — ↑ conduction velocity (T/F)
D. III — ↓ conduction velocity in AV node (T/F)
E. IB — ↑es APD (T/F)

31. Brugada:
A. RBBB with ST ↑ (T/F)
B. K^+channelopathy (T/F)
C. ICD is treatment of choice (T/F)
D. More common in Asia (T/F)
E. SCD during exercise (T/F)

32. ARVD:
A. Epsilon in early part of QRS (T/F)
B. LBBB + RAD–during VT (T/F)
C. RFA is good option of treatment (T/F)
D. CPVT having strong genetic basis (T/F)
E. Left ventricle never involved (T/F)

33. T/F:
A. PJRT–short RP (T/F)
B. VA = < 55 msec s/o AVNRT (T/F)
C. WPW with orthodromic tachycardia → IV procainamide is TOC (T/F)
D. Metoprolol metabolism is inhibited by quinidine → so it is not given in patient of AF (T/F)
E. Verapamil ↓es AV nodal ERP (T/F)
G. Postcardiac transplant heart show super-sensitivity to adenosine (T/F)

34. TDP:
A. AF is a risk factor (T/F)
B. LQT2 is most common (T/F)
C. LQT↓ death → SCD is less common in children (T/F)
D. For polymorphic VT diagnosis both variation in duration and axis of QRS is required (T/F)

35. QT dispersion < 50 ms is normal:
A. QRST angle < 60° (T/F)
B. QTC = QT (T/F)
C. QRS amplitude is more in African American (T/F)
D. QRS amplitude is more in male than female (T/F)
E. QRS amplitude is more in obese persons than thinner persons (T/F)

36. Voghun-Williams:
A. CCB = class III (T/F)
B. d-sotalol = class II (T/F)
C. Quinidine = 1B (T/F)
D. Morcizine = 1C (T/F)
E. Dofetilide = III (T/F)

37. APD:
A. Phase-4 = Na. exit (T/F)
B. Phase-2 = Slow Ca^{+2} entry (T/F)
C. Phase-1/3 = K^+ entry (T/F)

D. SAN/AVN → AP due to slow Ca^{+2} (T/F)
E. Atrial/Vent → AP due to K+ channel (T/F)

38. Cardiac tamponade without pulsus paradoxus, all *except:*
A. Rheumatic spondylitis (T/F)
B. AR (T/F)
C. Large PDA (T/F)
D. CCP (T/F)
E. OS-ASD (T/F)

39. CCP V/S RCMP → favoring CCP:
A. Prominent y descent (T/F)
B. PASP > 50 mmHg (T/F)
C. Interventricular interdependence (T/F)
D. EDP equal RV/LV (T/F)
E. Pulsus paradoxus (T/F)

40. IE prophylaxis → all *except*:
A. Ebstein'sanomoly (T/F)
B. Secondary ASD (T/F)
C. Cleft MV (T/F)
D. Muscular VSD (T/F)
E. PDA post op >3 months (T/F)

41. ABI:
A. ABI < 1 abnormal (T/F)
B. < 0.2 s/o tissue loss (T/F)
C. > 0.5 rest pain (T/F)
D. Doppler probe ideal (T/F)
E. Segmental volume plethysmography can be used for non-compressible vessel (T/F)

42. Case history:
Right arm BP - 180/90
Left arm BP - 210/100
Right ankle BP - 180/80
A. ABI = 1 (T/F)
B. PVD carries 1-2% risk of death in 5 years (T/F)
C. Normal = < 0.7 (ABI) (T/F)

43. Cardiac syndrome X:
A. Cardiac syndrome X and met. syndrome are synonymous (T/F)
B. More common in males (T/F)
C. Subendocardial ischemia is cause (T/F)
D. Can be trace of perfusion defect (T/F)
E. Does not affect prognosis in comparison to normal population (T/F)

44. Bio-prosthetic valve (BPV):
A. Aspirin is always indicated (T/F)
B. BPV less effective in CRF patients undergoing hemodialysis (T/F)
C. MV–INR = 2.5-3.5 (T/F)
D. AV–INR = 2.0-3.0 (T/F)

45. Prosthetic valve:
A. Star-Edwards less suitable for small cavity (T/F)
B. Omniscience = Ball caged valve (T/F)
C. Best hemodynamic = Bileaflet valve (T/F)
D. Ball-caged valve = Hemolysis (T/F)
E. Thromboembolism is not always due to valve (T/F)

46. Septal ablation T/F:
A. LBBB (T/F)
B. Complete RBBB (T/F)
C. Severe LV dysfunction (T/F)
D. VSD (T/F)
E. ↑ CPK-MB (T/F)

47. CFR = normal value seen in:
A. 39 years old female with strong family history of CAD (T/F)
B. 58 years male with 80% prox. LAD (T/F)
C. 75 years with HTN with LVH (T/F)
D. 60% mid LAD (T/F)
E. 75 years female with TVD (T/F)

48. MVO_2 requirement determined by:
A. Contractility (T/F)
B. RR interval (T/F)
C. EDP (T/F)
D. LV dimension/volume (T/F)
E. Diastolic relaxation (T/F)

49. CABG:
A. 7% renal dysfunction (T/F)
B. 30% AF (T/F)
C. 1st month = 10% SVG block (T/F)
D. Bilateral IMA = sternal dehiscence (T/F)
E. 2 months-1year → block of SVG due to atherosclerosis (T/F)

50. CABG:
A. LIMA can be closed or left open (T/F)
B. Minimal invasive CABG—always off pump (T/F)
C. Thickening of aorta-off pump required (T/F)
D. In patients with LV dysfunction pre-operative β-blocker should be stopped (T/F)

51. Pulsus alternans:
A. Brachial best (T/F)
B. Most common in HF with MR (T/F)
C. Due to variation in recovery of myocyte function (T/F)

52. ECG:
A. 1901—Einthoven discovered (T/F)
B. Wilson central terminal of precordial leads →–ve terminal is formed by 2 limb leads (T/F)

C. V_9-left spinal (T/F)
D. Einthoven law = I → II + III (T/F)
E. Augmented leads → –ve pole formed by other 2 limb leads (T/F)

53. Romhit testes criteria:
A. Intrinsicoid deflection—2 point (T/F)
B. LAD—3 point (T/F)
C. Digoxin with ST changes—No point (T/F)
D. Cornell criteria → Gender dependent (T/F)
E. QRS duration > 0.9 = 2 points (T/F)

54. PA:
A. > 1mm diameter = elastic art. (T/F)
B. > 1mm diameter = muscular art. (T/F)
C. After 1year PA diameter is less than 1/2 of aorta (T/F)
D. Left bronchus passes over left PA art. (T/F)
E. Normal PVR < 1–2 woods unit (T/F)

55. QRS voltage:
A. After septal activation → RV free wall next activated (T/F)
B. Intrinsicoid deflection s/o depolarization of epicardium below electrode (T/F)
C. QT indicates AP duration (T/F)

56. Coronary anomalies:
A. 2% of live birth (T/F)
B. LCx from right sinus is benign (T/F)
C. Most common anomaly is LCx from RCA (T/F)
D. Frequent cause of SCD (T/F)
E. MDCT → IOC (T/F)

57. Abciximab:
A. Shortest acting Gp IIa/IIIb (T/F)
B. Can persist upto 2 weeks in body (T/F)

58. True or False:
A. In isolated PS → RV curve is trapezoid (T/F)
B. ↑ LV dimensions ↑es afterload (T/F)
C. EDP is directly assessed by end diastolic fibre length (T/F)

59. True or False:
A. DT < 120 and EA > 1.5 → s/o severe pulmonary venous HTN (T/F)
B. Congenital MR not cor triatriatum (T/F)

45

SGPGI DECEMBER 2007

1. **Athlete's heart:**
   - **A.** Septal posterior wall ratio >1.3 : 1 (T/F)
   - **B.** ↑ LV mass (T/F)
   - **C.** LA enlargement (T/F)
   - **D.** ↑ RVEDV (T/F)
   - **E.** Paradoxical septal motion (T/F)
2. **Paradoxical S1:**
   - **A.** LV pacing (T/F)
   - **B.** LBBB (T/F)
   - **C.** LA myxoma (T/F)
   - **D.** Severe MS (T/F)
   - **E.** Ebstein's anomaly (T/F)
3. **Congenital PAV fistula:**
   - **A.** Muller maneuver more ↓ circulation (T/F)
   - **B.** Contrast echo not useful (T/F)
   - **C.** Mild dyspnea with cyanosis (T/F)
   - **D.** Lower zone affected more (T/F)
   - **E.** Cause brain abscess (T/F)
4. **Obligatory admixture in IC shunt:**
   - **A.** TA (T/F)
   - **B.** TAPVC (T/F)
   - **C.** PA (T/F)
   - **D.** CCTGA (T/F)
   - **E.** TGA (T/F)
5. **Situssolitus:**
   - **A.** Right bronchus shorter (T/F)
   - **B.** Right bronchus horizontal (T/F)
   - **C.** Right bronchus early (T/F)
   - **D.** Right hypoarterial (T/F)
   - **E.** Right epiarterial (T/F)
6. **Chronic malnutrition and starvation causes:**
   - **A.** Bradycardia with hypertension (T/F)
   - **B.** Pericardial effusion (T/F)
   - **C.** Ectopic rhythm (T/F)
   - **D.** MVP (T/F)
   - **E.** Heart block (T/F)
7. **IE with high risk:**
   - **A.** MVP with/without MR (T/F)
   - **B.** TV disease (T/F)
   - **C.** BT shunt (T/F)
   - **D.** COA (T/F)
   - **E.** ICD (T/F)
8. **Right side aortic arch associated with:**
   - **A.** CTGA (T/F)
   - **B.** Truncus arteriosus (T/F)
   - **C.** PS with VSD (T/F)
   - **D.** TAPVC (T/F)
   - **E.** Ebstein's anomaly (T/F)
9. **DM with CAD:**
   - **A.** Thrombolysis is more effective (T/F)
   - **B.** Revascularization any mode more helpful (T/F)
   - **C.** β blocker less helpful (T/F)
   - **D.** PCI vs. CABG better (T/F)
   - **E.** GPIIb/3a more beneficial (T/F)
10. **Tall U wave:**
    - **A.** Hypokalemia (T/F)
    - **B.** Hypertensive heart disease (T/F)
    - **C.** Regurgitant lesion (ch) (T/F)
    - **D.** Hypercalcemia (T/F)
    - **E.** CHB (T/F)
11. **Renovascular HTN:**
    - **A.** Aortoarteritis–Distal (T/F)
    - **B.** Atherosclerosis–Prox cm (T/F)
    - **C.** FMD most common in elderly F (T/F)
    - **D.** Atherosis> 50% cm (T/F)
    - **E.** FMD prox. (T/F)
12. **Open heart surgery:**
    - **A.** BT shunt (T/F)
    - **B.** Septectany (T/F)
    - **C.** Transmyocardial laser revascularization (T/F)

13. **Surgery in I/E:**
   A. Paravalvular abscess (T/F)
   B. ↑ Heart failure (T/F)
   C. Culture –ve/few > 10 days not response to antibiotics (T/F)
   D. Staph. excellent response to antibiotics (T/F)
   E. Relapse after in PV after successful therapy (T/F)

14. **Endothelin dysfunction True/False:**
   A. Smoking transiently ↑es contraction (T/F)
   B. NO acts by smooth muscle cell (T/F)
   C. NTG improves (T/F)

15. **AT II:**
   A. Vasoconstriction (T/F)
   B. ↑ thirst (T/F)
   C. ↓ k^+ (T/F)
   D. ↑ na^+ (T/F)
   E. ↑ Aldostern (T/F)

16. **EPS in sinus node disease:**
   A. SNRT < 550 (T/F)
   B. SACT < 150 (T/F)
   C. AH < 80 (T/F)
   D. HV < 25–55 (T/F)
   E. AAM < 25 (T/F)

17. **Antiplatal drug:**
   A. Clopidogrel reversible inhibitor (T/F)
   B. Low dose aspirin causes cox inhibition for 7 days (T/F)
   C. Aspirin + dipyradamole more effective (T/F)
   D. Mortality ↓n with aspirin is > ACE-I in acute MI (T/F)
   E. GPIIb/IIIa more effective in PCI (T/F)

18. **Cardiac tumor:**
   A. Leimyosarcoma is the most common tumor (T/F)
   B. Myxoma origin from posterior wall (T/F)
   C. Causes clubbing (T/F)
   D. Recurrence 10% (T/F)
   E. Calcification can lead to destruction of MV (T/F)

19. **Pacemaker code:**
   A. I and II sensing and pacing (T/F)
   B. IV and V programmability and anti-tachycardia pacing (T/F)
   C. In AF→ VDD is better (T/F)
   D. In bipolar cathode is distal to anode (T/F)
   E. ↑ skeletal muscle contraction ↓ output in asynchronous mode (T/F)

20. **Paradoxical septal motion:**
   A. TR (T/F)
   B. PR (T/F)
   C. Absent pericardium (T/F)
   D. Post CABG (T/F)
   E. RBBB (T/F)

21. **Example of reentra N^+ tachycardia:**
   A. Sinus tachycardia (T/F)
   B. A flutter (T/F)
   C. TDP (T/F)
   D. AIVR (T/F)
   E. WPW (T/F)

22. **Post MI–pericarditis:**
   A. Upto 5% (T/F)
   B. Not a C/I for anticoagulant (T/F)
   C. Poor prognosis (T/F)
   D. Depend on size of infarct (T/F)
   E. Incidence ↓ with thrombolysis (T/F)

23. **Drugs causing ↑ QT:**
   A. ↑ K^+ (T/F)
   B. Hypothermia (T/F)
   C. ↑ Mg has no role (T/F)
   D. Phenothiazine (T/F)
   E. Hypocalcemia (T/F)

24. **Regarding QT internal:**
   A. From start of QRS to start of T (T/F)
   B. Men > women (duration) (T/F)
   C. Can be calculated by Bazett formula (T/F)
   D. ↑ Catecholamines ↑ duration (T/F)
   E. ↑ QT related to DAD (T/F)

25. **Association of congenital syndrome:**
   A. Tuberous sclerosis-PS (T/F)
   B. NF-RAS (T/F)
   C. TAR-TOF (T/F)
   D. Noonan-HOCM (T/F)
   E. Friedreich's - Rhabdomyoma (T/F)

26. **TOF inheritance:**
   A. Retinoic acid ↑ (T/F)
   B. ↑ in diabetic mother (T/F)
   C. Associated with DiGeorge syndrome (T/F)
   D. Recurrent rates in TOF parent > TOF sibling (T/F)

27. **PS–ECG change:**
   A. Mild PS–ECG normal in 50% (T/F)
   B. Moderate PS abnormal 90% (T/F)
   C. R wave HT × 10 → PASP (T/F)
   D. Infant with PS can have LAD with LVH (T/F)
   E. Frontal plane axis > 110–150 in severe PS (T/F)

28. **Right heart endocarditis:**
   A. ↑ in elderly (T/F)

B. ↑ in drug addict (T/F)
C. Embolic rare other than lungs (T/F)
D. Unlikely with absent murmur (T/F)
E. Usually culture negative (T/F)

29. **Acute rheumatic fever T/F:**
A. Group A strept–skin infection (T/F)
B. Repeatedly throat culture rules out diagnosis (T/F)
C. Negative prophylaxis for at least 5 years (T/F)
D. Recurrence rate more in previous ARF/RHD (T/F)
E. Macrophage ↑ (+nt) in first drop from earlobe (T/F)

30. **Nitrate pharmacokinetics:**
A. Oral is more effective than sublingual (T/F)
B. Oral preparation totally degraded in liver (T/F)
C. Max oral dose 15 mg in 3-4 hours (T/F)
D. Ointment is most effective if applied on anterior (T/F)
E. Effect reversed by B_2 selective blocker (high dose) (T/F)

31. **BP measured:**
A. Adult cuff 3.5 cm by 8-9 cm (T/F)
B. Adult thigh cuff 18 cm/38 cm (T/F)
C. Deflation rate 3 mmHg/sec (T/F)
D. In infant stage IV correspond to DBP (T/F)
E. Auscultatory gap non relevant (T/F)

32. **Diuretic resistance (apparent):**
A. Loop diuretic with thiazide (T/F)
B. ↑ mg^{++} (T/F)
C. ↓ renal perfusion (T/F)
D. ↑ epinephrine (T/F)
E. Indomethacin (T/F)

33. **LV volume overload in valvular heart disease:**
A. Acute MR– ↑ stiffness (T/F)
B. Chronic AR– ↓ stiffness (T/F)
C. AS compensated– ↑ stiffness (T/F)
D. AS decompensated–stiffness ↓/↑ (T/F)
E. AS compensated volume ↓ (T/F)

34. **HF in first week:**
A. TGA (T/F)
B. AV fistula (T/F)
C. PAH (T/F)
D. Truncus arteriosus (T/F)
E. AVSD (T/F)

35. **Effect of respiration on murmur:**
A. OS of TS ↑ (T/F)
B. Hypertensive PR ↑ (T/F)
C. A2-P2-A2 shift less than P_2 (T/F)
D. Valsalva→ all murmur ↓ (T/F)
E. Presystolic murmur of Ebstein↑ in expiration (T/F)

36. **Fetal circulation:**
A. Major IVC blood goes 90se to LA (T/F)
B. RV-45% of CO (T/F)
C. IVC → descending aorta SVC→ASC (T/F)
D. Fetal pulmonary vasculature is ↑ed sensitive to hypoxia (T/F)
E. Ductus arteriosus close finally in 24 hours (T/F)

37. **Pacemaker syndrome:**
A. Vertigo, syncope common symptom (T/F)
B. VA conduction is mandatory (T/F)
C. More common with DDD (T/F)
D. Hysteresis and escape interval different (T/F)

38. **ST changes in TMT:**
A. Upsloping slow ST - is not suggest of CAD (T/F)

39. **β-blocker in CHF:**
A. Down regulation of B receptor (T/F)
B. ↓ NE return (T/F)
C. Improve baroreceptor reflex (T/F)
D. Potentiates kinin and vasodilatory action (T/F)
E. Metabolism shifts from carbohydrate to fatty acid (T/F)

40. **Framingham's:**
A. Radiograph cardiomegaly major (T/F)
B. Circulation time 25 sec (T/F)
C. LV S_4 (T/F)
D. CVP > 16 cm (T/F)
E. Two major or 1 major 2 minor (T/F)

41. **JVP:**
A. Contour of JVP and LA similar (T/F)
B. W shape in cardiac tamponade (T/F)
C. AF-A absent Y prominent (T/F)
D. Y descent in LV systole (T/F)
E. Cannon wave in APC (T/F)

42. **β-blocker as antiarrhythmia:**
A. Clsss I effect-due to anti-sympathetic effect (T/F)
B. Class III effect-due to k^+ channel (T/F)
C. ↑ AV node ERP (T/F)
D. In WPW acts on both antigrade and retrograde pathway (T/F)
E. Direct effect of catecholamines on SA node receptor (T/F)

43. **Prosthetic valve endocarditis:**
A. Thrombosis–0.1–6% (T/F)
B. Major embolism–4%/year without anti-coagulation (T/F)
C. Mortality–20–40% cate endocarditis (T/F)
D. Endocarditis–3.5% (T/F)
E. CHF–< 5% (T/F)

44. TDP:
- **A.** Triggered by short coupled beat after a pause (T/F)
- **B.** Triggered activity due to DAD (T/F)
- **C.** Giant T wave syncopal attack (T/F)
- **D.** Severe bradycardia predispose to TDA (T/F)
- **E.** Pacing prevents episode by QTC shortening (T/F)

45. Diagnostic CAG:
- **A.** Conus artery from right C.S.–/–50% (T/F)
- **B.** AV node by LCx –40–50% (T/F)
- **C.** Left ostia is lower and anterior than right ostia (T/F)
- **D.** IVUS is gold standard for thrombosis (T/F)
- **E.** Circles of vissuens–between LCx to AV node and posterior circulation (T/F)

46. BAV:
- **A.** Shock (T/F)
- **B.** Before causing major symptoms (T/F)
- **C.** Moderate LV dysfunction (T/F)
- **D.** Brut CA (T/F)
- **E.** Severity cannot be determined by provocative test (T/F)

47. Stunning and hibernation:
- **A.** Stunning ↓ coronary blood flow (T/F)
- **B.** Stunning ↑ lactate (T/F)
- **C.** Hibernation ↑ lactal (T/F)
- **D.** Hibernation spontaneous recovery (T/F)

48. Secondary HTN:
- **A.** Clonidine suppression test in 1° aldosteronism (T/F)
- **B.** Aldosterone/renin ratio < 200 →Dx of 1° aldosteronism (T/F)
- **C.** Renal vein renin ratio used to establish diagnosis of RAS (T/F)
- **D.** Adrenal vein epinephrine level > 1500 pg/ml (T/F)
- **E.** Captopril test/renin/12 (T/F)

49. Anti-arrhythmic drugs:
- **A.** Lignocaine ↑ APD (T/F)
- **B.** Adenosine ↑ APD (T/F)
- **C.** Quinidine ↑ APD (T/F)
- **D.** Phenytoin ↑ ERP (T/F)
- **E.** Disopyramide ↑ ERP (T/F)

50. Fatty acid:
- **A.** Oleic from olive oil (T/F)
- **B.** Linolic and alpha linolic are EFA (T/F)
- **C.** Coconut → linolenic (T/F)
- **D.** Tg↑ dense LDL (T/F)
- **E.** AHE step II diet, cholesterol < 100 mg/day (T/F)

46

SGPGI JUNE 2007

1. **Following trials are matched to their due:**
   A. HOT → Lipid control
   B. Life → Acute MI
   C. Rales→ HF
   D. Capture → PTCA in MI
   E. Replace → CMP

2. **Regarding embryonic development of heart:**
   A. Derived from mesoderm
   B. A 90° shift backward
   C. Atrial septum derived from dorsocephalic invagination
   D. Its rotation is a first e.g. of right and left asymmetry
   E. Sinus node derived from embryonic undiff. cell

3. **In HT:**
   A. JNC VII stage I-BP → 120-139
   B. β blockers recommended as first line therapy in NICE
   C. Guidelines changed after ALL HAT
   D. American guidelines tougher than European
   E. ABCD regimen based on renin index

4. **In HT:**
   A. Young patient < 55 years Doc → Beta blocker
   B. Elder patient > 55 years Doc → ACEI
   C. Diastolic BP increases more than systolic BP in elderly
   D. Lowering diastolic BP < 50 causes T shaped response
   E. Decreased BP decreases CVS risk

5. **In HT:**
   A. Diabetes w/o Proteinuria BP goal → less than 130/80
   B. Beta blocker causes diabetes mellitus
   C. Patient on beta blocker, not responding, add thiazide
   D. Causes micro albuminuria

6. **Regarding cholesterol:**
   A. Excess cholesterol in diet means decreased synthesis in liver
   B. Saturated fatty acid does not interfere in LDL receptor metabolism
   C. Plant sterol are significantly absorbed
   D. Plant sterol causes fat malabsorption
   E. Plant sterol competes with sterol in absorption from intestine

7. **Obesity:**
   A. Causes diastolic dysfunction
   B. Long QT interval
   C. Causes concentric hypertrophy
   D. LV systolic function is maintained even in severe cases

8. **CCTGA:**
   A. PS-15%
   B. Regurgitation-60%
   C. VSD-25%
   D. HB block-75%
   E. AV stenosis-15%

9. **Tachycardia and bradycardia:**
   A. TOF with AR B. PS
   C. Ebstein D. CTGA
   E. AS

10. **Cyanosis with holosystolic murmur:**
   A. TOF B. SV + PS
   C. DORV + PS D. Tricuspid atresia
   E. COA

11. **TOF with left ventricular apex:**
   A. Collateral circulation
   B. Severe anemia
   C. AV regurgitation
   D. Hypertension
   E. Elderly

12. **Symptomatic neonates:**
   A. Severe systemic AV fistula
   B. PDA
   C. SVT
   D. Severe PS
   E. CHB with low heart rate

13. **In precordial examination:**
A. Hyperkinetic apex indicate LV dysfunction
B. Skeletal deformity and absent left pericardium causes apex shift beyond mid clavicular line
C. Right supraclavicular pulsation caused by tortous right carotid
D. Double apex usually has 'a' wave at LV apex
E. Apex and carotid pulse felt synchronously

14. **In hypercalcemia:**
A. Upright T wave changes
B. In hypocalcemia causes long QT
C. Calcium and Mg^{+2} go hand in hand
D. Change correlate with ionic rather than nonionic
E. ST ↑ may occur in V_1–V_2

15. **Pulmonary HTN:**
A. > 50 in high altitude smaller
B. > 50% in newborns
C. 3.3 woods in high altitude is normal
D. Lung parenchyma has most extensive network of endothelium
E. Atrial

16. **Cyanosis:**
A. In cyanosis, iron deficiency cannot manifest Hct< 65%
B. Adult has cerebral arterial thrombosis
C. In Eisenmenger syndrome, pulmonary thrombus/hemorrhage in 1/3 of patient
D. In acute transplantation rejection, obliterative bronchilitis is most common
E. P_2 is due to pulmonary valve opening

17. **Radial artery catheterization:**
A. Radial artery is easily accessible and devoid of major nerves and vein in it
B. In lack patient Allen test can be done by oximetry
C. Sheath is removed immediately irrespective of Glrb/3A
D. Major complication is hemontuse and dissection
E. Dissection

18. **Catheterization:**
A. Angioberman catheter is balloon floatation catheter
B. Position of pulmonary vein in swanging identified by fluttering
C. O_2 setouch < 95% indicate pneumonitis
D. Pulmonary capillary wedge pressure 'a' and 'v' are delayed and dampened than left atrium
E. Left atrial O_2 saturation can be slightly less than PCW

19. **PVR:**
A. 10 dyne/cm/m^2
B. Measured by pressure gradient across arteriole, venule and capillary
C. PVR correspond to blood flow through pulmonary artery
D. Mean saturation valve is preferred than peak saturation
E. O_2 content is more important than O_2 saturation

20. **Catheterization:**
A. Femoral pseudo aneurysm compression of the expansile glowing mass guided by doppler ultrasound is acceptable therapy
B. Renal vein O_2 saturation is more than other vein
C. SVC > IVC O_2 sect
D. 7% step up between RA and PA significant
E. Determination of shunt can be done only if shunt flow > 20 between left and right ventricle

21. **Post surgical correction of VSD, any percutaneous intervention is indicated in:**
A. PHT
B. Volume overload
C. Dilated RA/RV
D. Q_p/Q_s <1.5 : 1
E. Residual VSD

22. **PVE:**
A. Duke criteria not applied
B. Less fever in early PVE
C. Streptococcal infection most common in late PVE
D. Early PVE in ↓ 90%
E. Flexible endoscopy and bronchoscopy–Ampi and grants 1 hour prior procedure

23. **RVMI:**
A. Normal RVEDP
B. Kussmaul syndrome common
C. Normal PA pressure
D. LA pressure not elevated
E. Arrhythmia more common in acute RVMI

24. **Jugular vein pressure:**
A. < 3 cm water normal
B. RV and LV feature most common cause
C. Steep Y descent associated with ↑CVP and RV volume overload and RV dysfunction

25. **Morphology of RV:**
A. Moderator bond
B. Crescent cavity with fine trabeculations
C. LV AV value lower than RV
D. Chorda of LV has setpal attachment

26. **IMA graft:**
A. > 90% patency at 10 years
B. Early patency < SVG
C. Early spasm is problem
D. Patency not related to recipient vessel size
E. Competitive flow cause of decreased patency

27. **Prizmetal angina:**
A. ↓ NO which is not corrected by nitrate
B. Myocardial bridge most common in Px RCA

28. **Neurocardiogenic syncope:**
A. Premonitory symptom most common than seizure
B. Fatigue more common after seizure
C. Palpitation uncommon in arrhythmia
D. Pallen less common associated with arrhythmia
E. Symptoms are more prolonged

29. **Peripartum CMP:**
A. > 30 years
B. 1st pregnancy
C. Mostly irreversible
D. Features of toxemic present
E. One month before to 5 months after delivery

30. **PCI preferred in:**
A. > 120 min
B. MI (> 3 days)
C. > 12 hours
D. In CVA
E. Class III killip

31. **Rheumatic MS:**
A. LVEDP is usually ↓ed
B. Usually associated with left ventricle hypokinesia
C. RV enlargement causes socalled silent MS
D. Murmur heard till gradient betweem LA and KV present
E. Intensity of murmur does not indicate severity

32. **Endomyocardial fibroelastosis:**
A. Within 1 year manifestation
B. ↓ LV size with features of DCMP
C. LV involved only
D. Although LV predominant involved diagnosis by RV biopsy
E. Common histopathological feature with different etiology

33. **Health care person vs lay person differences in CPR:**
A. Lay person not supposed to check pulse/resp.
B. Chest compression not allowed by lay man
C. If intubation not in hand, chest compression not done
D. CPR should be routinely measured
E. After 2 breadths, not more than 10 sec should be taken by health care person to fill pulse
F. Aortic diastolic pressure should be measured

34. **CPR:**
A. Central line is necessary
B. Peripheral line used then it take 2 min to reach central
C. Flushing necessary (5 ml fluid to be injected after bolus injection)
D. Limb elevated after injection
E. In vein collapse, interosseous access can be used but the level achieved is less than central line

35. **Coronary blood flow:**
A. Reversal flow in LV systole
B. Perfusion pressure measurement proximal to stenosis is different from distal
C. Flow pattern in right and left coronary artery are same despite high LV pressures

36. **Subclinical atherosclerosis diagnosed by:**
A. Carotid VSG
B. ABI
C. Inflammatory markers
D. EBCT
E. Ultrapast CT

37. **Multislice CT:**
A. Adventitial Cal^{+} does not cause interference
B. Coronary artery anomaly easily detected
C. Coil stent does not cause interference
D. Graft stenosis not seen

38. **Radiation:**
A. Fluoroscopy causes more radiation than cine-angiography
B. In 3 months, 3 REM permissibility
C. Cumulative effect
D. Oblique X-ray causes less exposure
E. Oblique X-ray causes more scatter

39. **Contrast induced nephropathy:**
A. Non-diabetic elderly
B. Frusemide given in treatment
C. Hydration is effective
D. NAC for prevention
E. > 24 hours → creatinine can rise

40. **In CHF:**
A. ↑ed sympathetic flow
B. β_1 receptor ↓ down regulates due to adrenergic flow
C. Adrenal-medullary suppression

41. **In Eisenmenger:**
A. Controlling uric acid decreases nephropathy
B. Glomerulonephritis caused by erythrocytes

42. **Digoxin:**
A. Not protein bound
B. Therapeutic level → 1-2 ug/ml
C. Half life—12 hours (36-48 hours)
D. Lipid insoluble
E. 30% non-reval clearance

43. **True/False:**
A. Aldactone causes ↓ed myofibrosis
B. Eplerenone causes less gynaecomastia
C. Most effective in NYHAI and II
D. Has anti-arrhythmic effect

47

SRICHITRA 2010

1. **Regarding heart failure with preserved ejection fracture – identify the true statement:**
   A. Prevalence increases with age
   B. More common in men
   C. Mortality more than with heart failure with reduced EF
   D. History of systemic hypertension is seen in 20-30%

2. **The apoprotein linked with Lp(a):**
   A. Apo B 100 B. Apo A
   C. Apo B48 D. Apo E

3. **The ideal period for collection of blood sample for estimation of lipid parameters for patient admitted 72 hours after AMI is:**
   A. On admission B. 2 weeks
   C. 8 weeks D. 16 weeks

4. **Ranolazine – Not true.**
   A. Inhibits late sodium current (I Na)
   B. Approved for use in stable angina
   C. Prolongs action potential duration
   D. Contraindicated in QT prolongation

5. **Which is a contraindication for diagnostic coronary angiography?**
   A. Recurrent admission for chest pain
   B. Morbidly obese, in whom coronary artery disease is suspected
   C. Known angina patient who survived sudden cardiac death
   D. Low probability of coronary disease with desire to establish diagnosis

6. **Diabetes is considered as a coronary artery disease equivalent because:**
   A. The modified natural history of type 2 diabetes with treatment has reduced the acute phase mortality and hence is decided by the macro vascular complications
   B. The modified natural history of type 1 diabetes with treatment has reduced the acute phase mortality and hence is decided by the macro vascular complications
   C. Natural history of patients with type 2 diabetes and an acute coronary event in non diabetic individuals is almost similar over the next 7 years
   D. All patients with diabetes will have acute coronary syndrome

7. **Which among the following is not useful in assessing cardiac dyssynchrony?**
   A. Color Doppler evaluation
   B. Pulse Doppler evaluation
   C. Tissue Doppler evaluation
   D. M-mode echocardiography

8. **Dose of tenecteplase for reperfusion therapy in acute myocardial infarction is:**
   A. Two bolus doses of 10 units
   B. Upto 100 mg as infusion over 90 minutes
   C. 30-50 mg depending on body weight
   D. 1.5 million units intravenously

9. **The wrong statement regarding Troponin I:**
   A. Found only in myocardial tissue
   B. Found in skeletal tissue during neonatal development S-1.50 Question Bank DM Cardiology Entrance Exam
   C. Not found in severely damaged skeletal muscle
   D. Heterotopic antibodies may be the cause of false positive elevations in cTnI

10. **Regarding Dressler's syndrome – Not true:**
    A. Usually occurs 1-8 weeks after MI
    B. Leukocytosis is a feature
    C. Aspirin is the drug of choice
    D. NSAIDs and steroids are helpful in refractory cases

11. **Abdominal aortic aneurysm – strongest risk factor:**
    A. Hypertension B. Age
    C. Smoking D. Gender

12. **Class I indication for valve replacement for chronic severe aortic regurgitation is:**
 A. NYHA Class II symptom, ejection fraction 55%
 B. Asymptomatic, left ventricular end-diastolic dimension >55 mm
 C. Left ventricular ejection fraction 22%
 D. Class III symptom, left ventricular ejection fraction 55%

13. **Which is false in aortic stenosis?**
 A. Angina occurs without coronary artery disease
 B. Sudden death occurs only in severe stenosis
 C. Surgery is indicated only in symptomatic patients
 D. Aortic valve area has to be reduced by 50% of normal before a measurable gradient is produced

14. **Which is true of infective endocarditis?**
 A. Most cases are attributable to an invasive procedure
 B. Erythromycin is an alternative drug in penicillin-allergic patients for prophylaxis
 C. Echocardiography is not cost-effect in patients with low pre-test probability
 D. Leukocytosis is a reliable manifestation

15. **Which of these conditions is the most likely to result is constant intensity first heart sound?**
 A. Isoarrhythmic AV dissociation
 B. Mobitzs' type 2, second degree AV block
 C. First degree heart block
 D. Infra Hisian complete heart block

16. **Systolic tenting of mitral valve with mitral regurgitation is characteristic feature of:**
 A. Mitral valve prolapse
 B. Rheumatic mitral valve disease
 C. Dilated cardiomyopathy with mitral regurgitation
 D. Chordal rupture

17. **Mitral valve closure to tricuspid valve closure interval can be negative in:**
 A. Atrial septal defect and large left to right sheet
 B. Severe form of Ebstein's anomaly of tricuspid valve
 C. Severe pulmonary hypertension
 D. Severe mitral stenosis

18. **Which among the following is not a contraindication for balloon mitral valvotomy?**
 A. Left atrial thrombus
 B. Severe mitral regurgitation
 C. Calcified mitral valve
 D. Atrial fibrillation

19. **The left atrial pressure trace and pressure likely to be seen in the presence of pathological S3:**
 A. Prominent V wave and elevated LA mean pressures
 B. Prominent V wave and normal LA mean pressures
 C. Prominent A wave and normal LA mean pressures
 D. Prominent A wave and elevated LA mean pressures

20. **Which clinical sign is suggestive of elevated pulmonary wedge pressure in mitral stenosis?**
 A. Loud S1
 B. Loud OS
 C. Short A2-OS interval
 D. Mid diastolic murmur

21. **The boundaries of 'Triangle of Koch' does not include:**
 A. Tendon of Todaro
 B. Coronary sinus
 C. Tricuspid annulus
 D. Crista terminalis

22. **Congenital heart disease not seen in rubella:**
 A. PDA
 B. Pulmonary valve stenosis
 C. ASD
 D. Coarctation of aorta

23. **Which is true of ventricular septal defects?**
 A. Aortic regurgitation occurs with large shunts
 B. Pulmonary vascular disease is generally reversible in first 12 months of life
 C. Single second sound is an indicator of large left to right shunt
 D. Large defects produce murmur on first day of life

24. **In transposition of great arteries:**
 A. Second heart splits normally in most patients
 B. Arterial switch is the best option in the presence of pulmonary obstruction
 C. Females are more commonly affected
 D. Cardiac catheterization is the investigation of choice

25. **Fontan circulation refers to:**
 A. The circulatory physiology of children born with functionally univentricular heart
 B. Artificially created circulation preventing admixture in children born with functionally univentricular hearts
 C. Both
 D. None of the above

26. **Paradoxical motion of interventricular septum is seen in:**
 A. Ventricular septal defect
 B. Mitral regurgitation
 C. Patent ductus arteriosus
 D. Total anomalous pulmonary venous connection

27. **Which of the following is not a contraindication for Fontan surgery?**
A. Pulmonary hypertension
B. Single ventricle physiology
C. Ventricular systolic dysfunction
D. Disconnected pulmonary arteries

28. **Surgical procedure of choice for a neonate with complete transposition of great arteries is:**
A. Atrial switch surgery
B. Arterial switch surgery
C. Rastelli operation
D. Fontan operation

29. **All four cardiac chambers will be volume overloaded in the following *except*:**
A. Aorta – LV tunnel
B. Complete endocardial cushion defect.
C. Gerbodies type VSD
D. Large systemic arterio-venous fistula

30. **Which of these suggest RV hypertrophy in the ECG of a neonate 7 days old?**
A. R/S ratio in V1 > 1
B. Right axis deviation
C. S waves in V_6
D. Upright T in V_1

31. **Which cardiac condition is not associated with left axis deviation?**
A. AV canal defects
B. Single ventricle
C. Tricuspid atresia
D. Ebstein's anomaly

32. **RV hypertrophy is not characteristic of:**
A. VSD with Eisenmenger
B. Simple TGA
C. Ebstein's anomaly
D. Mitral atresia

33. **Which feature is not seen in total anomalous pulmonary venous connection?**
A. Continuous murmur
B. Figure of 8 appearance on chest X-ray in infracardiac type of TAPVC
C. Right axis deviation on the ECG
D. Similar oxygen saturation in all the chambers

34. **The following statements regarding tetralogy of Fallot are true *except*:**
A. Left axis deviation on the ECG suggests associated AV canal defect
B. The RVOT gradient is proportional to the severity of the disease
C. JVP is usually not elevated in children with TOF
D. Good surgical outcome is primarily decided by the pulmonary anatomy

35. **The false statement regarding counseling parents with CHD:**
A. Recurrence risk in offsprings can be 4-10%
B. Recurrent heart defects in offsprings may be similar to parent
C. Fetal echocardiography recommended in first trimester
D. Recurrence risk can be higher if more than one relative is affected with CHD.

36. **Spot the wrong statement in transposed great arteries:**
A. TGA babies are predominantly males
B. Maternal diabetes may be associated
C. Birth weights are normal
D. Extra cardiac anomalies are frequent

37. **Regarding recording of routine normal ECG – which one is not true?**
A. The paper speed is 50 mm/sec
B. One small square represents 40 milliseconds
C. The bandwidth for ECG recording is 0.05-150 Hz for adults
D. 1 mV is depicted by 10 mm vertical displacement

38. **Ivabradine – Not true:**
A. Specific and selective inhibitor of If. channel
B. Reduces sinus rate
C. Increase time of angina
D. Side effect is negative inotropism

39. **Drugs not used for upright tilt table testing:**
A. Isoprenaline
B. NTG
C. Edrophonium hydrochloride
D. Atropine

40. **Dual chamber pacemaker (DDD) is not useful in patients with complete heart block and:**
A. Sinus node dysfunction
B. Atrial fibrillation
C. Left ventricular systolic dysfunction
D. Tricuspid regurgitation

41. **All of the following is a short RP narrow QRS tachycardia *except*:**
A. Orthodromic AVRT
B. Typical AVNRT
C. Junctional ectopic tachycardia (JET)
D. Permanent form of junctional reciprocating tachycardia (PJRT)

42. **A 25-year-old male present to OPD with a regular narrow QRS tachycardia rate 180/bpm with P waves following each QRS. During carotid sinus massage patient the tachycardia converts to**

RBBB morphology at a rate of 165/bpm. The most likely diagnosis:
A. AVNRT
B. Orthodromic AVRT using a right side bypass tract
C. VT with 1: 1 VA conduction
D. AVNRT and VT co-existing

43. **12 lead ECG has negative QRS deflections in leads 1, aVL and aVR. The frontal plane QRS axis is:**
A. Between +60 and +90
B. Between +90 and +120
C. Between +120 and +150
D. Can be anywhere between +60 and +150

44. **Which of the following is not a predictor of sudden death in an otherwise healthy individual with no structural heart disease or metabolic derangement?**
A. Markedly prolonged PR interval of 0.36 ms
B. QTc 0.245 ms
C. QTc 580 ms
D. Epsilon wave in right precordial leads

45. **Cardiac conduction defects are characteristic of:**
A. Emery-Dreifuss dystrophy
B. Fascioscapulohumeral muscular dystrophy
C. Carnitine palmitoyl transferase deficiency
D. Limb-Girdle muscular dystrophy

46. **Nitric oxide mediated vasodilatation is the property of:**
A. Carvedilol B. Bisoprolol
C. Nebivolol

47. **Hemodynamic changes in pregnancy include:**
A. Increase in systematic vascular resistance
B. Increase in cardiac output
C. Maximal increase in left atrial pressure in mitral stenosis in first trimester
D. Non-tolerance of regurgitant lesion

48. **Evaluation of a pregnant lady with hypertension and aortic coarctation should include:**
A. Chest X-ray, electrocardiogram and echo Doppler studies
B. Electrocardiogram, echo Doppler studies and CT angiogram
C. Electrocardiogram, echo Doppler studies and MR angiogram
D. Cardiac catheterization and assessment of hemodynamics systemic diseases affecting heart S-5.11

49. **The disorder where you would consider pregnancy to be contraindicated is:**
A. Mitral regurgitation
B. Aortic regurgitation
C. Atrial septal defect
D. Pulmonary arterial hypertension

50. **Most common primary cardiac tumor in infants:**
A. Rhabdomyoma
B. Fibroma
C. Myxoma
D. Pericardial teratoma

51. **After a person is infected with HBV, the first indicator is:**
A. HbsAg positivity
B. Transaminitis
C. Clinical symptoms
D. Presence of anti-HBs antibodies

52. **MRI (1.5 Tesla) is not useful in assessment of:**
A. Ventricular function
B. Severity of valve regurgitation
C. Myocardial viability
D. Extent and severity of coronary atherosclerosis

53. **Deposition of the basal ganglia contribute to the pathogenesis of hepatic encephalopathy:**
A. Magnesium B. Manganese
C. Copper D. Iron

54. **Serum amylase is elevated in all the following *except*:**
A. Acute pancreatitis
B. Acute sialadenitis
C. Intestinal perforation
D. Acute myocardial infarction

55. **Regarding pancreatic pseudocysts – not true:**
A. Develops 1-4 weeks after acute pancreatitis
B. Mostly seen in the head of pancreas
C. Second most common etiological factor is trauma
D. Serum amylase levels elevated in the majority

56. **Watermelon stomach is seen in:**
A. Sjögren's syndrome
B. Systemic sclerosis
C. Whipple's disease
D. Systemic lupus erythematosis

57. **Regarding pituitary adenoma – True statement:**
A. Hormone levels correlate with tumour size
B. All pituitary micro adenomas detected by CT need excision biopsy
C. Poly clonal in origin
D. One third are non-functioning

58. **Regarding candidal esophagitis – True:**
A. Can occur without any predisposing factors
B. Empirical therapy with amphotericin B is appropriate

C. Barium swallow is always abnormal
D. Diagnosis is confirmed by histopathological examination

59. Regarding hepatitis A virus infection – Not true:
A. Incubation period is around 4 weeks
B. It is a DNA virus
C. IgA antibodies persist indefinitely
D. Acute phase diagnosis is by IgM antibodies

60. The earlier epidemic of avian flu around the world was caused by:
A. H5N1 influenza virus
B. H2N3 influenza virus
C. H1N4 influenza virus
D. H3N1 influenza virus

61. Human cadaver pituitary as a source of growth hormone was banned because of the outbreak of:
A. Hepatitis B infection
B. Hepatitis C infection
C. Prion disease
D. HIV infection

62. The difference in insulin secretion for a given amount of glucose given orally and intravenously is known as:
A. Somogyi effect
B. Dawn effect
C. Incretin effect
D. Reactive hypoglycemia

63. Autoantibody is not involved in which of the autoimmune disease?
A. Type I diabetes mellitus
B. Hashimoto's thyroiditis
C. Insulin resistant diabetes mellitus
D. Pemphigus vulgaris

64. Which of the following are examples of genetically engineered mice?
A. Transgenic mice
B. Knock out mice
C. Hypomorphic mice
D. All of the above

65. Recently described paternal inheritance of diseases is mediated by:
A. Extra nuclear genetic material in sperm mitochondria
B. Extra nuclear genetic material in sperm centrosome
C. Extra nuclear genetic material in Golgi apparatus
D. Enzyme content of lysosome

66. The vaccines known to prevent cancers include:
A. Human papilloma virus (HPV) vaccine
B. BCG vaccine
C. Hepatitis B vaccine
D. All of the above
E. A and C
F. A and B
G. B and C

67. The following are bariatric surgical procedures *except*:
A. Calcium channel blockers
B. Beta blockers
C. Phosphodiesterase-5 inhibitors
D. Endothelin receptor blockers

68. Which among the following is not useful in treatment of pulmonary hypertension?
A. Calcium channel blockers
B. Beta blockers
C. Phosphodiesterase-5 inhibitors
D. Endothelin receptor blockers

69. Which of the following statements regarding Oseltamivir is false?
A. It is a prodrug
B. It is a hemagglutinin inhibitor
C. It is used for prophylaxis against influenza
D. Neuro psychiatric side effects can occur with therapy in pediatric population

70. Which of the following statement regarding stenotrophomonas maltophilia is false?
A. It is a nonfermentative gram negative bacteria
B. It is usually sensitive to carbapenems
C. Co-trimoxazole is an effective drug against this organism
D. Can be a colonizer in patients with cystic fibrosis

71. Which among the following bacteria cannot be detected by Gram's staining of sputum?
A. Mycoplasma pneumoniae
B. Listeria monocytogens
C. Hemophilus influenzae
D. Moraxella catarrhalis

72. Which of the following is false statement regarding Whipple's disease?
A. Presence of the bacteria outside macrophages is suggestive of active disease
B. T. Whippleii cannot be grown in culture
C. Trimethoprim / sulfamethoxazole is effective
D. PAS positive macrophage in intestinal biopsy is suggestive of the disease

73. Which of the following is not suggestive of alcoholic hepatitis?
A. Elevated gamma glutamyl transpeptidase
B. Elevated carbohydrate deficient transferrin
C. Low erythrocyte mean corpuscular volume
D. Elevated uric acid level

74. Most serious adverse effect of Herceptin therapy is:
A. Cardiomyopathy
B. Hepatic toxicity
C. Peripheral neuropathy
D. Pancreatitis

75. Which of the following first-line anti-tuberculous drugs is a prodrug?
A. Isoniazid B. Rifampicin
C. Pyrazinamide D. Ethambutol

76. Which of the following statements is incorrect regarding the use of desmopressin in the treatment of haemophilia?
A. Can cause hyponatremia
B. It can increase the factor VIII level in the recipient by 2-3 fold
C. It is recommended mainly for severe haemophilia as an adjuvant to Factor VIII infusion
D. It can precipitate thrombosis

77. Which of the antimetabolites is known to cause hearing loss as a side effect?
A. Cisplatin B. Anthracycline
C. Paclitaxel D. Irinotecan

78. Which of the transitions in cell cycle is considered as the critical regulator of cell proliferation?
A. M to G1 B. G1 to S
C. S to G2 D. G2 to M

79. Neutrophilic inclusion bodies called Dohle bodies, seen in acute infections are the remnants of:
A. Nuclear membrane
B. Endoplasmic reticulum
C. Mitochondria
D. Lysosomes

80. Which of the following is not a cause of isolated microscopic hematuria?
A. IgA nephropathy
B. Hereditary nephropathy
C. Hereditary nephritis
D. Membranoproliferative glomerulonephritis

81. The clinical manifestations of cretinism are worsened by the concomitant deficiency of:
A. Selenium B. Zinc
C. Chromium D. Magnesium

82. Nephrotoxicity is least with which of the following aminoglycosides?
A. Streptomycin
B. Gentamicin
C. Tobramycin
D. Amikacin

83. Rose spots in enteric fever are characterized by all of the following *except*:
A. Distribution predominantly in trunk and chest
B. Prevalence in only 30% of cases
C. Seen within the initial 2 weeks of illness
D. Salmonella can be cultured in less than 10% of cases only

84. The only recommended drug in the treatment of congenital syphilis in infancy:
A. Penicillin B. Cephalosporins
C. Doxycycline D. Azithromycin

85. The incubation period of chickenpox is usually between:
A. 3-8 days B. 8-13 days
C. 14-17 days D. 18-23 days

86. The most common presentation of syphilis in HIV infected patients is:
A. Lues maligna B. Condyloma lata
C. Neurosyphilis D. Unexplained fever

87. Which of the following complications of severe falciparum malaria is unusual in children as compared to adults?
A. Hypoglycemia B. Severe anemia
C. Renal failure D. Convulsions

88. The drug of choice for strongyloidosis stercoralis infection is:
A. Ivermectin B. Mebendazole
C. Albendazole D. Thiabendazole

89. Karnofsky algorithm is used in the assessment of change in tumor size in response to:
A. Chemotherapy
B. Radiotherapy
C. Surgical resection
D. All of the above

90. Primary lymphedema is known to be associated with all of the following *except*:
A. Turner's syndrome
B. Klinefelter syndrome
C. Down's syndrome
D. Yellow nail syndrome

91. Which of the following measurements of ventilator function cannot be determined by the use of spirometer alone?
A. Vital capacity
B. Functional residual capacity
C. Inspiratory capacity
D. Expiratory reserve volume

92. Hemothorax is diagnosed if hematocrit of the pleural fluid exceeds ..... that of the peripheral blood.
A. 10% B. 20%
C. 35% D. 50%

93. Which of the following ions need not be estimated to calculate anion gap?

A. Na^+ B. K^+
C. Cl^- D. HCO_3

94. Portal hypertension is said to be present when the pressure in portal vein is more than:

A. 5 mmHg B. 10 mmHg
C. 15 mmHg D. 20 mmHg

95. Which of the following immune system disorder is associated with mutations in apoptotic genes?

A. Juvenile-onset diabetes
B. Familial Mediterranean fever
C. Inflammatory bowel disease
D. Rheumatoid arthritis

96. Which of the following neoplasms is often associated with humoral hypercalcemia of malignancy?

A. Renal cell carcinoma
B. Leukaemia
C. Lymphoma
D. Multiple myeloma

97. The most common form of porphyrias is:

A. Porphyria cutanea tarda
B. Porphyria variegata
C. Acute intermittent porphyria
D. Erythropoietic porphyrias

98. Which of the following is a lower motor neuron disease with X-linked inheritance?

A. Adult Tay-Sach's disease
B. Multifocal motor neuropathy with conduction block
C. Werdnig-Hoffmann disease (Spinal muscular atrophy 1)
D. Kennedy's disease

99. Which is false in pulmonary function test?

A. Residual volume is increased in obstructive disease
B. Maximum inspiratory pressure is reduced in myasthenia gravis
C. Vital capacity is reduced in scoliosis
D. Total lung capacity is normal in parenchymal restrictive disease

ANSWERS

1	A	2	A	3	C	4	C	5	D	6	D	7	B
8	C	9	A	10	D	11	C	12	A	13	B	14	C
15	B	16	C	17	D	18	D	19	A	20	C	21	D
22	D	23	A	24	D	25	B	26	D	27	B	28	B
29	A	30	D	31	D	32	C	33	B	34	D	35	C
36	C	37	A	38	D	39	D	40	A	41	D	42	B
43	B	44	D	45	A	46	C	47	B	48	C	49	D
50	A	51	A	52	D	53	B	54	D	55	B	56	B
57	D	58	A	59	B	60	A	61	C	62	C	63	C
64	D	65		66	D	67	B	68	B	69	B	70	B
71	A	72	B	73	D	74	A	75	C	76	C	77	A
78	B	79	B	80	D	81	A	82	A	83	D	84	A
85	C	86	B	87	C	88	A	89	D	90	C	91	B
92	D	93	B	94	B	95		96	A	97	A	98	D
99	D												

48

SRICHITRA 2008

1. **Most common cause of sustained tachyarrhythmia:**
   A. Reentry **B.** ↑ EAD
   C. ↑ DAD **D.** ↑ automaticity
2. **Regarding kawasaki disease, all *except:***
   A. Occurs in children < 5 years
   B. Aneurysm develop after 6 weeks of fever onset
   C. Pathology shows acute vasculitis
   D. Small aneurysm resolves spontaneously
3. **Regarding AF, all *except:***
   A. ↑ incidence with age
   B. ↑ one AF aspirin sufficient to ↓ stroke risk
   C. Paroxysmal AF < stroke risk then persist AF
   D. AAI, DDD better than VVI for prevention
4. **True regarding anti-arrhythmic, all *except:***
   A. IV ibutilide approved for acute convention of AF
   B. Amiodarone ↓ post operative AF
   C. Digoxin loading dose to be ↓ in renal failure
   D. Sotalol should be avoided where β blocker contraindicate
5. **6 MET O_2 workload, peak O_2 consumption:**
   A. 21 **B.** 16
   C. 18 **D.** 30
6. **5L C/O with 25 mmHg aortic valve gradient AVA:**
   A. 1 **B.** 2
   C. 0.5 **D.** 3
   E. 4
7. **NYHA class-I can perform more than:**
   A. 12 **B.** 9
   C. 7 **D.** 5
8. **Positive QRS in aVR and lead-II axis:**
   A. 120-150 **B.** 150-180
   C. 0-30 **D.** 30-60
9. **V1–V9 negative terminal is:**
   A. Wilson central terminal
   B. Right arm
   C. Left arm
   D. Left leg
10. **V8 lies at:**
    A. Mid axillary line **B.** Post axillary line
    C. Post scapular line **D.** Left border spine
11. **LBBB with MI highest PPD:**
    A. 1 mm ST elevation with concordant QRS
    B. 1 mm ST depression V_1–V_2
    C. 5 mm ST ↑ in discordant QRS
    D. LAD
    E. Tall T V_5–V_C
12. **TAO, all *except:***
    A. Medium and small vessels
    B. Coronary involvement rules out diagnosis
    C. Pathology shows highly cellular thrombus occluded mostly
    D. 80% are male
13. **CT angio least useful in:**
    A. Post CABG graft evaluation
    B. Stent evaluation
    C. Pulmonary embolism
    D. Severity of obstructive CAD
14. **Regarding pericardial evaluation, all *except:***
    A. MRI better than CT for calcification
    B. CT detects thickness of 2 mm
    C. MRI 4 mm
    D. Inflammation ↑ses godolinium enhancement
15. **Tubercular pericarditis:**
    A. Caused only by lymph node rupture
    B. Evaluation of culture highly diagnostic
    C. Steroids prevent development of CCP
    D. Not treated → highly lethal
16. **Sestamibi Tc 95 mm detects:**
    A. Infarct size
    B. Hibernating myocardium
    C. Myocardium at risk

D. All
E. None

17. **Which of following in minor criteria for rheumatic fever?**
A. Prolonged PR
B. ↑ ASO filter
C. Syndertam chorea
D. Scarlet four
E. All
F. None

18. **ODD mon out:**
A. Acetazolamide B. Spironolactone
C. Thiazides D. Metalazone

19. **Tammhorsfall protein source:**
A. DCT B. PCT
C. 100P of ..... D. Mesengial cells

20. **Restrictive atrial septal defect in a cyanotic heart disease A/W pulmonary venous HTN in:**
A. Simple TGA
B. L-TGA
C. PA with infarct IVS
D. TA
E. TAPVC

21. **Ebstein's anomaly post operative issue is:**
A. CHB
B. Atrial arrhythmias
C. VT
D. Sick sinus syndrome

22. **All venous return traverses through defect:**
A. TA B. Truncus arteriosus
C. SV D. TAPVC

23. **Cyanosis seen in all *except:***
A. Truncus arteriosus
B. Mitral atresia
C. Sinus venous ASD with right PV unroofed
D. Left SVC with complete unroofed coronary sinus

24. **Gosseneck deformity on LV angiography:**
A. Complete AV septal defect
B. Truncus
C. TGA

25. **HOCM mode of inheritable:**
A. AD B. AR
C. X-linked

26. **HOCM, all *except:***
A. More gradient delays SAM
B. β-blocker ↓ses exercise induced gradient
C. LV systolic function normal
D. Children/young adults SCD common

27. **Holosystolic murmur seen typical of:**
A. Cleft mitral valve B. VSD
C. MVP

28. **Mitral valve renting:**
A. MVP B. HOCM
C. Functional MR D. PMD

29. **Cardiomyopathy caused by:**
A. Se B. Co
C. Mg D. Zn

30. **HOCM least likely:**
A. MR
B. Systolic dysfunction
C. Subaortic stenosis
D. SAM

31. **VSD true is:**
A. Incidence 8/1000
B. Shunt size determines development of AR
C. If ASD with VSD → large sized LA is seen
D. Offspring recurrence

32. **Aortic dissection, all *except*:**
A. DA most common site of intimal tear
B. Cystic medial necrosis most common cause
C. Chronic stable distal treated medically
D. Proximal dissection 50% AR

33. **Aortic dissection:**
A. W > M 2 times
B. 75% present with HT
C. Bicuspid aortic valve with AS determines severity of dissection

34. **AAA true is (Abdominal aortic aneurysm):**
A. Smoking most common cause
B. Suprarenal most common
C. Rupture more common in female
D. Rupture to peritoneum common

35. **TOF, all *except:***
A. Right AA 30%
B. RAH can be seen
C. Squalling in teenagers
D. Cour en sabot may not be seen in infancy

36. **Brugada channel:**
A. NA B. K
C. Cl D. Ca

37. **Autonomic influence suggested by all *except*:**
A. Baroreceptor sensitivity
B. QT dispersion
C. Heart rate variability
D. CBF

38. **ASD is a part of ECD:**
A. OP B. OS
C. SV D. OD

39. **Maximum vasodilatory effect on normal epicardial coronaries:**
A. Serotonin B. Nitrate
C. Adenosine D. Aminophyle
E. Dipyridamole

40. **PAH not used:**
A. Presternine B. Prostacyclin
C. Bosontan D. Sildenafil

41. **Most common primary cardiac tension in infancy:**
A. Myxoma B. Rhabdomyoma
C. Fibroma D. Angiosarcoma

42. **Regarding rhabdomyoma, all *except:***
A. Atria is most common site
B. 80% < 1 year
C. TS seen in 50%
D. Most common primary tumour of children

43. **SLE true is:**
A. Antism specific
B. 50% ANA +ve
C. Coronary ↓↓ in SLE
D. Cytotoxic drug do not ↓ development of ARF

44. **Oligopeptide reversible GP IIb/IIIa:**
A. Abciximab B. Tirotiban
C. Eptifibolide D. Prasugrel

45. **Reversible ADP platelet receptor antagonist:**
A. Prasugrel B. Congrelor
C. Clopidogrel D. Ticlopidine

46. **Thienopyridines acts on:**
A. GP-IIb/IIIa B. ADP receptor
C. Cyclooxygenase D. All

47. **Acute MI not given:**
A. IV mg
B. IV β blocker
C. IV thrombolysis
D. Angioplasty

48. **Cardiac tamponade, all *except*:**
A. Prominently descent in JVP
B. Equalization of diastolic pressure
C. Pulsus paradoxsus
D. Silent chest

49. **True pulmonary embolism *except*:**
A. ABG is very useful
B. CT is diagnostic chest
C. Proximal leg vein most common source
D. Alteplase approved by FDA for massive PE

50. **Warfarin act on, all *except* factor:**
A. 2 B. 7
C. 9 D. 11

51. **All antagonise the action of warfarin *except*:**
A. Phenytoin
B. Penicillin
C. Carbamazepine
D. Rifampicin

52. **Warfarin, all *except*:**
A. Inhibits epoxide reductase and Vitamin K reductase
B. Safe in first trimester
C. Loading dote delays attainment of INR

53. **A drug with half life of 4 hours given 4 hourly steady state plasma concentration in:**
A. 12 hours B. 8 hours
C. 20 hours D. 24 hours

54. **Drug contraindicated first trimester:**
A. Captopril B. Digitalis

55. **Earliest viral marker of hepatitis B:**
A. HBs Ag B. HBC Ag
C. Anti HBC D. HBC Ag

56. **Most severe life threatening hypocalcemia:**
A. Hypoparathyroidism
B. Vitamin D deficiency
C. ↑ dietary intake
D. Osteoblastic mets

57. **Most common cause of endogenous Cushing's:**
A. Adrenal adenoma
B. Adrenal hypoplasia
C. Pituitary adenoma
D. Ectopic ACTH syndrome

58. **Most common paraneoplastic syndrome:**
A. Acromegaly
B. Tumour related hypercalcemia
C. SIADH
D. Cushing's syndrome

59. **Graves' disease, all *except:***
A. ↑ most common of thyroidoxicosis
B. Ophthalmopathy nerve leads to visual impairment
C. Extrathyroid manifestation immunological
D. Pretibial myxodema

60. **All are causes of Rv volume overload *except*:**
A. PS B. TR
C. ASD D. TAPVC

61. **Not autoimmune:**
A. Postpartum thyroiditis
B. Graves'
C. Hashimoto
D. De quarrins

62. **Hypoglycemia ↑es, all *except:***
A. Epinephrine B. Cortisol
C. Glucagon D. GH
E. Amylin

63. **Delta cells secrete:**
A. Somatostatin B. PP
C. Amylin D. Glucagon

64. **Parkinson, all *except:***
A. Tendon jerks preserved
B. Lewy bodies are basophilic
C. Tremor frequency 4-6 Hz
D. On/off seen in levodopa

65. **Anti obesity drug not act on dopaminergic/ adrenergic/5HT:**
A. Orlistat
B. Sibutramine
C. Forfluramine
D. Dextroamphetamine

66. **Ab not act on ribosome:**
A. Macrolides B. Tetracycline
C. Daptomycin D. Linezolid
E. Aminoglycoside .

67. **Metabolic syndrome, all *except:***
A. LDL
B. HDL
C. Abdominal circumference
D. TG
E. Insulin resistance
F. IFG

68. **Most common cause of meningitis in HIV:**
A. Pneumococcus
B. Meningococcus
C. Cryptococcus
D. Coccidiodomycosis

69. **Epstein-Barr virus, all *except:***
A. Nasopharyngeal Ca
B. Kaposi
C. Burkitts
D. B-cell
E. Hodgkin's

70. **Multiple myeloma best prognostic marker:**
A. B_{12}-microglobulin
B. Serum Ca
C. HO
D. Creatinine

71. **Celiac disease, all *except:***
A. Anti endomyosal AO may be seen
B. Diet gluten is responsible
C. Duodenal biopsy normal
D. Predisposes to malignancy

72. **Pseudohyponatremia not seen in:**
A. Mannitol
B. Hyperproteinemia
C. Hypothyroidism
D. Hyperglycemia

73. **Cockcroft formula female correction factor:**
A. 0.85 B. 0.88
C. 1.17

74. **Normal conditions chemoreceptor stimulation in carotid body:**
A. O poisoning
B. Anemia
C. Met Hb
D. High altitude

75. **ARDS, all *except:***
A. ↑ permeability of capillaries
B. Septic common cause
C. Residual lung function deterioration > 50%
D. ↑ lung compliance

76. **More arterial thrombosis than venous:**
A. Antithrombin-III
B. Factor-V leiden
C. Protein deficiency
D. All
E. None

77. **Iron deficiency anemia true:**
A. ↑ TIBC
B. ↑ ferritin
C. ↓ protoporphyrin

78. **TLC-RV is:**
A. VC B. ERV
C. FRC D. TV

79. **Nephrolithiasis, all *except:***
A. Proteus cause for struvite
B. Ca PO_4/Ca oxalate more common
C. Uric acid crystal in alkaline
D. Papillary nephrocalcinosis in distal RTA

80. **Ascites in cirrhosis, all *except:***
A. SG > 1.016
B. Bilestain
C. Protein < 25
D. Mesothelial cell

81. **Bronchoalveolar lavage most common cell normally:**
A. Alveolar macrophages
B. Lymphocytes
C. PMN
D. Eosinophilia

82. **Cobalamin site of ABS:**
A. Illeum
B. Jejunum
C. Stomach

83. **All true about Ramsay Hunt syndrome *except*:**
A. Genicular ganglion involvement
B. Loss of sensation on anterior 2/3 tongue
C. Deafness common
D. Vesicular eruption on EAM
E. VZV causes it

84. **HRS, all *except:***
A. Biopsy shows eosinophilia
B. Intense intrarenal vasocervix
C. No sediment in urine
D. Urine Na < 5

85. **Eruptive xanthoma:**
A. Type-III
B. Hyperchylomicronemia
C. Hyper sitosterolemia
D. Low HDL

86. **OSA true:**
A. Polysomnography is definitive
B. All snoring ↓ investigation
C. Sleep ↓ses BP
D. Fluoxetine DOC in severe cases

87. **Enthesopathy seen in:**
A. Ankylosing spondylitis
B. RA
C. OA

88. **OA vs RA more in OA:**
A. DIP
B. Metacarpophalangeal
C. Metatarsophalangeal
D. Shoulder/Elbow

89. **All passes through lung *except*:**
A. Ascaris
B. Necator americanus
C. Trichuris trichiura
D. Strongyloides

90. **Trinucliotide repeat, all *except:***
A. Limb girdle MP
B. Friedreich's ataxia
C. Huntington's chorea
D. Fragile-X

91. **Single gene combiiation disorder mimics:**
A. Microdeletion syndrome
B. Mosaicism
C. Multigenic intervention
D. Mandesion introcitale

92. **CoA with HTN with pregnancy evaluation should include:**
A. ECG, X-ray, MRI angio
B. ECG, 2D-doppler with CT angio
C. ECG, doppler, MR angio
D. Catheterization with hemodynamics

93. **Wernicke's triad:**
A. Ataxia, ophthalmoplegia, confusion
B. Ataxia, ophthalmoplegia, seizures

94. **Reye's syndrome:**
A. Jaundice seen
B. USG shrunken liver diagnostic
C. Exclusively in < 15 years
D. Children mortality < 15%

95. **Major criteria of CHF:**
A. Hepatojugular reflux
B. Ankle edema
C. Pleural effusion
D. Hepatomegaly

96. **Vulnerable plaque suggested by all *except*:**
A. Angioscopy
B. IVUS
C. Doppler intracoronary
D Spectroscopy

97. **DTI are:**
A. Ximelagatron
B. Lepirudin
C. Bavarian
D. All of the above

ANSWERS

1	A	2	B	3	C	4	C	5	A	6		7	C
8	A	9	A	10	C	11	A	12	B	13	B	14	A
15	B	16	D	17	A	18	A	19	B	20		21	B
22	D	23	B	24	A	25	A	26	A	27	B	28	C
29	A	30	B	31	B	32	A	33	B	34	C	35	B
36	A	37	D	38	A	39		40	A	41	B	42	A
43	A	44	C	45	B	46	B	47	B	48	A	49	A
50	D	51	B	52	B	53	C	54	A	55	A	56	
57		58	A	59	B	60	A	61	D	62	E	63	A
64	B	65	A	66	C	67	A	68	C	69	B	70	A
71	C	72	C	73	A	74		75	D	76	E	77	A
78	A	79		80	B	81	B	82	C	83	E	84	A
85	B	86	A	87	A	88	A	89		90	A	91	
92	C	93	A	94		95	A	96		97	D	98	A

49

SRICHITRA 2007

CARDIOLOGY

1. **Coronary sinus:**
   A. RtHoin of SV
   B. Vein of Marshall
2. **Vent interdependence maximum in:**
   A. CCP B. RCMP
   C. C. tamponade D. RVMI
3. **Cardiac involvement least:**
   A. Beckers
   B. FSHD
   C. Emery drevifuss
   D. Myotonic
4. **BP = 110 (SBP), maximum PA pressure (syst.) in:**
   A. TR jet = 4
   B. PR jet = 4 end diastolic
   C. VSD jet = 4
5. **STEMI-least useful:**
   A. IV Mg B. IV βB
   C. Thrombolysis
6. **Cardiac tamponade least:**
   A. Parodoxes
   B. ↓ in systolic venous pressure with inspiratory
   C. Tachycardia
7. **RCM > CCP in:**
   A. PASP = 60
   B. Septal bounce
   C. Exaggerated respiratory variation
8. **McConnell sign:**
   A. Pulmmonary
9. **PTE → Thrombolysis not in:**
   A. Hypotension
   B. RVF
   C. Defect in < ½ of lobe
   D. Extensive DVT
10. **Takotsubo:**
    A. Stress induced CMP
11. **Brugada→ all *except*:**
    A. ST ↓ in anterior lead
    B. ICD treatment
12. **Best prognosis CMP:**
    A. Dilated B. Ischemic
    C. Peripartum D. HIV
    E. Doxo
13. **Radiation M. on:**
    A. Pericardium
14. **Reversal of diastolic how in both ascend and descend aorta:**
    A. ILVOT-aortic tunnel
    B. Eisenmenger with absent PV
    C. PDA with PR
    D. Large PDA with L → R
15. **To and fro:**
    A. Idiopathic pulmonary regurgitation
    B. TOF with pulmonary atresia
    C. TOF with APV
    D. VSD + AR
16. **Minimal chance of PDA:**
    A. TOF with APV
    B. TOF with pulmonary atresia
    C. PA + IVS
    D. TGA
17. **Masor likar modify all *except*:**
    A. LAD
    B. (RAD +nt)
18. **Cyanosis with equal blood across 4 valve:**
    A. PAVF
19. **No cyanosis equal blood flow across 4 valve:**
    A. RSOV → RA
    B. Gerbode
    C. PAPVC
20. **Maximum time of open valve:**
    A. MV B. TV
    C. PV D. AV

21. **RHD with mild PAH multi valve. Maximum get on doppler:**
A. AS B. MR
C. AR D. TR

22. **Holosystolic murmur:**
A. Cleft AMC
B. VSD

23. **HOCM—Post extra systolic all *except*:**
A. ↑ pulse pressure

24. **CHF with HTN not given:**
A. Diuretic B. ACEI
C. BB D. CcB

25. **Renin ↑↑ in which anti-HTN:**
A. ARB B. α-Methyl dopa
C. Clonidine D. BB

26. **Most C/E pregnancy:**
A. PAH B. CMP
C. LVOTO

27. **II, III, aVF negative of wave:**
A. Posteroseptal path

28. **Narrow QRS atrial rate < ventricular:**
A. Junctional ectopic tachycardia
B. Post fascicle reenterant VT
C. PJRT

29. **Unipolar chest leads—Neutral:**
A. Einthoven B. Wilson central
C. V_1 D Right leg electrode

30. **LDL:**
A. Friendwald
B. Friedrickser formula

31. **Neutral—CAD:**
A. Lavrie B. Stearin
C. DHA D Oleic

32. **Amyloid of heart all *except*:**
A. Secondary > primary amyloid
B. Diffuse low voltage

33. **Pulmonary art spoz = 90:**
A. D-TGA

34. **Sub-pulmonary VSD + DORV like:**
A. D-TGA + VSD

35. **Neonatal IE—most common:**
A. Staph aureus
B. E viridans
C. GNG

36. **Methicillin sensitive staph arteriosis:**
A. Nafollon + Refam + Gents
B. Ampi + Genta
C. AVnco + Refam+ Genta

37. **Least atrial—mixed venous O_2 difference:**
A. Syst. AV fistula B. TOF
C. Anemia D Low CO

38. **Paradoxical split S_2 not:**
A. MR without PAH B. LBBB
C. PDA D RV pace

39. **Acute MI → 0% of narrowing on CAG:**
A. > 90 B. 20-50
C. 50-90 D < 10%

40. **Prone for rupture all *except*:**
A. Thick fibrous cap B. Macrophage
C. Lipid rich core D. SMC in atherome

41. **IVUS:**
A. 20-40 B. 6-8
C. 2-3 D < 10

42. **TOF operated → SCD max risk:**
A. Older ages + RBBB
B. Older ages + Wide QRS > 180 ms
C. Older ages + Residual lesion
D Newborn + older age

43. **SACT how to detect by APC on EPS?**
A. Interpolation B. Collision
C. Reset

44. **DDI:**
A. Pacing, sesong, inhibita
B. Intermittent AF DDZ not useful
C. P wave V tracking in DDI

45. **Sinus rate intrinsic:**
A. Slowest rate in sleeping
B. Peak exercise rate
C. Autonomic blockade rate
D. Vagolytic rate
E. Totally denervated heart rate

46. **Left axis deviation—all *except*:**
A. Eisenmenger
B. TA
C. ECD
D. Pulmonary atresia without (IUS)

47. **Most common tumor in infant in heart:**
A. Myoxoma
B. Rhabdomycoma

48. **Tricuspid atresia with ventricular-arterial discordance—true is (Br/IV/1517):**
A. Presentation with cyanosis
B. Presentation with pulmonary HTN and HF
C. No relation with pulmonary arterial flow
D. In tricuspid atresia there is no ventriculoarterial discordance

49. **All are true *except* (B/500) Table:**
A. E-deceleration time
B. Filling rate 300 ml/sec

MEDICINE

50. **Linezolid:**
A. Thrombocytopenia
B. Laxopenia
C. Anemia
D. Hemolyse

51. **Thyroid radioactive T.T.:**
A. 1 month before T.T. → start antithyroid drug
B. 3 days before T.T. → stop
C. Young male early relapse
D. Retreatment-Extra dose after 3 months

52. **RV apical hypokinetic:**
A. PTE

53. **Li induced nephrotoxicity:**
A. Amiloride
B. Chlorpropamide

54. **AD all *except*:**
A. α→anti-trypsin B. Deficiency
C. Marfan's syndrome D. ASPKD

55. **Anion gap mettabolic acidosis all *except*:**
A. Diarrhea-Meta-analysis
B. DKA
C. Alcohol
D. Starvation

56. **Anion gap:**
A. Na – (cl + HCO_3)
B. Na + k – (a⁺ + HCO_3)
C. Na –

57. **Lepra reaction all *except*:**
A. Type IV HS reaction
B. Steroid TT
C. Thalidomide in refractory
D. Seen in borderline

58. **Syphilis—late change is:**
A. I keratitis
B. Bone changes
C. Syphilis pemphigus
D. Snuffle

59. **Tuberous sclerosis brain tumor:**
A. Meningocele
B. Acoustic nervous
C. Astrocytomesangial

60. **Fulminant hepatic failure by overdose of:**
A. Niacin/Vitamin A B. Vitamin A
C. Vitamin B_6 D. Vitamin E

61. **Folic acid daily required:**
A. 1 mg B. 50 mg
C. 50 mg D. 1 mg

62. **SLE not by:**
A. Propafenone B. Disopyramide
C. Bocainamide D. Mexicletine

63. **Polycythovera all *except*:**
A. Hypoxia +
B. EPO ↓↓
C. Myeloproliferative disorder
D. Severe pruritus may present

64. **Aldosteronism:**
A. F > M
B. Unilateral adenoma most common
C. LUV absence

65. **Isolated hemature all *except*:**
A. Thin GBM disease
B. Herenephritis
C. MPGN
D. IgA nephro

66. **Amyloid involve of spleen. Splenectomy:**
A. Thrombocytopenia
B. Factor X deficiency
C. Hemdysia

67. **Glycemic disturbance:**
A. Gati B. Oflox
C. Ciplox

68. **Sensitivity—TP:**
A. TP + FN

69. **Y. Pesting:**
A. Gram negative coccobacilli
B. Gram the coccobacilli
C. Gram negative bacilli
D. Gram positive

70. **TB pleural effusion uncommon:**
A. ↓ Sugar
B. Abundant mesothelial cells
C. AFB

71. **Klinefelter germ cell tumor:**
A. Mediastinin
B. Retroperitoneum
C. Testis

72. **Ankylosing spondylitis all *except*:**
A. B-27 essential for diagnosis
B. Bamboo spine
C. Square vertebrae
D. Osteoporosis

73. **Pulmonic (Meta) resection curative in:**
A. Colon carcinoma
B. Thyroid carcinoma
C. Nephroblastoma
D. Osteosarcoma

74. **Sarcoidosis all *except*:**
A. Lung involve common
B. Hemoptysis rare
C. BAL is normal in most cases

75. **Sarcoidosis all *except*:**
A. Hemoptysis common
B. Paratracheal LN + CN
C. Gen LAP +
D. Waldenstorm → AC sarcoidosis chain in Alport syndrome

76. **Goodpasture:**
A. Bimodal age
B. Elderly – Lung non-collagenous domain of α_3 chain of collagen IV hemorrhage common
C. Collagen α_3 chain (Ag)
D. F > M

77. **Cerebellar involve:**
A. Dimethyle mercury
B. Cd
C. Tetraethyl lead
D. AS

78. **Chikungunya incubation:**
A. 2 – 3 days B. 8 – 9 days
C. 10 – 14 days D. 2 – 3 weeks

79. **Molluscum contangiosum like lesion in HIV seen is:**
A. HSV-1 B. CMV
C. Cryptococcus

80. **Radiation to brain characteristic rate ↑:**
A. Iherimitte sign

81. **Purpura fulminans:**
A. Meningococci

82. **Chancroid DOC →:**
A. Azithoro B. PnG
C. Tetra D. AGS

83. **Phenochromocytoma all *except*:**
A. α blockade → β (sequence of drugs given)
B. P blockade → α (sequence of drugs given)

84. **Bone resorption marker all *except*:**
A. N-Telo
B. C-Telo
C. TRAP
D. Bone specific AU phosphatase

85. **Hepatitis A → DNA virus:**
A. Once jaundice → virus shedding stop
B. Asymptomatic in adult
C. Incubation = 4 months
D. Despite presence of viral shedding in focus and presence of virus in liver : infectivity dimension once jaundice appears

86. **OSA + CAD:**
A. CPAP B. Fluoxetone
C. UP3 D. Sertraline

87. **PGAII:**
A. HLA asso B. AR
C. F > M D. Graves can be present

88. **Hyper Mg^{+2}:**
A. DTR ↑↑
B. IV carcinoma in treatment
C. CRF + ↑ Mg
D. Excess Mg can be excreted by kidney

89. **→ Broad cast seen:**
A. CRF

90. **Brush border loss and flat mucosa:**
A. Whipple
B. Apeta
C. Lymphangiectasis
D. Agammaglobulinemia

91. **Anticipation seen in:**
A. Trinucleotide repeat disorder

92. **All are true about MCT:**
A. Not through lymphatic by portal vein absorption

93. **↑↑ Paternal age not a risk factor in:**
A. Marfan
B. NF
C. Achondroplasia
D. HD Huntington

94. **Classic complement mediated action only:**
A. Iglglin = alternative pathway
B. A
C. M
D. D

95. **K^+ infusion rate that can be given by both central/ peripheral vein:**
A. 20 mmo and per hour
B. 40 mmo and per hour
C. 60 mmo and per hour
D. 80 mmo and per hour

96. **Serum O_2 carry:**
A. 1 gm Hb→ 1.34 ml O_2 transport in blood 20 mc/d
B. Plasma → 0.003 ml/al/mmHg PO_2 0.3 ml/d
C. 1.34
D. 13.4 ml

97. **Saris gas is a derivative of:**
A. Organophosphorus compounds

98. **When there is no need for investigation of thrombophilic conduction:**
A. Thrombosis is less than 50 years age growth
B. Thromboembolism major surgery
C. Recurrent thromboembolism

99. **Drug that can be given safely in porphyria is:**
A. Carbamazepine B. Alcohol
C. Aspirin D. Barbiturate

ANSWERS

1	A	2	C	3	B	4		5	A	6	B	7	
8		9		10	A	11	A	12	C	13		14	
15		16		17	A	18	A	19		20	B	21	
22	B	23	A	24	D	25		26	A	27	A	28	
29	A	30		31		32	A	33	A	34	A	35	A
36	A	37	A	38	A	39	B	40	A	41	D	42	B
43		44	A	45	C	46	A	47	B	48	B	49	
50		51		52		53		54		55		56	A
57		58		59		60		61		62		63	
64		65		66	B	67	A	68		69	A	70	B
71		72		73		74	C	75	A	76	D	77	
78	A	79	C	80		81		82	A	83	B	84	D
85	C	86	A	87	B	88	A	89		90	D	91	A
92		93	D	94	C	95	B	96	B	97		98	B
99	C												

50

UPDM 2009

1. **ST elevation is not seen in:**
   A. MI
   B. Ventricular aneurysm
   C. Coronary spasm
   D. Chronic const. pericarditis

2. **Isotope for myocardial perfusion:**
   A. Xe **B.** I131
   C. Hg **D.** Th201

3. **Mortality benefit in LV dysfunction is by all drugs all *except*:**
   A. ACEI **B.** Spironolactone
   C. Digoxin **D.** Nitrates – hydralazine

4. **SCD in all *except*:**
   A. DCMP **B.** HOCM
   C. VSD **D.** Eisenmenger

5. **Raynaud's phenomenon is:**
   A. Tingling and numbness to cold exposure
   B. Paresthesia of feet
   C. Paresthesia of hand
   D. None

6. **Digitalis toxicity least manifestation:**
   A. Atrial flutter **B.** AT
   C. Junctional tachy **D.** Bigeminy

7. **Aschoff nodule in:**
   A. Rheumatic carditis
   B. SLE
   C. CKD
   D. Hepatocellular carcinoma

8. **Bisferiens pulse is seen in all *except*:**
   A. AS + AR
   B. HOCM
   C. AR
   D. Pulmonary embolism

9. **Fixed split S2 in all *except*:**
   A. ASD **B.** LBBB
   C. Pulmonary embolism **D.** PS

10. **Acute pulmonary embolism most common ECG finding is:**
    A. Sinus tachycardia
    B. S1Q3T3 pattern
    C. Right axis deviation
    D. Left axis deviation

11. **AF in MS which is not used:**
    A. I.V. lignocaine **B.** I.V. digoxin
    C. I.V. esmolol **D.** Cardioversion

12. **Med. management of TOF:**
    A. I.V. prostaglandin
    B. Nitroglycerin
    C. S/L nifedipine
    D. Digoxin

13. **True about PDA:**
    A. L to R shunt
    B. Ligation done by Ross procedure
    C. Not present at birth in all individuals
    D. Connected to RPA

14. **Embryology true is:**
    A. PDA from 6th arch
    B. Aortic arch from 5th
    C. 3rd arch disappears
    D. Pulmonary from 5th

15. **TOF true is:**
    A. Aortic override present
    B. ASD required for survival
    C. VSD - muscular
    D. Pulmonary artery – normal

16. **Kent bundle, Mahaim and Jones bundles present in:**
    A. Heart **B.** Liver
    C. Kidney **D.** Brain

17. **Programmed cardioversion on:**
    A. P **B.** Q
    C. R **D.** T1 wave

18. **Digoxin toxicity all used for treatment *except* all:**
A. Lignocaine B. Potassium
C. Fab particle D. Hemodialysis

19. **Recent treatment of digoxin toxicity:**
A. Hemodiafiltration
B. Sequential dual filtration
C. Fab Ab
D. Exchange transfusion

20. **Sensitive and specific screening test for reno-vascular HT:**
A. MRI B. CTA
C. HRCT D. Captopril test

21. **Complication of eplerenone in HTn + DM + Albumin use:**
A. Acute renal shutdown
B. Increase K^+
C. Incresae blood sugar
D. Increase Ca^+ levels

22. **Hypokalemia worsens toxicity of:**
A. Insulin B. Digoxin
C. Warfarin D. None

23. **Not used in treatment of hyperkalemia:**
A. Glucose B. Insulin
C. Digoxin D. Dialysis

24. **Routine IV fluid in neonate:**
A. 3.5 Eq Na, 5 K+, 3 mg Cl, 5 mg glucose
B. 3 mEq Na, 5 K+, 3 mg Cl, 5 mg glucose
C. 3 mEq Na, 3 mEq K+, 3 mg Cl, 5 mg glucose
D. 3 mEq Na, 2 mg K+, 3 mg Cl, 5 mg glucose

25. **Hyrgian cap is:**
A. Congenital GB anomaly
B. Normal radiologic duodenum appearance
Suprarenal gland abnormal
Kidney tumor

26. **Hepatocellular ascites diuretic of choice:**
A. Frusemide B. Spironolactone
C. HCTZ D. Mannitol

27. **Statistic test to compare more than 2 methods of choice:**
A. ANOVA B. Poor – HOC test
C. Paired *t* test D. Unpaired *t* test

28. **Not a coronary catheter:**
A. Multipurpose B. Judkins
C. Sonnes D. Gensini

29. **True:**
A. Apoptosis is reversible
B. Stunned is irreversible
C. Hibernating improved on reperfusion
D. Stunned and hibernating both irreversible

30. **Local swelling after 1 week of femoral catheterization caused by:**
A. Pseudoaneurysm
B. A-V fistula
C. Hernia
D. Infection

31. **CRP marker of:**
A. Infection
B. Albuminuria
C. Nephritic syndrome
D. Hyperthyroid

32. **Urine pH:**
A. 2 B. 5
C. 7 D. 10

33. **Increase ferritin, increase transferrin, increase total iron saturation, diagnosis:**
A. Hemochromatosis
B. IDA
C. Chronic anemia
D. CKD

34. **Most common cause of meningitis in HIV in India:**
A. Cryptococcal meningitis
B. TBM
C. PML
D. Toxoplasmosis

35. **Hemoglobinuria all *except*:**
A. Thalassemia
B. $CuSO_4$ poisoning
C. Snakebite
D. Mismatched transfusion

36. **Hb electrophoresis in sickle cell anemia all *except*:**
A. HbA B. HbA2
C. HbS D. HbF

37. **Dexa-suppression test in elderly +ve in:**
A. Schizophrenia
B. Dementia
C. Major depression
D. DI

38. **Best Ix for GFR estimation:**
A. DTPA B. DMSA
C. IVP D. MAG-3

39. **Hyokalemia with hypertension:**
A. CRF
B. Cushing's
C. DM
D. 2' hyperaldesteronism

40. **True about CMV:**
A. First done by tubbs
B. Can be done by right thoracotomy
C. Overcome by BMV

41. **APLAS all *except*:**
A. Pancytopenia
B. Rec. abortion
C. Venous thrombosis
D. PHT

42. **Metabolic alkalosis:**
A. Base excess B. Incresae K^+
C. Acid excess D. Base loss

43. **Reference of a work in a text by:**
A. Asterisk + footnote
B. Name (first and last) of author
C. Name, date and citation method
D. Entire work in parenthesis

44. **Sarcoidosis all *except*:**
A. Often cavitates
B. Tuberculin test –ve
C. Bilateral hilar lymphadenopathy
D. Spontaneously regresses commonly

45. **Regression coefficient-Y= 25 +(0.5X1 + 10X2) X1 = 10 year (duration of training), X2 = 5 (score at previous test) cal. post test score:**
A. 80 B. 50
C. 35 D. 25

46. **Pneumothorax associated with all *except*:**
A. Marfan's syndrome
B. Eosinophilic granuloma
C. ABPA
D. Assisted ventilation

47. **Kasabach Meritt's syndrome:**
A. Watery diarrhoea decrease K^+, carcinoid
B. Decrease platelet, CCF, vascular tumor
C. Wilm's, horse shoe kidney, reflux

48. **SD = 1 is equal to:**
A. 68 B. 95
C. 35 D. 99

49. **Increase S. ACE in all *except*:**
A. Sarcoidosis B. Silicosis
C. Berylliosis D. Bronchogenic Ca

50. **Central cyanosis is seen in all *except*:**
A. Chronic asthma
B. Alv. hypoventilation
C. CCF
D. Congenital PS

51. **Apple Jelly nodules in:**
A. Syphilis B. TB
C. Leprosy D. Sarcoidosis

52. **Pancytopenia + hypercellular marrow is seen in all *except*:**
A. G6PD B. Megaloblastic anemia
C. MDS D. PNH

53. **Denominator in Z score:**
A. Mean B. SD
C. Range D. Mean - observed data

54. **Oral ulcer in all skin diseases *except*:**
A. Lichen planus
B. Pemphigus
C. Lupus vulgaris
D. Erythema multiforme

55. **FBS, PPBS normal with U. sugar +++, diagnosis:**
A. Renal glycosuria
B. Alimentary glycosuria
C. Pancreatic insufficiency

56. **50th percentile of orderly arranged values?**
A. Median B. Mode
C. Mean D. Range

57. **Scleroderma all *except*:**
A. Collagen disease
B. Upper 1/3rd esophagus involved
C. G.E. reflux present
D. Dysphagia–solids + liquid

58. **Hemoptysis least in:**
A. Pneumonia B. Empyema
C. MS D. Bronchiectesis

59. **Frederick's sign:**
A. CCP
B. Cor pulmonale

60. **ASD with MS:**
A. Holt Oram
B. Lutembacher

61. **Most common type of ASD:**
A. O. primum
B. O. secundum
C. Sinus venosum

62. **M shaped 'P' wave:**
A. LAH B. RAH
C. LVH D. RVH

63. **IWMI + Cardiogenic shock most common:**
A. Cardiac rupture
B. Septal rupture
C. RVMI
D. Papillary muscle rupture

64. **True about coronary artery surgery:**
A. 1st arterial anastomosis by claude
B. PK sen – IMA to coronary artery
C. Cervical and dorsal sympathectomy for angina
D. Coronary endartectomy first performed by

65. **ECG suggestive of RCA involvement:**
A. T inversion in V4R
B. Tall R in V1
C. ST depression in V1-V3
D. ST depression in I, aVL

66. **Dyspnea with decrease cardiac output due to:**
A. Diastolic dysfunction
B. CCP
C. A.V. fistula
D. Hyperthyroidism

67. **Cardiogenic shock most likely:**
A. CO 6 L/min SvO2 85% hypovolemia
B. CO 3 L/min SvO2 65% hypovolemia
C. CO 3 L/min SvO2 65% hypervolemia
D. CO 3 L/min SvO2 25% hypovolemia

68. **Radiological sign of coarctation of aorta are all *except*:**
A. Dock's sign (Notched Rib)
B. E3 sign on barium
C. Brunevell sign
D. Rotch's sign

69. **Thermoneutral zone in newborn with appropriate for gest age:**
A. 34-37 B. 30-36
C. 28-32 D. 32-34

70. **Most useful nonspecific marker of neonatal sepsis:**
A. Total leukocyte count
B. Total neutrophil count
C. Band cell count
D. Ratio - Immature to total count

71. **NHL (Non-Hodgkin's lymphoma) true is:**
A. LDL > 500 = low tumor burden
B. CT is diagnostic
C. Prophylactic cranial irradiation
D. Prognosis depends on tumor load

72. **Not a cause of 1° AV block (Prolonged PR):**
A. Aging
B. Increase sympathetic activity
C. AR
D. Digoxin

73. **S4 is seen in all *except*:**
A. HOCM
B. Hyperthyroidism
C. AF
D. MI

74. **Most common viral sialidenitis in child not immunized with mumps vaccine:**
A. Echo virus B. CMV
C. Coxsackie virus D. Para myxo virus

75. **Septic shock, true is:**
A. Mortality 10-20%
B. Exclusively gram -ve
C. Common in elderly
D. Most common source - alimentary tract

76. **Total body water in newborn:**
A. 75 B. 90
C. 60 D. 50

77. **Barbiturate neuroprotection is in all *except*:**
A. Post cardiac arrest
B. Carotid endartectomy
C. Thoracic aneurysmectomy
D. Thiopentone with CABG

78. **Unexplained cyanotic spells in newborn:**
A. Congenital cardiac disease
B. H fistula
C. Intestinal obstruction
D. Lung cyst

79. **Blood supply of bundle of His:**
A. Interventricular branch of RCA
B. Intermittent branch of LCA
C. Left marginal
D. Right marginal

80. **Conducting system is:**
A. Connective tissue
B. Modified heart cell
C. Modified nerve
D. Smooth muscle

81. **Highest plasma proteins binding:**
A. Propranolol B. Atenolol
C. Bisoprolol D. Metoprolol

82. **Sotalol-route of elimination is:**
A. Renal B. Hepatic
C. Cytochrome D. G.I.

83. **Best management for retaining exposed pacemaker:**
A. Skin graft B. Under skin

84. **Sildenafil not used in:**
A. PPH
B. PAH 2° to COPD
C. PAH 2° to connective tissue
D. Erectile dysfunction with prior MI
E. Under muscle
F. Ethylene oxide

85. **Cardioplegia true is:**
A. Calcium used for cardioplegia
B. Neonatal heart stiffer than adult
C. Blood now used as cardioplegic solution
D. Crystalloid solution for cardioplegia

86. **Failure to thrive:**
- A. >2 SD below normal body weight
- B. < 2 SD below normal body weight
- C. <3 SD below normal body weight
- D. >3 SD below normal body weight

87. **Post cardiac surgery acceptable parameter:**
- A. UO >0.5 m/kg/hr
- B. K+ more than 5.0
- C. HR < 70/min
- D. Elective for ventilation for 24 hours

88. **Aphasia is seen in:**
- A. Left cerebral hemisphere
- B. Right cerebral hemisphere
- C. Lacunar infarct
- D. None

89. **Most common lobe in infantile lobar emphysema:**
- A. RUL
- B. RLL
- C. LUL
- D. LLL

90. **Roser's cyst:**
- A. Vitelline
- B. Urachus
- C. Intestinal duplication
- D. Meconium

91. **40 years male 65 kg, ICU, postop, 24 hours, convulsions. S.NA+ = 118, Rx.**
- A. IV 0.9% NaCl
- B. 3% NaCl
- C. Hemodialysis
- D. AVP

ANSWERS

1	D	2	D	3	C	4	C	5	A	6	A	7	A
8	D	9	C	10	A	11	A	12	C	13	A	14	A
15	A	16	A	17	C	18	D	19	C	20	A	21	B
22	B	23	C	24	C	25	A	26	B	27	A	28	D
29	C	30	A	31	A	32	C	33	A	34	B	35	A
36	A	37	C	38	A	39	D	40	C	41	A	42	A
43	C	44	A	45	A	46	C	47	B	48	A	49	D
50	C	51	B	52	A	53	B	54	C	55	A	56	A
57	B	58	B	59	A	60	B	61	B	62		63	
64		65		66		67		68		69		70	
71		72		73	C	74		75		76		77	
78		79		80		81		82		83		84	
85		86		87		88		89		90		91	

51

MISCELLANEOUS

1. **Statin therapy reduces mortality by 33% (72% vs 8%) no. of subjects needed to reduce one death:**
   A. 25
   B. 33
   C. 100
   D. Not possible to calculate

2. **HIT – all *except*:**
   A. Warfarin
   B. Lepuridin
   C. Danaperoid
   D. Argatoban

3. **Ankle Brachial Index is associated with all *except*:**
   A. <0.5 – critical limb ischemia
   B. Smoking more with PUV >Co
   C. ABI doesnot change with exercise
   D. A - Arginine endothelial

4. **AC-MI not suggested:**

	RA	RV	PCWP	CI
A.	12	30/6	10	1.8
B.	10	50/12	20	2.1
C.	6	30/6	22	2.2
D.	15	50/15	10	1.8

5. **Asympt AS with – 60 mmHg gradient at rest. TMT at 11 min. – stopped due to fatigue. Management:**
   A. CAG
   B. Med follow up
   C. AVR
   D. Ballooning

6. **Definition of MI all *except*:**
   A. SCD may be due to MI
   B. Post CABG Trop > 3 times
   C. Re-infarction trop T increases 5-7% on serial examination
   D. New RWMA

7. **UA/NSTEMI true all *except*:**
   A. Prev. CAD history and risk factors positive
   B. Red thrombi common
   C. Women NSTEM I > STEMI
   D. 10~15% CAG – normal

8. **Patient comes within 1 hour of MI; PCI > thrombolysis all *except*:**
   A. Young smoker
   B. Elderly with anterior wall MI
   C. Middle age male within wall MI with previous CABG
   D. Women with card-shock

9. **Post thrombolysis all true *except*:**
   A. High risk patient routinely transformed for PCI
   B. Clopidogrel to all patients
   C. LMWH better than UFH in case of fibrinolysis with fibrin spec.
   D. Low dose prehosp. fibrinolysis + Gp2B /3A into in high risk cases

10. **Goal of revascularization all *except*:**
    A. T1 M 1 - 3 4 not T1 M1 - 2 is goal
    B. Infarct related artery- occlusion
    C. Spontaneous late patency of IRA
    D. OAT trial benefits after 3 days

11. **Patient with MI-chest clear, hypoxia increased cause could be:**
    A. RVMI　**B.** VSD
    C. Infarct extension　**D.** MR

12. **CCU-in MI all true *except*:**
    A. LVEBP - 12-18　**B.** K - 3.8
    C. Mg - 2　**D.** H.R. - 60-80

13. **ECG - STiina VR > V_1 ST .J..I, aVL, V_4 - Vflll, aVFLAD - Artery involved is:**
    A. LMA
    B. LCX
    C. LAD after SC
    D. Post lat. branch of RCA

14. TMT - LBBB at peak exertion is S/o of:
A. TVD with left main
B. TMT should not be done
C. May not indicate ischemia
D. VT

15. Pre-operative evaluation all false *except*:
A. Pre-operative revascularization not useful
B. Pre-operative PCI not useful
C. Smoking to stop 2 weeks before
D. $FEV_1 < 1$ Lis not an absolute C.I.

16. Instead of heparin and abciximab all true *except*:
A. Decrease 30 days mortality
B. Decrease bleeding risk
C. Decrease 24 hours instent thrombosis
D. Does not cause HIT

17. All are correctly matched *except*:
A. Tadafi 1-PDEs inhibit
B. Ranolazine Ca channel blocker
C. Bilaviridin - Direct thrombin inhibitor
D. Fondapaurinaux - Anti X-a

18. Prasugrel vs clopidogrel:
A. Increase bleeding risk
B. Reduced stent thrombosis
C. Rapid onset of action
D. Reduced MI

19. In ischaemic stroke right PA is contraindicated in all *except*:
A. L.P. < 7 days
B. MI < 3 months
C. Rapidly improving symptoms
D. On oral anticoagulants

20. M.I. Kilip class III PCl not available. STK given- + patient becomes hemodynamically stable best option is:
A. Continue monitoring
B. CAG after 7 days
C. TMT > 7 days
D. Shift to PCI

21. Atorvastatin decreases in all *except*:
A. Stroke
B. New onset diab.
C. Periprocedural complications in PCI
D. Non fatal MI

22. Periprocedural complications in chronic stable angina are reduced by:
A. Aspirin
B. Clopidogrel
C. Eptafibatide
D. Atorvastatin

23. LP(a) decrease by all *except*:
A. Gemfibrozil
B. Fenofibrate
C. Atorvastatin
D. Rosuvastatin

24. Lipid disorder in DM all *except*:
A. Increase LDL
B. Increase small dense LDL
C. Increase TG
D. Decrease HDL

25. All are used in right heart catheterisation *except*:
A. NIH B. Pigtail
C. Burrnan D. GL

26. Percent of HTN in urban males in India:
A. 25.5 B. 29
C. 10.8 D. 22.2

27. Young 30 years male had severe substernal pain at night, took s/c sorbitrate from father's room had shock. ECG, echo and angio were @ cause could be:
A. Erectile dysfunction
B. Vasospastic angina
C. PVD
D. PPH

28. 2 hours after cocaine ingestion, ECG showed ST elevation in II, III, aVF and V_1 and ST depression in I, aVL. Best line of management is:
A. tPA B. CART
C. NTG D. Phentolamine

29. Patient with severe pulmonary embolism was treated with heparin. On 2nd day platelet fall from 2,20,000 to 16,000, asymptomatic, best approach is:
A. Normal reaction and is transient continue heparin
B. Lepirudin (DTI)
C. Switch to LMWH
D. E

30. Pre-hospital thrombolytic:
A. Reteplase B. Alteplase
C. STK D. Urokinase

31. LMCA on angio, best view:
A. AP caudal
B. Lateral
C. LAO cranial
D. RAO cranial

32. CT coronary angiogram true is all *except*:
A. High positive predictive value
B. High negative predictive value
C. Accurately measure bypass patency
D. Over estimates severity of stenosis

33. **MRI true are all *except:***
A. Infarct detection
B. Measure accurately Cor A. stenosis
C. RWMA
D. Viability

34. **Metabolism marker in PET:**
A. Flourine B. Oxygen
C. Rubidium D. Nitrogen

35. **In myocardial repair, cell therapy true is:**
A. GCSF may cause angina in patients of ischemic CMP
B. GCSF ± intracoronary infusion
C. Can cause restenosis
D. BMCs can cause arrhythmia

36. **All are useful in symptomatic claudication in PAD *except:***
A. Pentoxifylline B. Cilostazol
C. Statin D. CCB

37. **Myocardial preconditioning is a/wall *except:***
A. CoX-2 upregulation
B. Dow regulation in adenosine receptor
C. Increase NO synthesis

38. **Direct thrombin inhibitor are all *except:***
A. Danaparoid B. Ximelagatran
C. Bivalirudin D. Hirudin

39. **In massive acute pulmonary thromboembolism all are to be done *except:***
A. Thrombolysis
B. Thrombolysis + IVC filter
C. IVCfilter
D. Unfractionated heparin

40. **Absolute C/I of thrombolytic are all *except:***
A. Ischemic stroke < 3 hours
B. Stroke 24 hours after rTP A
C. Cerebral AV malformation
D. Closed head trauma 3 months

41. **All are true for atheroma initiation *except:***
A. Intracellular accumulation of lipid
B. Extracellular accumulation of lipid
C. Oxidation of LDL
D. None of the above

42. **All indicate oxygen demand supply ratio all *except:***
A. $ScvO_2$ B. Arterial lactate
C. CO D. O_2 consumption

43. **Most common cause of coronary ischemia:**
A. Split RCA
B. Ectopic RCA from left
C. Coronary artery fistula
D. Ectopic RCA from right

44. **SCD true are all *except:***
A. Coronary AV fistula
B. ARVD
C. PHT
D. All of the above

45. **CABG all are true *except:***
A. 10% at discharge had blocked venous graft
B. 50% block at 10 years
C. Statin decrease progression of graft disease
D. Long term anticoagulant can prevent graft failure

46. **CEA is prefered over CAS in all *except:***
A. Visible thrombus
B. Tortous aortic arch
C. Lesion, calcification
D. C/L carotid artery occlusion

47. **Torcetrapib (CETP inhibitor) is a/wall *except:***
A. Transaminase elevation
B. Macro HDL increases cholesterol influx
C. Hypertension
D. Abdominal symptoms

48. **Stent thrombosis increases in all *except:***
A. Long stent
B. Aspirin resistance
C. BMS
D. Clopidogrel non-compliance

49. **Primary PCI is preferred over thrombolysis in all *except:***
A. Presentation < 3 hours
B. Late presentation
C. Elderly
D. Post CABG

49. **Anticoagulant in stroke (mod to severe) is not given in all *except:***
A. IE with stroke
B. Moderate to severe ischemic stroke
C. Stroke within 24 hours tPA
D. None of the above

50. **Least useful in CAD:**
A. Lowfat
B. Whole diet
C Increase PUFA
D. Increase 0 mega - 3 fatty acid

51. **Drug for orthostatic hypetension:**
A. Clonidine
B. Fludrocortisone
C. Esmolol (esmolol)
D. Phenylaphrine

52. **Metabolic syndrome:**
A. Increase LDL
B. Increase triglyceride

C. Abdominal obesity
D. Increase fasting sugar

53. **CCB, β blocker, nitrates ranolazine is added:**
A. ↓ MVO_2
B. ↓ intracellular Na load
C. CPT -1 inhibitor
D. Heart metabolism FF A → glucose

54. **Late gadolinium enhancement abnormal is seen in:**
A. Myocardial scar
B. Hibernated myocardium
C. Stumed myocardium
D. Iron overload

55. **Viable myocardium – suboptimal result with:**
A. Rest redistribution thalium
B. Stress thalium
C. FDGPET
D. Rubidium tracer

56. **LMWX after PTCA after sheath removal - Hypotension, RA collapse what should not be done?**
A. Pericardiocentesis
B. BT
C. Protamin
D. I/V fluid + vasodepresser

57. **Global hypokinesia - 12 years EF 30% HR - 200/m which is not possible D. AV node a situated in the triangle of Koch?**
A. Sinus tachycardia
B. Left fascicular VT
C. AVRT
D. Ectopic atrial tachycardia

58. **Chest pain 3 days at rest ECHO/ECG normal what next?**
A. Line NSAID and send home
B. EVal. for cervical spondyl
C. TMT
D. Troponin assay

59. **Patient with hypokinesia of anterior wall, improves with low dose of dobutamine and sickens with high dose of dobutamine. Which is correct?**
A. Viable ischaemic myocardium
B. Viable non-ischaemic myocardium
C. Scarred myocardium

60. **Not used as oral antiplatlet agent:**
A. Congrillar
B. Tica grollar
C. Clopidogrel
D. Prasugrel

61. **Aortogram bilateral RAS which is not true?**
A. Urgent RAS stenting
B. ACE inhibitors are initial drug of choice
C. Can develop less involvement of pulmonary artory in India

62. **STK – 90 min patency rate:**
A. 30%
B. 50%
C. 75%
D. 20%

63. **28 weeks pregnancy with PE what is true (BP – 90 systolic)?**
A. UFH better than STK
B. D Dimer false positive pregnancy
C. CT angio not done because of fetus
D. STK is DOC

64. **Which is not a contraindication of CAG:**
A. Digoxin toxicity
B. VT
C. Hypokalemia
D. Decompensated HF

65. **Feature of complicated atheromatous plaque are all *except*:**
A. Surface erosion
B. Thrombotic deposition
C. Calcifications
D. Hematoma

66. **OCT can diagnose *all except*:**
A. Fibrous and lipid core content
B. Thrombus
C. Macrophage content
D. Fibrous cap

67. **Patient on warfarin post MVR ~ MI ~ PCI done with - Sirolimus what should be done?**
A. Warfarin+ ASP
B. Warfarin + ASP + Clopidogrel
C. Warf + ASA + Progrel
D. Warfarin

68. **Which is not a atherosclerotic marker?**
A. Calcium
B. Brachial artery flow med dilatation
C. Carotid intima media
D. Aortic velocity

69. **Which is not a athero-marker?**
A. CD40 ligand
B. Preg. induced phospholipid A
C. Placental growth factor
D. Lipid binding protein

70. **2 days after husbands death a wife with non DM/ non HTN, has STEM. In precordial leads, Trop T positive with apical hypokinesia:**
A. ACS
B. Phaeochromocytoma induced CMP
C. All of the above

71. **Right gastroepiploic artery used in:**
A. LCX B. LAD
C. OM D. PDA

72. **Regarding heart failure with preserved ejection fracture - identify the true statement:**
A. Prevalence increases with age
B. More common in men
C. Mortality more than with heart failure with reduced EF
D. History of systemic hypertension is seen in 20 - 30%

73. **The apoprotein linked with Lp(a):**
A. Apo B 100 B. Apo A
C. Apo B 48 D. Apo E

74. **The ideal period for collection of blood sample for estimation of lipid parameters for patient admitted 72 hours after AMI is:**
A. On admission B. 2 weeks
C. 8 weeks D. 16 weeks

75. **Ranolazine - Not true:**
A. Inhibits late sodium current (INa)
B. Approved for use in stable angina
C. Prolongs action potential duration
D. Contraindicated in QT prolongation

76. **Which is a contraindication for diagnostic coronary angiography?**
A. Recurrent admission for chest pain
B. Morbidly obese, in whom coronary artery disease is suspected
C. Known angina patient who survived sudden cardiac death
D. Low probability of coronary disease with desire to establish diagnosis

Diabetes is considered as a coronary artery disease equivalent because:
A. The modified natural history of type 2 diabetes with treatment has reduced the acute phase mortality and hence is decided by the macro vascular complications
B. The modified natural history of type 1 diabetes with treatment has reduced the acute phase mortality and hence is decided by the macro vascular complications
C. Natural history of patients with type 2 diabetes and an acute coronary event in non-diabetic individuals is almost similar over the next 7 years
D. All patients with diabetes will have acute coronary syndrome

78. **Which among the following is not useful in assessing cardiac dyssynchrony?**
A. Color Doppler evaluation
B. Pulse Doppler evaluation
C. Tissue Doppler evaluation
D. M-mode echocardiography

79. **Dose of tenecteplase for reperfusion therapy in acute myocardial infarction is:**
A. Two bolus doses of 10 units
B. Upto 100 mg as infusion over 90 minutes
C. 30-50 mg depending on body weight
D. 1.5 million units intravenously

80. **The wrong statement regarding Troponin I:**
A. Found only in myocardial tissue
B. Found in skeletal tissue during neonatal development
C. Not found in severely damaged skeletal muscle
D. Heterotopic antibodies may be the cause of false positive elevations in cTnl

81. **Halitosis is seen in:**
A. Nitrates B. Bad breath
C. ACCI D. Cubes

82. **1st CABG done by:**
A. Matric
B. Frosinon correct, delakey's
C. Preloid
D. Kolessor

83. **NYHA f/a I, MS, 10 years survival:**
A. 100% B. 85%
C. 50% D. 30%

84. **Coronary blood flow:**
A. 30-50 B. 50-89
C. 90-110 D. E

85. **Optimal KV in cardiac fluoroscopy:**
A. 30-50 B. 50-70
C. 70-90 D. 90-120

86. **Asian middle age male TMT positivity:**
A. 5-10% B. 10-20%
C. 2-5% D. E

87. **Female proneuparisal, 3 mm ST depression, atypical chest pain, TMT positive in:**
A. 50% B. 70%
C. 80% D. 90%

88. **LV diastolic dysfuntion earliest in AMI:**
A. > 8% B. > 15%
C. > 25% D. > 40%

89. **MI - Prexisting LBBB - 65 years male treated with TLT, Heparin, NTG - BP 140/80, HR 80/min regular - all should be given *except*:**
A. I/V metoprolol F/B oral
B. TPI
C. ACEI
D. Statins

90. Anorexia neurosa all seen *except*:
A. HTN
B. Bradycardia
C. MVP
D. Hypocholesterolemia

91. 19 years boy- F/H/0 sudden death with some heart disease-murmur SM 2/6, which increase on standing decrease on squatting, BP normal HR 64 ECG with LVH – advise:
A. Avoid competitive sports
B. Competitive sport with beta blocker
C. A void contact

92. Post C ABG not true:
A. ± decrease fibrinolysis
B. Decrease AT ill
C. Platelet dysfunction
D. Protamine reaction

93. COMET trial:
A. Carvidalol better than metoprolol
B. Metoprolol better than carvidalol
C. Equal effective
D. Inconclusive

94. False is:
A. APSAC is not more fibrin specific than STK
B. tPA and STK has equal early angio patency rate
C. tPA repeat dose can be given but not STK and APSAC
D. GISSI 2 trial show equal mortality

95. Prognosis in MI:
A. Primary VF in initial 6-12 hours worsen prognosis than 6-12 days
B. Social deprivation and depression has worse prognosis
C. Large myocardial damage has high long term mortality

96. All *except*:
A. Physiological shunting can be corrected with 100% oxygen
B. Oxymetry has less sensitive but clinical relevant in diagnosis of most case of L to R shunt
C. Blood oxygen saturation less in valves thunder which drain in to RA
D. Shunt can be detected by oxymetry, echo, MRI and radionucleide

97. True in an angina patient:
A. PTCA improve symptom and decrease mortality
B. Bypass arterial graft improve prognosis in LMCA
C. Coronary angioplasty can not be done in streched bypass
D. 90% patient are symptom free at 5 years after CABG

98. HTN decrease all *except*:
A. Isometric exercise
B. Decrease Na intake 2 gm/day
C. Calorie reduction to 1000
D. Ca + supplimentation

99. Renal athero emboli diagnosed clinically:
A. RBC cast in urine
B. Eosinophilia
C. Proteinuria massive
D. Pulmonary embolism

100. Trans fatty acid:
A. Increase CAD risk
B. Decrease HTN
C. Decrease hyperlipidemia
D. Insulin resistance

101. In ICD patient all may be harmful *except*:
A. MRI
B. RV catheterization
C. Exercise test
D. CT

102. GP II b III a inhibitors are all *except*:
A. 40-80,000 receptors/platelet
B. Full dose Abcix and ~ TPA found equal to full dose RTPA
C. Oral GP II b III a inhibitors are effective and safe

103. CRT all *except*:
A. LBBB
B. Afibrillation
C. PR> 150 mB
D. NYHA III, IV

104. IWMI most likely complication are all *except*:
A. Myocardial rupture
B. Septal rupture
C. LV thrombus
D. MR

105. TMT and BP all *except*:
A. Hypotension during rest period suggest poor prognosis
B. Diastole BP no significant change
C. Increase in systolic BP is more in young than in elderly
D. Systolic BP increase is proportionate to work load

106. TMT all *except*:
A. ASx male no risk factors, +ve TMT
B. ASx male > 2 risk factors, +ve TMT
C. ASx female false +ve TMT upto 50%
D. +ve TMT is less suggestive in females than males

107. Earliest sign of PVHT:
A. Cephalisation
B. Peribronchial cuffing
C. Perihilar cuffing
D. Kerly B lines

108. RVD @ SBP, acute pulmonary emboli, treatment of choice:
A. TLT (Thrombolytic therapy)
B. Warfarin
C. Surgery
D. LMWH

109. Drug found to have mortality benefit with thrombolytic therapy are all *except*:
A. Clopidogrel
B. Beta-blocker
C. Aspirin
D. Telmisartan

110. D-dimer all true *except*:
A. Most sensitive
B. Most specific
C. Helps in diagnosis of pulmonary embolism
D. Depends on endogenous fibrinolysis and clot formation

111. Atherosclerosis most common site:
A. MCA
B. Proximal LAD artery
C. Carotid bifurcation
D. Proximal renal artery

112. For a patient having Duke score of ←11 on TMT, five-year survival is:
A. 97% B. 72%
C. 60% D. 50%

113. Which is not a LV assist device?
A. Paracor B. Novacor
C. Abiocor D. Heart mate

114. Which is not seen with torcetrapib?
A. Abdominal pain
B. Cholesterol influx
C. Hypertension
D. Abnormal LFT

115. Which is not associated with side effect?
A. Mercury – CAD
B. Arsenic – Pericardial effusion
C. Fluorouracil – ACS
D. Granisterone – AV block

116. Drug of choice in atrial fibrillation with normal heart:
A. Fleicanide B. Sotalol
C. Amiodarone D. Quinidine

117. Which is to be used in aortic dissection?
A. Nitroprusside B. Nitroglycerine
C. IV esmolol D. Diazoxide

118. Increase BNP is not seen in:
A. Acute MR B. Cirrhosis
C. Sepsis D. RCMP

119. Intervention against which of the following risk factor has maximum benefit on CVD mortality?
A. Obesity
D. DM
C. Physical inactivity
D. LVH

120. Least effective diet approach in reducing CVD risk is:
A. Low fat diet
B. High PUFA diet
C. Whole diet approach
D. Omega 3-fatty acid

121. Treatment of pulmonary embolism is all *except*:
A. IVC filter
B. Heparin
C. Thrombolysis
D. IVC filter with thrombolysis

122. Which is true regarding HT in old age?
A. Goal BP is 160/90
B. Carcinoma intake has favourable effect on BP control
C. No role of restrictive salt in take in elderly
D. Use of anti-hypertensive causes dementia in old age

123. Which of the following virus causes myocarditis?
A. Hepatitis A B. Hepatitis B
C. Hepatitis C D. Hepatitis G

124. Which is not used in RV angiography?
A. GL catheter B. Berman catheter
C. Pig tail D. NIH

125. Coronary collaterals are not seen in:
A. Anemia B. COPD
C. LVH D. None

126. POTS syndrome, all are seen *except*:
A. Systolic BP decreases in 20 mm after 1 min
B. Standing norepinephrine > 600 pg/ml
C. Orthostatic symptoms
D. Orthostatic tachycardia

127. All are indications for mitral valve replacement in MR *except*:
A. Pulmonary HT
B. New onset AF
C. LV dysfunction
D. None

128. Bidirectional tachycardia is seen in:
A. Digoxin toxicity
B. CPVT
C. Anderson syndrome
D. All of the above

129. On lateral chest X-ray heart border is not formed by:
A. LA
B. Right atrial appendage
C. RV
D. Aorta

130. Radiofrequency ablation for atrial fibrillation does not cause:
A. Pulmonary artery stenosis
B. Pericardium effusion
C. Myocardial perforation
D. Esophageal perforation

131. Cocaine induced coronary spasm is treated by:
A. Phentolamine B. NTG
C. Amlodipine D. Adenosine

132. Best prognosis is seen in:
A. Peripartum cardiomyopathy
B. Alcoholic cardiomyopathy
C. Amyloid cardiomyopathy
D. HIV cardiomyopathy

133. In an asymptomatic patient having VSD Eisenmenger syndrome with a hematocrit of 68%, the best management would be:
A. Phlebotomy
B. Immediate surgery
C. Nothing to be done at present
D. Call the patient after one month

134. Regular canon waves are seen in all *except*:
A. CHB
B. Ventricular tachycardia
C. AVNRT
D. AVRT

135. CHB is not seen in:
A. Lithium toxicity
B. Hyper magnesemia
C. Yellow oleander poisoning
D. Hypokalemia

136. All are reperfusion induced arrhythmia *except*:
A. Primary VF
B. NSVT
C. Slow junctional rhythm
D. Multiple VPC

137. In a diabetic patient having NSTEMI which of the following is irrational combination?
A. Bivaluridin + Fondaparinaux
B. Prasugrel + Eptifibatide
C. Enoxaparin + Abciximab
D. Clopidogrel + Eptifibatide

138. Which is not used in PTMC?
A. Fogarty balloon
B. Inoue balloon
C. Mullins sheath
D. Brokenbrough needle

139. 'No added' salt diet refers to a daily salt intake of:
A. 0.5 to 1 gm/day
B. 3-4 gm/day
C. 6-8 gm/day
D. 8-10 gm/day

140. In a patient who develops ST segment elevation in inferior leads during TMT, all are true *except*:
A. Ventricular aneurysm
B. MI
C. Coronary spasm
D. RCA dominance

141. Which shunt is unlikely associated with continuous murmur?
A. Modified BT
B. Glenn shunt
C. Potts shunt
D. Waterston shunt

142. Maximum oxygen saturation in a fetus is seen in:
A. Ductus venosus
B. Ductus arteriosus
C. Ascending aorta
D. Descending aorta

143. Oasis 6 trial involved patients with:
A. Unstable angina
B. STEMI
C. CHF
D. VT

144. Counter clockwise rotation in ECG is seen in all *except*:
A. ECD
B. DORV
C. Tricuspid atresia
D. TOF with absent pulmonary valve

145. Narrow vascular pedicle in chest X-ray is seen in all *except*:
A. TGA
B. Truncus arteriosus
C. Pulmonary atresia
D. Ebstein's anomaly

146. Earliest marker of myocardial ischemia:
A. ProBNP
B. Ischemia modified albumin
C. Choline
D. Myoglobin

147. Mexilitine can be used in:
A. LQT_1 B. LQT_2
C. LQT_3 D. LQT_7

148. AF is associated with:
A. LQT_1 B. LQT_2
C. LQT_3 D. LQT_4

149. Nocturnal angina may occur in all *except*:
A. Severe AR
B. Severe MR
C. Left main disease
D. Prinzmetal's angina

150. Bicuspid aortic valve, β blocker to be given when aortic root diameter is:
A. >3 cm B. >4 cm
C. >4.5 cm D. >5.5 cms

151. Infant with mild cyansis, CHF, with a collapsing pulse with single S_2 with decrescendo early diastolic murmur, likely diagnosis is:
A. VSD with severe AR
B. TOF with PA with collaterals
C. Ruptured sinus of valsalva
D. Truncus arteriosus

152. Systolic coronary perfusion occurs in:
A. HOCM
B. Supravalvular AS
C. IABP
D. ALCAPA

153. Primary PCI trials of DES vs BMS are all *except*:
A. Typhoon B. React
C. Passion D. Sesami

154. Most common pathological changes in MS:
A. Commissural fusion
B. Cuspal fusion
C. Chordal fusion
D. Papillary muscle fusion

155. Pulmonary valve dysplasia is characterized by all *except*:
A. 3 cusps
B. Family history
C. Commissural fusion
D. No pulmonary artery dilatation

156. TOF with pulmonary atresia, which subset has best prognosis:
A. Confluent and normally distributed PA
B. Confluent but abnormally distributed PA
C. Non confluent pulmonary artery
D. Confluent pulmonary artery with collaterals from right subclavian

157. β blockers have underperformed in recent hypertension trials because of:
A. ↓ contractility
B. Reflected waves
C. Diabetes
D. Impotency

158. Most likely ECG finding in TGA at birth is:
A. RAD +RVH B. Normal
C. LAD+RVH D. RAD+LVH

159. Characteristic ECG changes after alcohol septal ablation in HOCM:
A. LBBB
B. ↑ PR
C. LVH regression
D. RBBB

160. Criss-cross heart means:
A. AV inflow tracts are at 90°
B. Great arteries at 90°
C. RVOT and LVOT at 90°
D. Aortic and mitral valve at 90°

161. Most important contraindication of Fontan principle:
A. LV dysfunction B. MR
C. Severe PAH D. AF

162. All are echo indicators of CRT *except*:
A. Septal posterior wall delay >130 msec
B. RV-LV interventricular delay >40 msec
C. Aortic pre ejection time > 40 msec
D. Dyssynchrony index > 32 msec

163. Prognostic determinant of C-TGA are all *except*:
A. L to R shunt
B. AV block
C. AV valve regurgitation
D. SaO_2 <85%

164. In CoA, ECG showing deep T wave inversion in left precardial leads is suggestive of:
A. Gradient >40 mmHg
B. 100% occlusion
C. Bicuspid AoV with AS
D. Berry aneurysm

165. All can be seen in ECG of ALCAPA *except*:
A. Q in 1 aV_l and V_6
B. LVH
C. LAE
D. RAD

166. Brugada criteria of VT diagnosis include all *except*:
A. RS complexus
B. QRS >P
C. R to S nadir >70msec
D. Fusion beats

167. In Fontan classification of PAD, nocturnal pain is a feature of:
A. Stage IIa B. Stage IIb
C. Stage III D. Stage IV

168. Best imaging test for pulmonary embolism in hospitalized patients is:
A. Spiral CT
B. MRI
C. Ventilation perfusion scan
D. Echocardiography

169. Risk of venous thromboembolism is increased by OCP use in patients with factor V Leiden mutation by:
A. 2 times B. 5 times
C. 10 times D. 20 times

170. Marked increased in inspiratory SVC systolic forward flow velocity occur in:
A. CP
B. COPD
C. Both A+B
D. None of the above

171. Carcinoid syndrome like valvulopathy is seen with:
A. Cobalt B. Cisplatin
C. Mitomycin D. Pergolide

172. P mitrate for LA enlargement has:
A. High sensitivity, low specificity
B. High specificity, low sensitivity
C. High sensitivity, high specificity
D. Low specificity, low sensitivity

173. Combination of relatively low limb voltage and prominent precordial voltage seen in:
A. DCMP
B. HOCM
C. RCMP
D. Adrenal insufficiency

174. Absolute contraindication to exercise testing include all *except*:
A. Acute MI (3-5 days)
B. Acute pericarditis
C. High risk unstable angina
D. Pulmonary embolism

175. Renovascular hypertension, true is:
A. Serum K^+ - low
B. Serum Na^+ - high
C. Family history of hypertension
D. Low plasma rennin activity

176. For sulfonamide sensitive patients, diuretic of choice is:
A. Indapamide
B. Ethacrynic acid
C. Hydrochlorthiazide
D. Spironolactone

177. Dietary sodium restriction, decreases the effectiveness of:
A. Resserpine B. Amlodipine
C. Aliskiren D. Hydralazine

178. Uricosuric ARB is:
A. Losartan B. Telmisartan
C. Candesartan D. Irbesartan

179. Drug used for prehypertension in TROPHY trial:
A. Telmisartan
B. Candesartan
C. Losartan
D. Hydrochlorthiazide

180. In TIMI risk score of STEMI, 2 points given to all *except*:
A. Systolic BP <100 mmHg
B. Age 65-74 years
C. HR > 100 bpm
D. Killip class II

181. Fondaparinux, true is:
A. ↑ catheter thrombosis
B. Oasis - 6 trial – NSTEMI
C. Oasis - 5 trial – STEMI
D. Direct thrombin inhibitor

182. After successful thrombolysis, >50% residual stenosis remains in:
A. 30% B. 50%
C. 70% D. 90%

183. Reocclusion rate after successful thrombolysis is:
A. 5-10% B. 15-20%
C. 25-30% D. 35-40%

184. Risk of intracranial haemorrhage with PCI is:
A. 0.01% B. 0.05%
C. 0.1% D. 0.5%

185. Fexofenadine is used for:
A. Brugada syndrome
B. LQT2
C. LQT3
D. LQT7

186. Drug of choice for sitosterolemia:
A. Niacin B. Ezetimibe
C. Atorvastatin D. Fenofibrate

187. Brugada syndrome, treatment include all *except*:
A. Quinidine B. Tedisamil
C. Cilostazol D. Mexiletine

188. Most common symptom of pericardial malignancy is:
A. Dyspnea
B. Non-productive cough
C. Orthopnea
D. Unexplained chest pain

189. After PTCA and stenting, reendothelialization occurs in 4-6 weeks. What is the source of endothelial cells?
A. Media
B. Intima
C. Adjunct endothelium
D. Circulating blood and adjunct endothelium

190. Commotio cordis:
A. Is concussion of heart caused by blunt trauma
B. Usually occurs in young people
C. Death is usually uncommon
D. All of the above

191. Patent foramen ovale is found in how much percentage of cases?
A. 5% B. 15%
C. 25% D. 35%

192. Osmotic diuresis, urine osmolality:
A. >350 B. 600
C. 750 D. 400

193. ACEI hyperkalemia all *except*:
A. DM
B. Unilateral RAS
C. Bilateral RAS
D. ↓ in trans volume

194. Above C5 spasticity appears at:
A. 3 days –3 weeks
B. 3 weeks – 3 months
C. 1 – 3 days
D. 6 months

195. FSF dorsal interonei supply:
A. CBT B. T1T2
C. C7C8

196. Lissauers Trait:
A. Pain
B. Propsoieptosis
C. Spindle afferent
D. Motor

197. Bladder in multiple sclerosis:
A. Premature emptying
B. Small maximum bladder volume
C. ↑ed residual volume
D. Loss of voluntary control

198. OPCA (Olivopont cerebellar atrophy):
A. Familial
B. Neurotoxin
C. Post infections

199. Gille de La Tou syndrome:
A. Copropalia
B. Motor ties
C. >1 year persistence
D. Paranoid delusion and hallucinations

200. Migraine visual field defect:
A. Homomyomas
B. Centrocacial
C. Bivascul
D. Sickle

201. ESR related with:
A. Age B. Both
C. Weight D. None

202. LVH criteria in avF R ht:
A. >20 B. >15
C. >25 D. >30

203. ABPA all *except*:
A. Bronchial asthma
B. Pulmonary infiltrates
C. IgE
D. >1500 peri roxins

204. The proteinuria all *except*:
A. CCBs B. ARBs
C. ACEIs D. NSAIDs

205. Ulcerative colitis severe all *except*:
A. <6 stools/days
B. Bleeding
C. Tachy >130
D. Fever >37°C

206. Trigeminal neuralgia all *except*:
A. Basilar aneurysm
B. Acoustic schwannoma
C. Posterior fossa messinger
D. Tolura Hunt syndrome

207. SLE prognostic factor all *except*:
A. Hypocomplementia
B. HS <12.4 gm%
C. Proteinuria >2.5 gm
D. Severe creatinine >1.5

. Pneumatoid arthritis:
A. CLL B. B cell
C. T cell D. AML

209. Amiodarone transient:
A. ↑ce T4 B. ↓T4
C. ↑T3 D. ↓T3

210. Myopathy drugs all *except*:
A. Chloroquine B. CCB
C. Zidovudine D. Coledine

211. JU fluids in metabolic alkaline:
A. ½ NS B. RL
C. NS D. 5% Dex

212. Hodgkin's infection:
A. Staph B. Strepto
C. Histeria D. Pneumary carinii

213. Ti Hepra reaction:
A. Cortico
B. Clofaznuni
C. Thaliclouid
D. Cortio+Thalido

214. I matinis all *except*:
A. Oedema
B. Periph neuro
C. Hepato toxi
D. Skin manifest: scalable hicheriform skin emption

215. Bulivia nervosa all *except*:
A. Hyponatremia
B. Hypokalemia
C. Hypocholemic alkaton
D. Normal renal function

216. Incorrect about HIV and TB:
A. ↑ AFB sputum positivity
B. ↑ cavitary feroni
C. 40-60% extrapulmonary
D. Meningitis and mycobacterium common

217. correct about ascariasis:
A. More in jejunum
B. Percutaneous route of infection
C. 15-40 cm
D. Egg is infective

218. Amoebiasis:
A. IgG ab prevent infection for life
B. IgA good for infectional immunity
C. Disrar is the most common worldwide
D. For serologic testing is +ve only with r. histology

219. Gametocyte destroyed by:
A. Meffoquine B. Chloroquine
C. Primaquine D. Halofamin

220. Toxoplasma all *except*:
A. Congenital infection may be asymptomatic
B. May be associated with chori rectinitis
C. Not by organ transplant
D. Avail in all organs except RBCs
E. Tachyrout is infection in all organ except HBC

221. Giardiasis:
A. Most common cause of malabsorption in India
B. Nitrox in treatment
C. Stool Ag equivalent to macroscopic test in stool

222. Wegeners granulomatosis:
A. ANCA in pathogenesis
B. Respiratory and renal hamp
C. Predis to rec. staph

223. Sarcoidosis:
A. ACE in >2/3
B. Segment of Krein feit very imporn
C. Erythema modern
D. Uncommon

224. Hyperprolactinemia all *except*:
A. Metoclopro
B. Mozapride
C. Fluoxatine
D. Chlorpromazine

225. Rheumatoid neochrome:
A. 0.1% HT cases
B. 10% malign term
C. 10% hereditaty
D. >10 cm size

226. Nephrogenic diab susp all *except*:
A. Hypoxia B. Hypohalem
C. Amphot B D. Lithium

227. AF with stroke all *except*:
A. <65 years B. CHF
C. Prior TA D. HT

228. AC pancreatitis poor risk factors:
A. Apache >8
B. >130 min HR
C. Rantec score <3
D. GI bleed

229. Chronic hepatitis C diagnosis:
A. Hamivuden + Fufe
B. PEG fuster + Riban
C. Adefour
D. 50 interferon

230. ASF male incorrect:
A. Sickle cell trait resistant to Vmax
B. Hyperglycemia due to IgM ab
C. Stable transmission round the year
D. Buffalo low icom sporadic

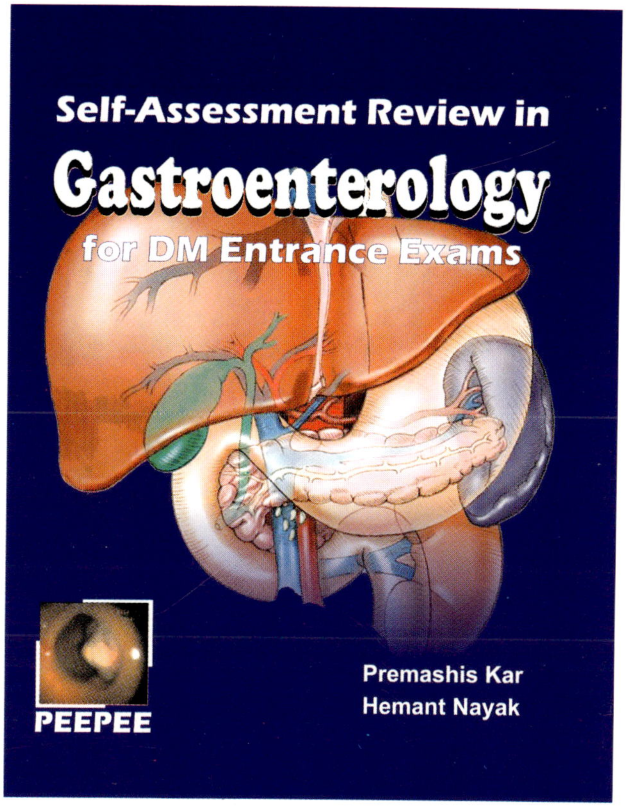

Premshis Kar
1st Edition 2012
978-81-8445-116-0
170 pg, Rs. 250.00
Code No: 160

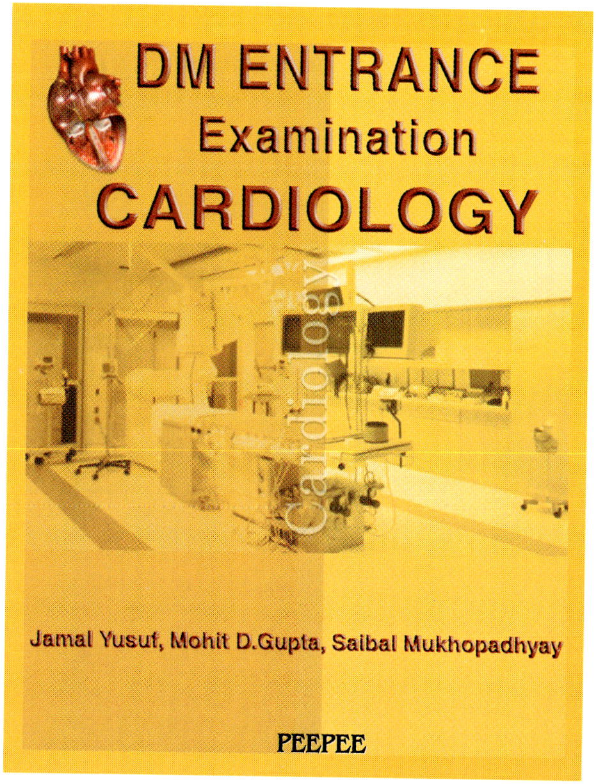

Jamal Yusuf
1st Edition 2005
81-88867-35-7
535 pg,
Code No: 357

DM ENTRANCE EXAMINATION
CARDIOLOGY - 2

The idea of this book came because of lack of a comprehensive question bank on cardiology questions for DM entrance. This book is based on memory recall so there may be some missing options or phrases. The purpose of this book is to help DM Cardiology aspirants, in understanding the nature and variety of questions asked in various entrance examinations. As a beginner it is very hard to get a set of question papers which may help in orientation of mind for different entrance examinations. This book may just help you to find right direction.

ISBN: 978-81-8445-123-8

9 788184 451238

Code: 238

PEEPEE

Publishers and Distributors (P) Ltd.
7/31, First Floor, Ansari Road, Daryaganj
New Delhi - 110002 (India)